*P*atient Care in Radiography

With an Introduction to Medical Imaging

SIXTH EDITION

Patient Care in Radiography

With an Introduction to Medical Imaging

Ruth Ann Ehrlich, RT (R)
Senior Instructor, Radiology
Western States Chiropractic College
Portland, Oregon

Ellen Doble McCloskey, RN, MN
Consultant, Private Practice
Oregon City, Oregon

Joan A. Daly, RT (R), MBA
Faculty/Clinical Coordinator
Radiography Program
Portland Community College
Portland, Oregon

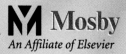 Mosby
An Affiliate of Elsevier

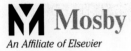
Mosby

An Affiliate of Elsevier

11830 Westline Industrial Drive
St. Louis, Missouri 63146

NOTICE

Radiography is an ever-changing field. Standard safety precautions must be followed, but as new research and clinical experience broaden our knowledge, changes in treatment and drug therapy may become necessary or appropriate. Readers are advised to check the most current product information provided by the manufacturer of each drug to be administered to verify the recommended dose, the method and duration of administration, and contraindications. It is the responsibility of the licensed prescriber, relying on experience and knowledge of the patient, to determine dosages and the best treatment for each individual patient. Neither the publisher nor the author assumes any liability for any injury and/or damage to persons or property arising from this publication.

Previous editions copyrighted 1981, 1985, 1989, 1993, 1999

ISBN-13: 978-0-323-01937-8
ISBN-10: 0-323-01937-4

Publisher: Andrew Allen
Executive Editor: Jeanne Wilke
Senior Developmental Editor: Linda Woodard
Publishing Services Manager: John Rogers
Senior Project Manager: Cheryl A. Abbott
Book Design Manager: Amy Buxton

Printed in the United States of America

Last digit is the print number: 9 8 7 6 5 4

Robin G. Avison, CNMT, RT (N)(MR)
Chief MR Research Technologist
University of Kentucky
Lexington, Kentucky

Robert F. George, MA, CNMT, RT (N)
Lecturer III
University of New Mexico School of Medicine
Albuquerque, New Mexico

Charles Francis, MEd, RT (R)(QM)
Department Chairperson and Associate Professor
Idaho State University
Pocatello, Idaho

M. Elia Flores, RT (R), MEd
Program Director
Blinn College
Bryan, Texas

Sandra D. Ostresh, MEd, RT (R)
Professor/Program Director
Radiologic Technology Program
Quinsigamond Community College
Worcester, Massachusetts

Suggestions by students, instructors, colleagues, and reviewers have contributed greatly to this edition and are acknowledged with our thanks. We deeply appreciate the gracious assistance of Dr. Elizabeth Olsen in revising the material on grieving, hospice, death, and other end-of-life issues. We are also especially grateful to Dr. Lorraine Ginter for adding insight to the discussion of diversity and cultural attitudes toward health care and to Dr. Dennis Hoyer for his expert guidance on the subject of clinical laboratory procedures. It has again been a privilege and a pleasure to work with the fine editorial staff at Elsevier. Jeanne Wilke, Allied Health Executive Editor, Linda Woodard, Senior Developmental Editor, Editorial Assistant Melissa Kuster, and Cheryl Abbott, Senior Project Manager for Production, have all made significant contributions and have been great to work with. Special thanks to Linda Woodard for her patience and her positive attitude throughout the process.

Ruth Ann Ehrlich
Ellen Doble McCloskey
Joan A. Daly

During the past 23 years, *Patient Care in Radiography* has expanded to meet the changing needs of students and technologists in radiography and other medical imaging modalities. It is a resource that provides an introduction to these professions and an orientation to the hospital environment. First and foremost, however, it is a fundamental text on patient care, designed and written to help radiographers meet patient needs. The reader learns to care for the patient effectively while functioning as a responsible and valuable member of the health care team, from the introduction to the patient, through routine procedures and emergency situations, to the final recording of events in the medical record.

While the primary goal is centered on patient care, concern for those who provide that care is also an essential focus in this text. Important self-care concepts are incorporated into the sections on radiation safety in Chapter 1; career planning, malpractice, and legal considerations in Chapter 2; professional attitudes and dealing with burnout and grief in Chapter 3; environmental and ergonomic safety in Chapter 4; and Standard Precautions for infection control in Chapter 5. Applying these principles is critical to your ability to provide good care to others.

Changes in standards for professional practice, health care, and technologist education since publication of the previous edition have affected the content of this, the sixth edition. The American Society of Radiologic Technologists (ASRT) has drafted new curriculum guidelines, revised its Code of Ethics, and has replaced its Scope of Practice statements and Position Descriptions with new Practice Standards. The Centers for Disease Control and Prevention (CDC) has issued new guidelines for minimizing the spread of infectious diseases, including new isolation guidelines and new information and recommendations on hand hygiene. The Occupational Safety and Health Administration (OSHA) has also issued new guidelines. These will increase the well-being of radiographers by raising ergonomic standards in the workplace and by minimizing risks of exposure to bloodborne pathogens through modifications of equipment for medication administration and recommendations for institutional management of needlestick injuries. The Health Insurance Portability and Accounting Act (HIPAA) has been enacted to protect the privacy rights of patients and is having a significant impact on the management of medical information and records. This edition is updated throughout in response to these changes. Every effort has been made to address the content of the new ASRT curriculum that falls within the general scope of the text.

Changes in this edition include expansion of the ethics discussion in Chapter 2 and discussion of ethical analysis as a problem-solving method. Chapter 3 is reorganized and expanded as well, including more information on human diversity and cultural attitudes toward health care. Chapters 5 and 7 contain the latest information from both the CDC and OSHA with respect to infection control and bloodborne pathogen safety. The information on patient assessment in Chapter 6 is improved with a discussion of clinical laboratory tests and convenient reference tables of normal values for both vital signs and laboratory tests.

If you have used this text previously, we hope you will like the new order of chapters in this edition. Chapters 5 and 6 have been reversed in position, placing infection control before patient assessment. This change enables students to utilize their newly-acquired infection control skills while practicing patient evaluation procedures. Material on contrast radiography procedures has been separated from the discussion of other imaging modalities. Chapter 10 is now devoted exclusively to the discussion of contrast agents for radiography and the procedures that involve their use. This information has been updated and is supplemented by revised tables of contrast procedures and contrast media. Chapter 12 has been added to feature updated material on imaging modalities other than radiography. This new chapter introduces imaging and patient care concepts involved in mammography, computed tomography (CT), magnetic resonance imaging (MRI), nuclear medicine, and sonography. Cutting-edge advancements in these technologies, including CT angiography, MR angiography, MR spectroscopy, positron emission tomography (PET) scanning, single photon emission computed tomography (SPECT) imaging, and three-dimensional sonography are described and illustrated in this chapter.

Again, we have done our best to retain those features that readers have appreciated in previous editions. Step-by-step procedures are shown in photo essays, and patient care is integrated with procedural skills. The reading level is comfortable for the student radiographer without being overly simplistic, and each chapter is supplemented with learning objectives, vocabulary lists, illustrations, tables, boxes, and review questions. We have responded to reviewer suggestions by revising the review sections at the ends of the chapters. Instead of open-ended questions, each chapter now has five or more multiple choice questions and three to six critical thinking exercises. These features can be used to enhance the effectiveness of individual study or incorporated into classroom objectives and activities.

The chapters of this text were designed to be used consecutively; each section builds on the preceding information. A basic glossary is included for quick reference, but please bear in mind that it is not meant to replace the more detailed definitions and discussions found in a good encyclopedic medical dictionary.

We hope this book proves to be a valuable resource to you as you care for patients in the challenging field of medical imaging.

TEACHING AIDS FOR THE INSTRUCTOR
Instructor's Curriculum Resource

The instructor's electronic resource to accompany *Patient Care in Radiography* consists of an instructor's manual, a computerized test bank, and an electronic image collection on CD. The instructor's manual and computerized test bank are also available as a print product. The instructor's manual is a guide for the instructor to be used in the development of class presentations, clinical experiences, and evaluations of student learning. Included in this manual are course design, classroom activities, chapter summaries and outlines, audiovisual supplements, plus answers and key concepts to support the study questions and critical thinking exercises in the text. The computerized test bank offers over 300 multiple choice questions that can be sorted by subject matter. The electronic image collection includes all the images from the text, and each can be printed out or transferred to other files as presentaion graphics.

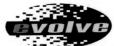

Evolve—Online Course Management

Evolve is an interactive learning environment designed to work in coordination with *Patient Care in Radiography*. Instructors may use Evolve to provide an Internet-based course component that reinforces and expands the concepts presented in class. Evolve may be used to publish the class syllabus, outlines, and lecture notes; set up "virtual office hours" and e-mail communication; share important dates and information through the online class calendar; and encourage student participation through chat rooms and discussion boards. Evolve allows instructors to post exams and manage their grade books online. For more information, visit http://www.evolve.elsevier.com or contact an Elsevier sales representative.

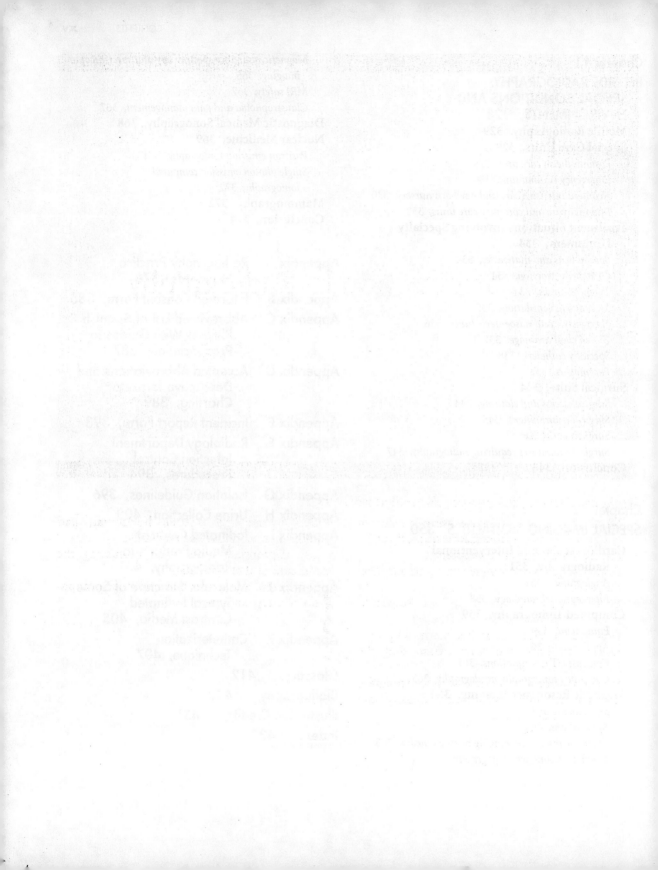

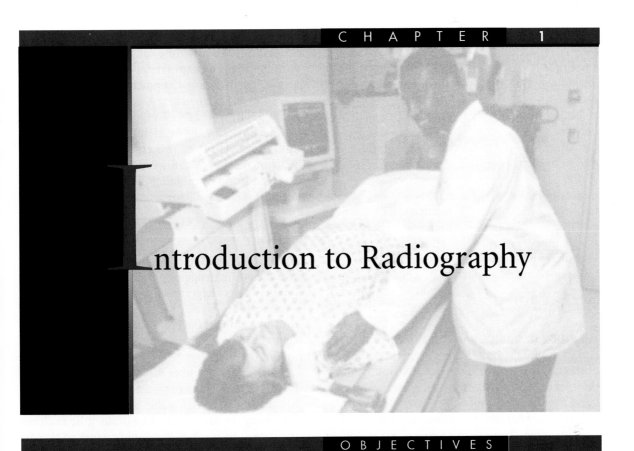

Introduction to Radiography

At the conclusion of this chapter, the student will be able to:

- Name four pioneers in the development of radiography and describe their contributions.
- List six characteristics of x-radiation.
- Draw a diagram of a simple x-ray tube and label the parts.
- Explain the significance of mAs with respect to image quality and patient exposure.
- Describe the effects of an increase in kVp with respect to both the x-ray beam and the radiographic image.
- Explain the effect of an increase in source-image distance on both radiographic density and radiographic definition.

- Demonstrate the vertical, horizontal, and angulation motions of an x-ray tube.
- Use appropriate units when discussing the measurement of x-radiation.
- Demonstrate practices that minimize occupational x-ray exposure.

THE STUDY OF RADIOGRAPHY includes many topics, and each topic is best understood when a host of others has already been mastered. Obviously, something has to come first. As you progress in your radiography education, you will discover that learning occurs somewhat like the peeling of an onion—one layer at a time. You will visit topics again and again, each time building a broader understanding based on prior learning and experience. The topics in this chapter are treated on an introductory level to provide a starting place for your radiography education. All these topics will be presented in depth at a later time in your program; some are the subjects of entire courses in the radiography curriculum. Eventually, the knowledge of these many topics will be woven together to provide a sound basis for clinical practice and decision making. Have patience and confidence in yourself as you take the first steps in your new profession.

Some radiography programs combine the topic of patient care with an introduction to radiography and find that this chapter provides a suitable beginning. The curriculum design of other schools may include the material in this chapter under a different course heading. Regardless of whether the content of this chapter is a part of your current course, it may serve as a useful resource.

Entering a hospital radiology department as a student for the first time can be both exciting and bewildering. The equipment, language, and activities unique to this environment require some guidance for comprehension. A good way to introduce radiography would be to walk the student through a medical imaging department to explore and point things out. Think of this chapter as the textbook version of such a tour. But before we enter the modern world of radiology, let's take a moment to see how it all began over a century ago.

HISTORY

In the 1870s and 1880s research involving electricity was the cutting edge of physical science, and many physicists were experimenting with a device called a Crookes tube (Fig. 1-1), a cathode ray tube that was the forerunner of the fluorescent lamp and the neon sign. Although Crookes tubes also produced x-rays, no one detected them.

Then, on November 8, 1895, Wilhelm Conrad Roentgen, a German physicist (Fig. 1-2), was working with a Crookes tube at the University of Wurzburg. In his darkened laboratory, he enclosed the tube with black photographic paper so that no

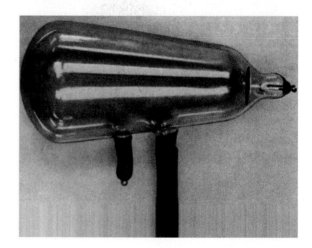

FIG. 1-1 Pear-shaped Hittorf-Crookes tube used in Roentgen's initial experiments.

light could escape. Across the room, a plate coated with barium platinocyanide crystals, a fluorescent material, began to glow. Roentgen noted that the plate fluoresced in relation to its distance from the tube, becoming brighter when the plate was moved closer. He placed various materials, such as wood, aluminum, and his hand, between the plate and the tube, noting variations in the effect upon the plate. He spent the next few weeks investigating this mysterious energy that he called "x ray," *x* being the symbol for the unknown. By the end of the year Roentgen had identified nearly all of the properties of x-rays known today. In recognition of his discovery he was awarded the first Nobel Prize in physics in 1901.

During his early experimentation with x-rays, Roentgen produced the first anatomical radiograph, an image of his wife's hand. The first documented medical application of x-rays in the United States

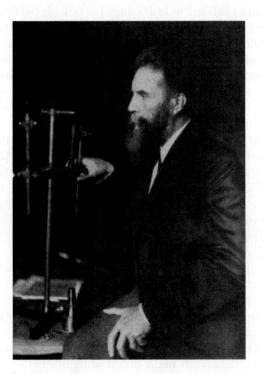

FIG. 1-2 Photograph of W. C. Roentgen, the discoverer of x-rays, taken in 1906.

was an examination performed at Dartmouth College in February of 1896 of a young boy's fractured wrist.

Early radiography required up to 30 minutes to create a visible image. Over the years many advances in this technology have reduced the time and radiation exposure involved in radiography. The early sources of electricity were not powerful enough to be efficient and could not be easily adjusted until H. C. Snook, working with an alternating current generator, developed the interrupterless transformer. William Coolidge designed the "hot cathode" x-ray tube to work with Snook's improved electrical supply. The Coolidge tube (Fig. 1-3), introduced in 1910, was the prototype for the x-ray tubes of today.

Roentgen used a glass plate coated with a photographic emulsion to create the first radiograph. Soon after Roentgen's discovery was published, Pupin demonstrated the radiographic use of fluorescent screens, now called intensifying screens. He used light given off by fluorescent materials when activated by x-rays to expose photographic plates.

In 1898, Thomas Edison began experiments with more than 1800 materials to investigate their fluorescent properties. He invented the first fluoroscope and discovered many of the fluorescent chemicals used in radiography today. Edison abandoned his research when his assistant and longtime friend, Clarence Dally, became severely burned on his arms by the x-rays. Dally's arms had to be amputated, and in 1904 he died. This was the first recorded x-ray fatality in the United States.

Until World War I, glass photographic plates were used as a base for x-ray images. During the war manufacturers of photographic plates for radiography could not get high-quality glass from suppliers in Belgium, and the U.S. government turned to George Eastman, founder of the Eastman Kodak Company, for help. Eastman had invented photographic film using cellulose nitrate, a new plastic material, as a substitute for glass. He produced the first radiographic film in 1914.

Early in the twentieth century, radiation injuries such as skin burns, hair loss, and anemia began to appear in both doctors and patients. Measures were

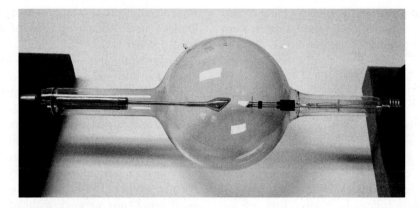

FIG. 1-3 Coolidge "hot cathode" tube, prototype of modern tubes, was introduced in 1910.

taken to monitor and limit exposures, a process that is still ongoing. Lead apparel and protective barriers have substantially reduced the exposure received by equipment operators. Today, because of improved technology and safety precautions, x-ray examinations are much safer for patients and radiography is considered to be a very safe occupation.

The first radiographers were physicists familiar with the operation of the Crookes tube. As x-ray-generating equipment was installed in hospitals and physicians' offices, physicians learned to take radiographs and soon developed techniques for the demonstration of many different anatomical structures. Physicians who used x-rays began to train their assistants to develop the photographic plates and to assist with x-ray examinations. In time, many of these assistants became skilled in radiography.

On-the-job training of "x-ray technicians" in hospitals evolved into hospital-based educational programs. Formal classes and clinical experience were combined to provide students with the knowledge and skills needed to take radiographs and to assist with radiation therapy (x-ray treatments). As the fields of diagnostic and therapeutic radiology became more complex and specialized, education for radiation therapy technologists was separated from that for radiographers.

Colleges were first involved in radiographers' education because hospital-based radiography programs took advantage of the academic offerings at local colleges. Radiography students often attended college part-time to learn basic science subjects such as anatomy and physiology.

Following World War II, with many returning soldiers wanting to attend college on the GI Bill, junior colleges were developed to provide the first 2 years of academic education for university-bound students. In the 1960s, these institutions expanded and multiplied into the community college system that is a significant part of national public education in the United States today. In the process of this expansion, more emphasis was placed on vocational education. Community colleges formed effective partnerships with companies and institutions that provided on-the-job training. Following this trend, many hospital-based radiography programs became affiliated with community colleges to provide the necessary academic courses. Some 4-year colleges and universities also began to offer educational programs in radiologic technology.

As the requirements for accreditation of educational programs in radiography have increased over the years (see Chapter 2), the organizational structure of colleges has proved to be well suited to the management of these programs. Today, colleges and hospitals still cooperate to provide education in radiography. The majority of programs are based in colleges, but many outstanding hospital-based programs still exist and in some areas proprietary vocational schools offer radiography education.

OVERVIEW OF RADIOGRAPHIC PROCEDURE

To take a typical radiograph, the radiographer positions the patient on the x-ray table and places a **cassette** or other image receptor into the cassette tray located under the table surface (Fig. 1-4). The cassette tray is aligned to the anatomical area of interest, and the x-ray tube position is adjusted to align the x-ray beam to the film. The radiographer then goes to the control booth, sets the exposure factors on the control console, and activates the exposure switch. During the exposure, x-rays from the tube pass through the patient. Some of the x-rays are absorbed by the patient, and others are not, resulting in a pattern of varying intensity in the x-ray beam that exits on the opposite side of the patient. The radiation then passes through the table-top and the cassette and exposes the film. The film now has a pattern of exposure, a **latent image.** The cassette is then removed from the tray. The patient's identification is stamped on the film before it is placed in an automatic processing machine. The processor develops the film, changing the latent image into a visible image.

As you may have suspected, many details were omitted from the previous paragraph. Memorizing the paragraph will not qualify you to be a radiographer! This is only the first layer of the onion. Next, we consider how x-rays are produced, their physical nature, and how their various characteristics relate to the process of radiography.

X-RAY PRODUCTION

There are four basic requirements for the production of x-rays:

1. A vacuum
2. A source of electrons
3. A target for the electrons
4. A high potential difference (voltage) between the electron source and the target

The container for the vacuum is the x-ray tube itself (Fig. 1-5), sometimes referred to as a "glass envelope." It is made of Pyrex glass to withstand heat and is fitted on both ends with connections for the

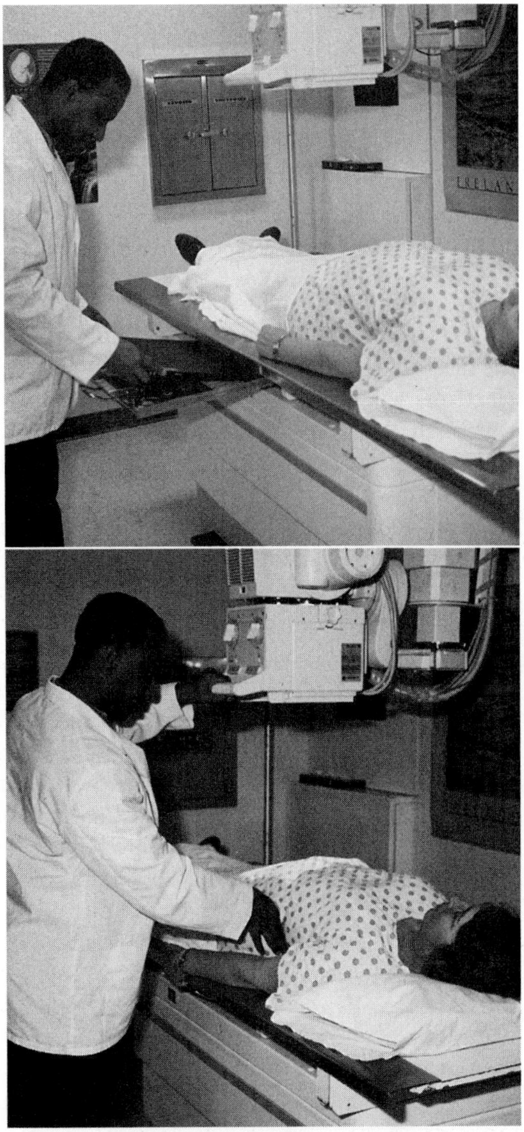

FIG. 1-4 **A,** Radiographer places cassette in bucky tray. **B,** Radiographer aligns x-ray tube to patient and cassette.

electrical supply. All of the air is removed from the tube so that gas molecules will not interfere with the process of x-ray production.

The source of electrons is a wire filament at one end of the tube. It is made of the element tungsten, a large atom with 74 electrons in orbits around the nucleus. An electric current flows through the filament to heat it. This speeds up the movement of the electrons and increases their distance from the nucleus. Electrons in the outermost orbital shells get so far from the nucleus that they are no longer held in orbit, but are flung out of the atom, forming an "electron cloud" around the filament. These free electrons, called a *space charge*, provide the needed electrons for x-ray production.

The target is at the opposite end of the tube from the filament. This smooth, hard surface to which the electrons will travel is the place where x-rays are generated. It is also made of tungsten.

The voltage required for x-ray production is provided by a high-voltage transformer. The two ends of the x-ray tube are connected in the transformer circuit so that during an exposure, the filament or cathode end is negative and the target or anode end is positive. The high positive electrical potential at the target attracts the negatively charged electrons of the electron cloud, which move rapidly across the tube, forming an electron stream. When these fast-moving electrons collide with the target, the kinetic energy of their motion must be converted into a different form of energy. The great majority of this kinetic energy is converted into heat (99+%),

but a small amount is converted into the energy form that we know as x-rays.

CHARACTERISTICS OF RADIATION

X-rays are among several types of energy described as **electromagnetic energy,** or electromagnetic wave radiation. They have both electrical and magnetic properties, changing the field through which they pass both electrically and magnetically. These changes in the field occur in the form of a repeating wave, a pattern that scientists call a sinusoidal form or sine wave.

Several characteristics of this waveform are significant. The distance between the crest and valley of the wave (its height) is called the **amplitude** (Fig. 1-6). More important to radiographers is the distance from one crest to the next, or **wavelength** (Fig. 1-7). The **frequency** of the wave is the number of times per second that a crest passes a given point.

Since all electromagnetic energy moves through space at the same velocity, approximately 186,000 miles per second, which is 30 billion (3×10^{10}) centimeters per second, it is apparent that a relationship exists between wavelength and frequency. When the wavelength is short, the crests are closer together, so more of them will pass a given point in a second,

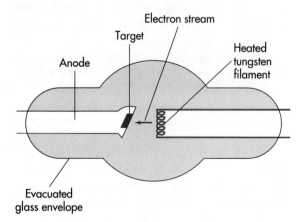

FIG. 1-5 Diagram of Coolidge tube simplifies understanding of x-ray production.

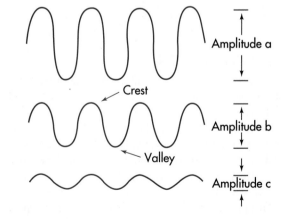

FIG. 1-6 These three sine waves are identical except for their amplitudes.

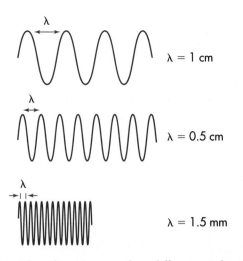

FIG. 1-7 These three sine waves have different wavelengths. The shorter the wavelength, the higher the frequency. (Note symbol for wavelength is Greek letter, lambda—λ.)

resulting in a higher frequency. Longer wavelengths will have a lower frequency. This may be expressed mathematically:

$$\text{Velocity } (v) = \text{Wavelength } (\lambda) \times \text{Frequency } (f)$$

The more energy the wave has, the greater will be its frequency and the shorter its wavelength. We can therefore use either wavelength or frequency to describe the energy of the wave. In radiologic science, wavelength is more often used to describe the energy of the x-ray beam. The average wavelength of a diagnostic x-ray beam is approximately 0.1 nanometer, which is .00000000001 (10^{-10}) meters, or about a billionth of an inch.

The wavelength of electromagnetic radiation varies from exceedingly short, even shorter than that of diagnostic x-rays, to very long, more than 5 miles. This range of energies is known as the electromagnetic spectrum. It includes x-rays, gamma rays, visible light, microwaves, and radio waves (Fig. 1-8). Radiation with a wavelength shorter than one nanometer (10^{-9} meters) is said to be ionizing radiation, because it has sufficient energy to remove an electron from an atomic orbit. X-rays are one type of ionizing radiation.

The smallest possible unit of electromagnetic energy (analogous to the atom with respect to matter) is the **photon,** which may be thought of as a minute "bullet" of energy. Photons occur in groups or "bundles" called **quanta** (singular, **quantum**).

Since x-rays and visible light are both forms of electromagnetic energy, they share some similar characteristics. Both travel in straight lines, and both have an effect on photographic emulsions. The photographic effect of x-rays is significant in the production of radiographs. It is also important to remember because accidental exposure can occur when film is placed near x-ray sources.

Both x-rays and light have a biological effect; that is, they can cause changes in living organisms. X-rays are capable of producing more harmful effects than light because of their greater energy.

Unlike light, x-rays cannot be detected by the human senses. This fact may seem obvious, but it is important to consider. If x-rays could be seen, felt, or heard, we would have an increased awareness of their presence and radiation safety might be much simpler. As it is, safety requires that you learn to know when and where x-rays are present without being able to perceive them.

X-rays can penetrate matter that is opaque to light. This penetration is differential, depending on the density and thickness of the matter. For example, x-rays penetrate air very readily. There is less penetration of fat or oil, even less of water, which is about the same density as muscle tissue, and still less of bone. X-rays that have passed through the body are referred to as remnant radiation or exit radiation. Remnant radiation has a pattern of intensity that reflects the absorption characteristics of the body. It is this pattern that is recorded on the radiograph.

X-rays cause certain crystals to fluoresce, giving off light when exposed. Among crystals that respond in this way are barium platinocyanide, barium lead sulfate, calcium tungstate, and several salts from rare earth elements. These crystals are used to convert the x-ray pattern into a visible image that can be viewed directly, as in fluoroscopy, or recorded on photographic film. The use of fluorescent intensifying screens to expose radiographs greatly reduces the quantity of radiation needed.

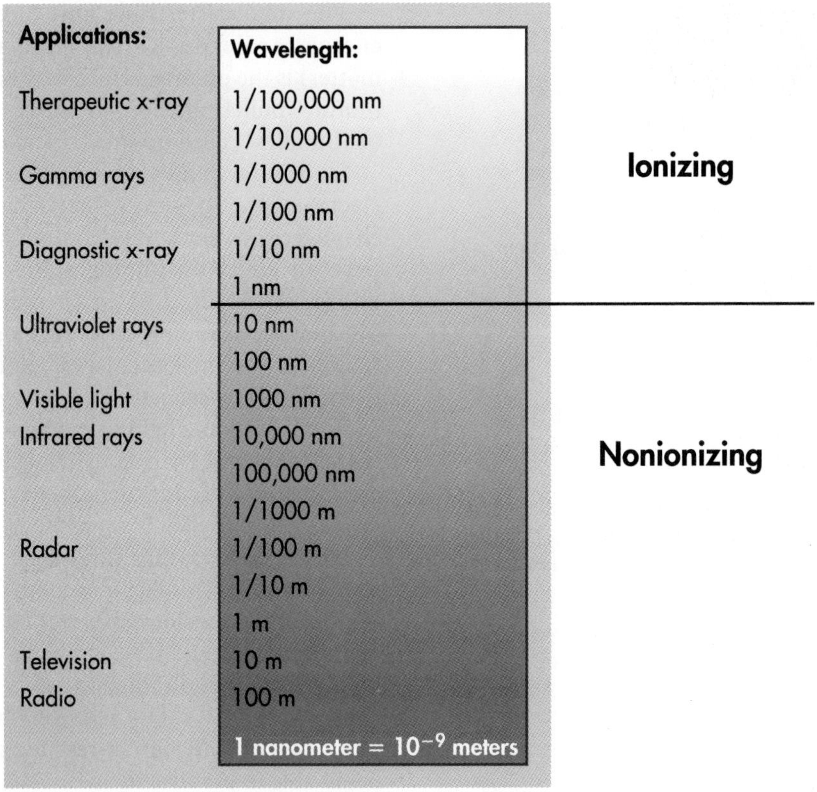

Applications:	Wavelength:	
Therapeutic x-ray	1/100,000 nm	**Ionizing**
	1/10,000 nm	
Gamma rays	1/1000 nm	
	1/100 nm	
Diagnostic x-ray	1/10 nm	
	1 nm	
Ultraviolet rays	10 nm	
	100 nm	
Visible light	1000 nm	
Infrared rays	10,000 nm	**Nonionizing**
	100,000 nm	
	1/1000 m	
Radar	1/100 m	
	1/10 m	
	1 m	
Television	10 m	
Radio	100 m	
	1 nanometer = 10^{-9} meters	

FIG. 1-8 Electromagnetic spectrum.

Unlike light, x-rays cannot be refracted by a lens. The x-ray beam diverges into space from its source until it is absorbed by matter.

THE X-RAY BEAM

X-rays are formed within a very small area on the target. The actual size of the largest focal spot is no more than a few millimeters in diameter. From this point, the x-rays diverge into space, forming the cone-shaped *primary x-ray beam* (Fig. 1-9). The cross section of the x-ray beam at the point where it is utilized is called the *radiation field.* A photon in the center of the primary beam and perpendicular to the long axis of the x-ray tube is called the *central ray.*

The x-ray beam size is restricted by the size of the port, the opening in the tube housing. Attached to the housing is the **collimator,** a device that enables the radiographer to control the size of the radiation field.

Scatter Radiation

When the primary x-ray beam encounters matter, such as the patient, the x-ray table, or the cassette, a portion of its energy is absorbed within the matter. This results in the production of scatter radiation (Fig. 1-10). This radiation generally has less energy than the primary x-ray beam, but it is not easily controlled. It emanates from the source in all directions, causing unwanted exposure on the film and posing a radiation safety hazard to anyone in the room.

The characteristics of primary radiation, scatter radiation, and remnant radiation are summarized for comparison in Table 1-1.

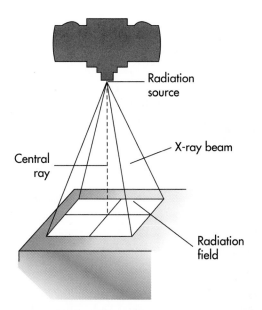

FIG. 1-9 Cross section of x-ray beam is called the radiation field; an imaginary perpendicular ray at its center is called the *central ray*.

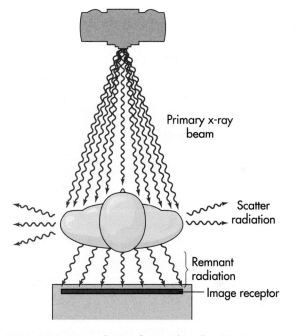

FIG. 1-10 Scatter radiation forms when the primary x-ray beam interacts with matter.

RADIOGRAPHIC EQUIPMENT
The X-Ray Tube

The x-ray tube is the source of the radiation. Modern multipurpose x-ray tubes (Fig. 1-11) are dual focus tubes. They contain two filaments, one large and one small (Fig. 1-12). Each is situated in a focusing cup that directs its electrons toward the same general area on the target. When the small filament is activated, its electrons are directed to a tiny focal spot on the target. The small filament and focal spot provide finer image detail when a relatively small exposure is appropriate. The large filament

TABLE 1-1		
X-RAY BEAM ATTENUATION		
PRIMARY RADIATION	**SCATTER RADIATION**	**REMNANT (EXIT) RADIATION**
The x-ray beam that leaves the tube and is unattenuated except by air.	Radiation scattered or created as a result of the attenuation of the primary x-ray beam by matter.	What remains of the primary beam after it has been attenuated by matter.
Its direction and location are predictable and controllable.	It travels in all directions from the scattering medium and is very difficult to control.	Since the pattern of densities in the matter results in differential absorption, this pattern is inherent in remnant radiation.
Its energy is controlled by the kilovoltage setting.	Generally, it has less energy than the primary beam.	The pattern of intensity of remnant radiation creates the radiographic image.

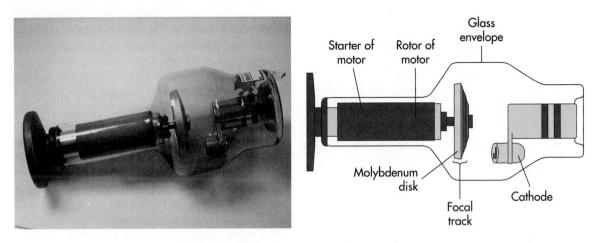

FIG. 1-11 Modern rotating-anode x-ray tube.

provides more electrons and is aimed at a larger target area. The combination of large filament and large focal spot is used when a large exposure is required, because the large filament provides more electrons and the large focal spot can better handle the resulting heat at the anode. The anode is disk-shaped and rotates during the exposure (Fig. 1-13), distributing the anode heat over a larger area and increasing the heat capacity of the tube. It is the rotation of the anode that causes the whirring sound just before and after the exposure.

X-Ray Tube Housing

The x-ray tube is located inside a protective housing (Fig. 1-14). The housing incorporates shielding that

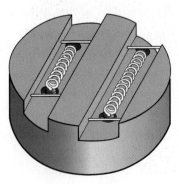

FIG. 1-12 Dual focus x-ray tube has focusing cups with large and small filaments.

absorbs radiation that is not a part of the useful x-ray beam. The housing protects and insulates the x-ray tube itself, while providing a base for attachments that allows the radiographer to manipulate the x-ray tube and to control the size and shape of the x-ray beam.

X-Ray Tube Support

The tube housing either may be attached to a ceiling mount ("tube hanger") or on a tube stand. Both types of mountings provide support and mobility for the tube. A tube hanger (Fig. 1-15) is suspended from the ceiling on a system of tracks to allow positioning of the tube at locations throughout the room. This ceiling mount is useful when positioning the tube over a stretcher or when moving the tube for use in different locations. A tube stand (Fig. 1-16) is a vertical support with a horizontal arm that supports the tube over the radiographic table. The tube stand rolls along a track that is secured to the floor (and sometimes also the ceiling), allowing horizontal motion.

A system of electric locks holds the tube support in position. The control system for all, or most, of these locks is an attachment on the front of the tube housing. To move the tube in any direction, the locking device must be released. Moving the tube without first releasing the lock may damage the lock, making it impossible to secure the tube in position. *Do not attempt to move the tube without first releasing the appropriate lock.*

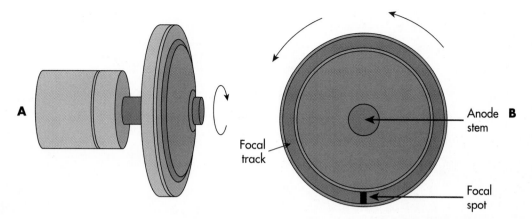

FIG. 1-13 Rotating anode. Electrons strike the anode in the tiny focal spot area, but the heat is spread around the entire focal track of the spinning anode face. **A,** Side view. **B,** View from cathode.

Typical tube motions (Fig. 1-17) include the following:

- Longitudinal—along the long axis of the table
- Transverse—across the table, at right angles to longitudinal
- Vertical—up and down, increasing or decreasing the distance between the tube and the table
- Rotation—allows the entire tube support to turn on its axis, changing the direction in which the tube arm is extended

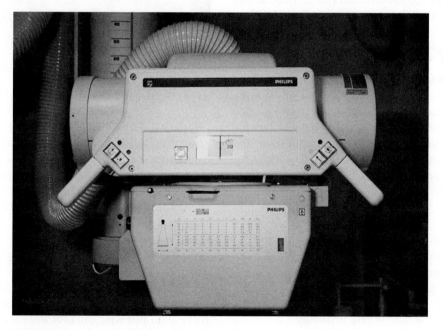

FIG. 1-14 Tube housing shields the tube and provides mounting for tube motion controls and collimator.

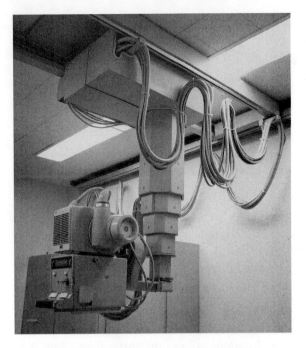

FIG. 1-15 Ceiling-mounted tube support.

- Roll (tilt, angle)—permits angulation of the tube along the longitudinal axis and also allows the tube to be aimed at the wall rather than the table

A **detent** is a special mechanism that tends to stop a moving part in a specific location. Detents are built into tube supports to facilitate placement at standard locations. For example, a vertical detent will indicate when the distance from tube to film is 40 inches, a common standard distance. Other detents provide "stops" when the transverse tube position is centered to the table and when the tilt motion is such that the central ray is perpendicular to the table or to the wall.

Collimator

Another attachment to the tube housing is the collimator, a boxlike device mounted beneath the port, the opening of the housing. Collimators allow the radiographer to vary the size of the radiation field and to indicate with a light beam the size, location, and center of the field. There is usually a centering light that helps align the cassette tray as well

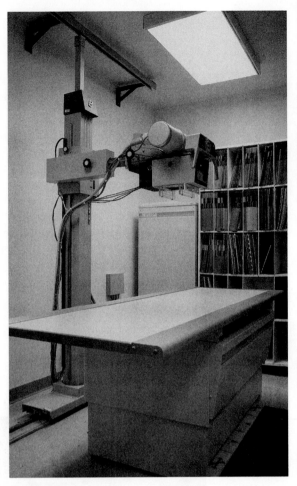

FIG. 1-16 Floor-mounted tube stand.

(Fig. 1-18). Controls on the front of the collimator allow the radiographer to adjust the size of each dimension of the radiation field. The collimator also has a scale that indicates each dimension of the field at specific source-image distances. A timer controls the collimator light, turning it off after a certain length of time, usually 30 seconds. This helps to avoid accidental overheating of the unit by prolonged use of its high-intensity light.

Radiographic Table

The radiographic table is a specialized unit that is more than just a support for the patient. While the table is usually secured to the floor, it may be capable

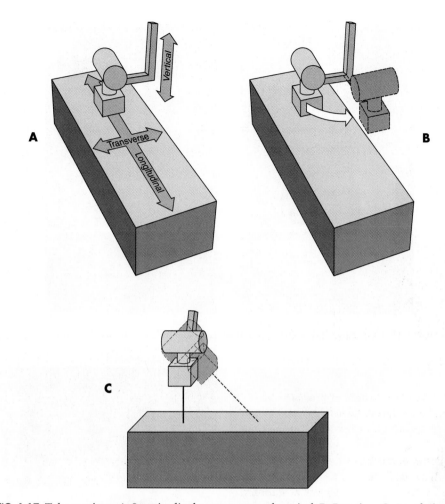

FIG. 1-17 Tube motions. **A,** Longitudinal, transverse, and vertical. **B,** Rotation. **C,** Angulation.

of several types of motion: vertical, tilt, and "floating" tabletop.

For vertical table motion a hydraulic motor, activated by a hand, foot, or knee switch, raises or lowers the height of the table. This allows lowering of the table so the patient can sit down on it easily and also permits the table to rise to a comfortable working height for the radiographer. Adjustments to exact stretcher height can be made to facilitate patient transfers. There will be a detent or standard position for routine radiography. This standard table height corresponds to indicated distances from the x-ray tube. Since it is important that standard tube/film distances be used, it is necessary to return the table to the detent position after lowering it for patient access. Not all tables are capable of vertical motion.

A tilting table (Fig. 1-19) also uses a hydraulic motor to change position. In this case, the table turns on a central axis to attain a vertical position. This allows the patient to be placed in a horizontal position, a vertical position, or at any angle in between. The table may also tilt in the opposite direction, allowing the patient's head to be lowered at least 15° into the Trendelenburg position. A detent stops the table in the horizontal position. The ability

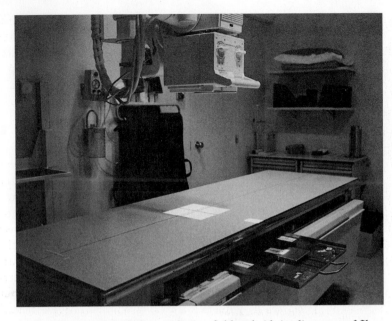

FIG. 1-18 Collimator light defines radiation field and aids in alignment of film tray.

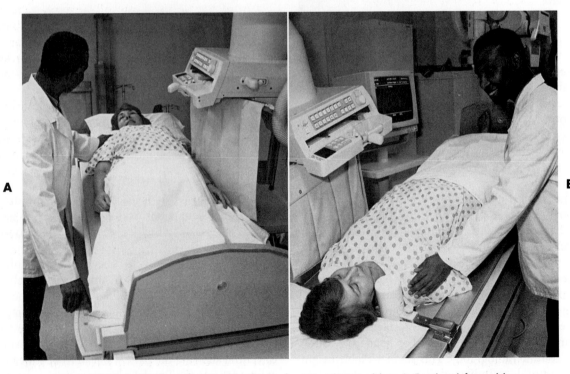

FIG. 1-19 Hydraulic fluoroscopic table tilts to change patient position. **A,** Semiupright position. **B,** Trendelenburg position.

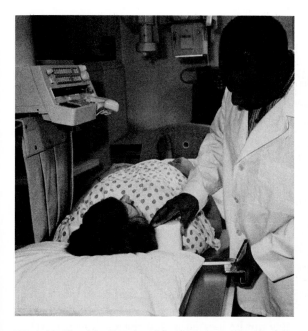

FIG. 1-20 Shoulder guard and footboard must be carefully secured for patient safety before tilting table.

to tilt is an essential feature of most fluoroscopic tables and may also be a feature of a radiographic unit.

Special attachments for the tilting table include a footboard and a shoulder guard to provide safety for the patient when tilting the table (Fig. 1-20). Pay particular attention to the attachment mechanisms so that you will be able to apply these attachments correctly when needed. Before tilting a patient on the table, always test the footboard or shoulder guard to be certain that it is securely attached.

The motor that tilts the table is quite powerful and can overcome the resistance of obstacles placed in the way. Many step stools and other pieces of moveable equipment have been damaged because they were under the end of the table and out of view when the table motor was activated. Such a collision can also damage the table motor. Be certain that the spaces under the head and foot of the table are clear before activating the tilt motor.

A floating tabletop allows the top of the table to move independently of the remainder of the table for ease in aligning the patient to the x-ray tube and the image receptor. This motion may involve a mechanical release, allowing the radiographer to shift the position of the tabletop, or the movement may be power-assisted, activated by a small control pad with directional switches. The latter case is common for fluoroscopic tables.

Grids and Buckys

Beneath the table surface is a moving grid device called a **bucky** (Fig. 1-21). The bucky device incorporates the cassette tray that holds the film. The entire unit can be moved along the length of the table and locked into position where desired. The **grid** is situated between the tabletop and the film. It is a plate made of tissue-thin lead strips, mounted on edge, with radiolucent interspacing material (Fig. 1-22). The grid or bucky's purpose is to protect the film from being fogged by scatter radiation that emanates mainly from the patient. The strips must be carefully aligned to the path of the primary x-ray beam, so precise alignment of the x-ray tube is essential. The purpose of moving the grid is to blur its image so that it is not visible on the radiograph. When the table has a floating tabletop, the bucky mechanism and film tray do not move with the tabletop.

Stationary grids that do not move during the exposure serve the same purpose as a bucky. A grid may also be incorporated into the front of a special cassette called a grid cassette, which is useful for mobile radiography and other special applications.

Grids or buckys are generally used only for body parts that measure more than 10 to 12 cm in thickness. (The average adult's neck or knee measures 12 cm.) When a grid is not needed, the cassette is placed on the tabletop.

Upright Cassette Holders

The upright cassette holder, as its name implies, is a device to hold the film in the upright position for radiography (Fig. 1-23). It is adjustable in height and may incorporate a bucky or grid. When a grid is included, this device may be referred to as a grid cabinet; when the grid is a moving grid, the device

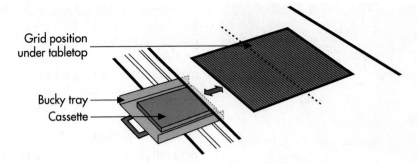

Grid position
under tabletop

Bucky tray
Cassette

FIG. 1-21 Bucky device for scatter radiation control incorporates cassette tray and is mounted under tabletop. Note that lead strips are parallel to long axis of table.

is called an *upright bucky*. Even when the table tilts to the upright position, it is usual to have a separate upright cassette holder for some examinations such as cervical spines and chests. When the patient is sitting or standing at the upright cassette holder, the tube is angled to direct the x-ray beam toward the cassette. The distance may be adjusted to 40 or 72 inches, depending on the requirements of the procedure.

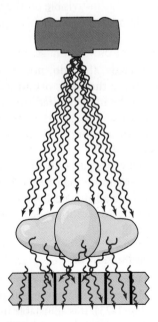

FIG. 1-22 Lead strips in grid absorb scatter radiation emitted from patient; remnant radiation passes through grid and exposes film.

Transformer

Cables from the tube housing connect the x-ray tube to the transformer, which provides the high voltage necessary for x-ray production. Some transformers look like a large box or cabinet, which may or may not be located within the x-ray room. Newer transformer designs are much smaller and may be incorporated into the control console.

Control Console

The control console, located in the control booth, is the access point for the radiographer to determine the exposure factors and to initiate the exposure (Fig. 1-24). Radiographic control consoles have buttons, switches, dials, or digital readouts for some or all of the following functions:

- Off/On—controls the power to the control panel
- mA—allows the operator to set the milliamperage, the rate at which the x-rays are produced; determines the focal spot size
- kVp—controls the kilovoltage, and thereby the wavelength and penetrating power, of the x-ray beam
- Timer—controls the duration of the exposure
- mAs—some units have an mAs control instead of mA and time settings. The mAs (the product of mA and time) determines the total quantity of radiation in an exposure
- Bucky—activates the motor control of the bucky device so that the grid will move during the exposure

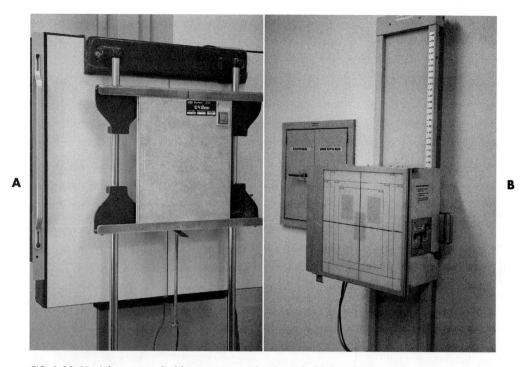

FIG. 1-23 Upright cassette holders. **A,** Nongrid cassette holder with cassette in place. **B,** Upright bucky.

- Automatic exposure controls—special settings available on certain units that allow termination of exposure when a certain quantity of radiation has reached the image receptor
- Meters or digital readouts to indicate the status of the settings
- Prep (ready or rotor) switch—prepares the tube for exposure and must be continuously activated until exposure is complete
- Exposure switch—initiates the exposure and must be continuously activated until the exposure is complete
- Accessories—other controls may also be present, depending on the equipment and its specific features

FLUOROSCOPIC UNITS

A **fluoroscope** is an x-ray machine designed for direct viewing of the x-ray image. Fluoroscopy

permits the viewing of x-ray images in motion. Early fluoroscopes consisted simply of an x-ray tube mounted under the x-ray table and a fluorescent screen mounted over the patient. The physician watched the x-ray image on the screen while turning the patient into the desired positions to view various anatomical areas. The fluoroscopic image was very dim, dark adaptation was required, and the procedure was carried out in a dark room.

Today's equipment is far more sophisticated. Most fluoroscopic units are properly called *radiographic/fluoroscopic (R/F)* units because they can be used for both radiography and fluoroscopy. This is convenient because most fluoroscopic examinations also have a radiographic component. "Spot films" are taken during fluoroscopy to record the image as seen on the fluoroscope. Depending on the equipment, cassettes, roll film, or digital systems may be used to record fluoroscopic images. The fluoroscopic tube is used to expose spot films and image

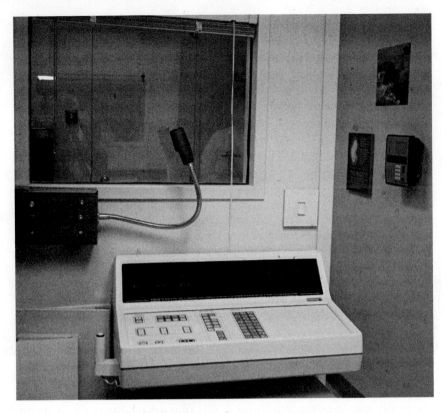

FIG. 1-24 Computerized x-ray control console.

areas of interest. After the fluoroscopic portion of the study is completed, radiographs may be taken for comprehensive visualization of the entire anatomical region.

The radiation required for a fluoroscopic study has been greatly reduced by the use of the **image intensifier**. This electronic device is in the form of a tower that fits over the fluoroscopic screen (Fig. 1-25). Inside is a series of photomultiplier tubes that brighten and enhance the image formerly seen by looking directly at the fluoroscopic screen. The enhanced image is digitized or photographed by a video camera to provide direct viewing on a video monitor. A computer or video tape recorder can be used to make a record of the entire study. Some towers can be removed from the fluoroscope and moved away from the table when it is not

needed. The fluoroscope and spot film device can also be moved out of the way when the table is used for radiography.

The control console of an R/F unit is more complex than that of a basic radiography unit. There may be separate mA and kVp settings for the control of the radiographic (overhead) and fluoroscopic (under table) tubes, and special settings for spot film radiography. A timer on the control advances when the fluoroscope is on, and an alarm sounds after a preset period, usually 5 minutes.

For a fluoroscopic examination, the duties of the radiographer include the following:

- Taking the patient's history, including information on the success of preparation
- Getting the patient gowned
- Explaining the procedure to the patient

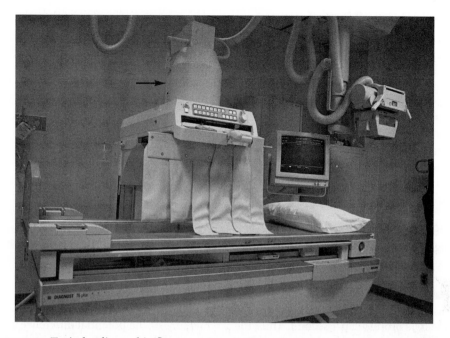

FIG. 1-25 Typical radiographic/fluoroscopic unit. Tower *(arrow)* contains image intensifier.

- Taking and processing any required preliminary radiographs
- Setting the control panel correctly for fluoroscopy and spot film radiography
- Positioning the patient for the start of the procedure
- Preparing the equipment for fluoroscopy
- Entering patient data into the computer for digital imaging, if applicable
- Loading the spot film device
- Preparing contrast agents as needed
- Assisting the radiologist as needed. This may involve helping the patient assume various positions; assisting the patient and/or the radiologist with the contrast medium; changing spot film cassettes as needed; or loading, unloading, and identifying roll film, or electronically sending digital images for laser printing.
- Taking follow-up radiographs
- Providing patient care as needed when the procedure is complete

Your orientation to the fluoroscopy suite may be to observe or assist with fluoroscopic studies of the gastrointestinal tract. These x-ray examinations of the stomach or the bowel are described in detail in Chapter 9. Other examinations involving fluoroscopy are discussed in Chapters 10 and 11.

FACTORS OF RADIOGRAPHIC EXPOSURE
Exposure Time

Exposure time is simply a measure of how long the exposure will continue and is measured in units of seconds, fractions of seconds, or milliseconds (thousandths of seconds). Electronic timers provide a wide range of possible settings, allowing the operator to precisely control the length of exposure. Together with milliamperage (see below), exposure time determines the total quantity of radiation that will be produced. When a variation in the quantity of exposure is desired, the exposure time is varied. Since a longer exposure time results in the production of more x-rays, all other factors being equal, a longer exposure time will produce a darker radiograph. A decrease in exposure time will result in less radiation exposure and a lighter film. Patient dose is directly proportional to exposure time.

Possible exposure time settings may vary from as little as 1 millisecond (0.001 second), to as much as several seconds. Some units have automated exposure devices (AEDs). These automated exposure timers terminate the exposure when a specific quantity of radiation has reached the image receptor. These features are often referred to by their commercial trade names, Phototimer or Iontomat.

Milliamperage

Milliamperage (mA) is a measure of the current flow in the x-ray tube circuit. It determines the number of electrons available to cross the tube, and thus the rate at which x-rays are produced. You can think of mA as an indication of the number of x-ray photons that will be produced per second. Thus, the mA setting will determine how much exposure time is required to produce a given amount of exposure. High mA settings are used to shorten the needed exposure time when motion during a longer exposure would likely cause blurring of the radiographic image.

The number of possible mA settings is limited and is usually in whole numbers that are divisible by 50 or 100. For example, a typical radiographic unit may have the following mA settings: 50, 100, 200, 300, 400, and 500. Some x-ray machines are capable of producing as much as 1000 or 1500 mA.

The relationship between milliamperage and exposure time is simple. The product of mA and time is **milliampere-seconds (mAs),** which is an indicator of the total quantity of radiation produced in the exposure. This relationship is represented by the mAs formula:

$$mA \times Time \ (seconds) = mAs$$

Most control consoles today provide the option of setting the mAs directly, while older models usually require the operator to set mA and exposure time separately. The mAs settings for various applications commonly range between 1 and 100.

Changing the mA has other effects as well. In dual focus tubes, specific mA stations control each filament. In general, mA settings of 150 or less utilize the small filament and the small focal spot, while mA settings of 200 or more are associated with the large filament and large focal spot. On controls that permit the operator to select the mA setting, each setting will have an indication of which focal spot is associated with it. Controls that provide mAs selection without specific mA settings will have a separate means of selecting focal spot size.

In addition to varying the focal spot size, changes in mA will affect the amount of heat that accumulates in the anode during the exposure and will be cause for concern when large exposures are required. As a rule, an x-ray tube can handle larger exposures when the desired mAs is obtained with a lower mA setting and a longer exposure time.

Kilovoltage

The kilovoltage or **kilovoltage peak (kVp)** is a measure of the potential difference across the x-ray tube and determines the speed of the electrons in the electron stream. This determines the amount of kinetic energy each electron has when it collides with the target and thus determines the amount of energy in the resulting x-ray beam. This energy is expressed by the wavelength of the photons. X-ray photons with shorter wavelengths have more energy and are more penetrating than those with longer wavelengths. For this reason, an increase in kVp results in a more penetrating x-ray beam. This will cause more exposure on the film, since a higher percentage of the x-rays produced will pass through the patient and reach the film. An increase in kVp will therefore produce a darker film, and a kVp decrease will produce a lighter one.

Changes in kilovoltage will cause other changes to the film as well. Since the differential penetration that forms the image will be affected by wavelength, the contrast on the film will also change. This means that the degree of difference between the darker and lighter areas of the image will be affected. Somewhere between no penetration and total penetration of the subject is the optimum amount of differential penetration that will show a contrast in exposure between the various features of the subject. The amount of kVp that produces optimum penetration varies with the examination. This concept is further discussed in the section on image quality.

Kilovoltage settings for typical radiographic units range between 40 kVp and 150 kVp in increments of 1 or 2 kilovolts. Low kVp settings are used for small body parts. For example, 50 to 60 kVp is commonly used for x-ray examinations of the hand, wrist, or foot. Spine radiography typically utilizes settings between 75 and 100 kVp, while settings above 100 kVp may be used for chest radiography and for barium studies of the digestive tract.

Distance

The distance between the source of the x-ray beam (the tube target) and the imaging plane (film) is referred to as the **source-image distance (SID).** This distance is a prime factor of exposure because it affects the intensity of the x-ray beam. Since the x-ray beam diverges from its source, the size of the beam expands as the distance from the source increases. As the total quantity of x-ray photons in the beam spreads out, there are fewer photons in any given area (Fig. 1-26).

The change in x-ray beam intensity that results from changes in the SID is expressed by the inverse square law, which states that the intensity of the radiation is inversely proportional to the square of the distance. You will note in Fig. 1-26 that as the distance is doubled, each dimension of the radiation field is doubled; so the radiation field is four times greater in area and the intensity is one fourth of the original amount. Likewise, if the distance were tripled, the field area would be nine times as large (3^2), and the radiation intensity would be one ninth of the original amount.

Of course, as the radiation intensity decreases, exposure to the film will also decrease. If it is desired to maintain the same film density when the SID changes, the mAs must be adjusted correspondingly.

Technique Charts

A technique chart located near the control console usually provides the radiographer with a listing of recommended mAs and kVp settings, as well as the SID, for each of the various body parts for different sizes of patients. Some control consoles have

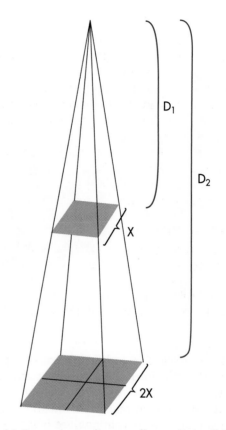

FIG. 1-26 Source-image distance affects radiation field size and radiation intensity.

"anatomical programming." These computerized units are preprogrammed with the required exposure settings for the selected body part and size.

IMAGE RECEPTOR SYSTEMS
Cassettes and Intensifying Screens

The cassette (Fig. 1-27) serves as the film holder during the radiographic procedure. It provides a light-tight, rigid structure to protect the film and also houses the intensifying screens. Most cassettes contain two intensifying screens, one front and one back, and the film is placed between them. Intensifying screens are plates coated with phosphors (fluorescent crystals) that give off light when exposed to x-rays. Their purpose is to reduce the amount of exposure required. Without intensifying

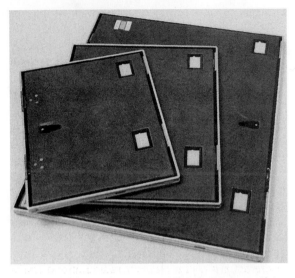

FIG. 1-27 Radiographic cassette is lined with intensifying screens that are held in contact with both sides of the film.

screens, as much as 50 to 100 times more exposure would be needed. Intensifying screens greatly reduce patient dose and also reduce the output capacity requirements of x-ray generators and x-ray tubes.

Most phosphors in common use today are salts from one of the rare earth elements. When exposed to x-rays, they give off green, blue, or blue-violet light, depending on the specific phosphor. The size of the crystals and the thickness of the phosphor layer determine the amount of exposure required. Larger crystals and/or thicker layers require less exposure. Screens with finer crystals and thinner layers produce sharper image detail. Most radiography departments have at least two types of screens: "fast" screens with larger crystals for routine use, and "detail" or "extremity" screens that have smaller crystals and require more exposure. The detail screens are used only for relatively small parts, such as hands and feet, where fine detail is most important. They are used only on the tabletop, not with grids or buckys.

Each cassette has a small area where there is no intensifying screen and where exposure is blocked from the film by lead foil. This area is reserved for the photographic imprint of the patient identification. It is indicated on the front of the cassette by the position of the identifying label.

It is important that you become familiar with the types of intensifying screens used in your department so that you can select cassettes correctly and use them with the appropriate exposure factors. Cassettes are marked according to the type of screens they contain, and the technique chart will state which screens are appropriate with a given set of exposures.

Intensifying screens are quite expensive and are easily damaged. Damaged areas, dirt, or stains on the screens prevent light from exposing the film and result in artifacts on the image. For these reasons, it is important to avoid touching the screens and to keep the film processing area free of dust and dirt.

Film

Radiographic film is manufactured with a particular sensitivity to the light emitted by intensifying screens. Green sensitive film is used with screens that emit green light, and blue sensitive film is matched with blue-emitting screens. Film for routine radiography has emulsion coated on both sides of the base so that the film responds to the light from both intensifying screens. This system decreases the exposure required by half. Both sides of the film are therefore identical; there is no "right" or "wrong" side to a sheet of double-emulsion film.

Film and cassettes come in standard sizes. You will work more effectively in the clinical area when you have learned to recognize them at a glance. The most common sizes are the following:

- 8 × 10 inches (20 × 25 cm)
- 9 × 9 inches (23 × 23 cm)
- 10 × 12 inches (25 × 30 cm)
- 11 × 14 inches (28 × 35 cm)
- 7 × 17 inches (18 × 43 cm)
- 14 × 14 inches (35 × 35 cm)
- 14 × 17 inches (35 × 43 cm)

Film Processing

Film must be stored correctly to avoid fog, a generalized exposure that reduces film contrast. A good storage area is clean, cool, and dry, protected from radiation and processing chemical fumes. Film boxes should stand on edge with the expiration date visible. This date is checked to be sure older film is used before its expiration date.

To avoid artifacts from improper film handling, be sure your hands are clean and dry and touch only the corner of the film when removing it from the cassette. Avoid bending and crimping the film by allowing it to hang vertically when holding it with only one hand. To place it horizontally, use both hands and hold by opposite corners.

Processing may involve darkroom procedures or a "daylight processing" system. In a conventional darkroom system, the exposed cassette is taken to the darkroom where the film is removed, identified, and fed into the automatic processor in near darkness. The cassette is then reloaded with fresh film from the film bin, a storage unit located under the counter. A safelight provides just enough illumination for you to see where things are located. A tone or a red light on the processor will indicate when it is safe to feed another film or to turn on the lights.

Cassettes are often passed to and from the darkroom without opening the door by using a passbox. This compartment is installed in the darkroom wall and has two sets of doors, one set inside the darkroom and one set in the outside wall. Since the inner and outer doors cannot be opened at the same time, cassettes can be transferred while the darkroom remains dark. The passbox has two compartments, one for exposed cassettes awaiting processing, and one for the unexposed cassettes that have been reloaded and are ready for use. Correct locations for cassettes are essential, since it is not possible to determine by looking at the cassette whether the film is exposed. Only by following the established routines can radiographers be confident that a cassette is unexposed and ready for use.

Daylight processing systems enable radiographers to process film without a darkroom. These systems include a special film processor, a daylight film identification camera, and special cassettes. Films can be identified while still in the cassette, and then the entire cassette is fed into the processor. The processor removes and processes the film and reloads the cassette.

Filmless Radiography

Computed radiography (CR) is a radiographic imaging system that does not use film. An imaging plate, similar to an intensifying screen, is exposed in a special cassette using conventional x-ray equipment. The radiographer inserts the exposed cassette into a special processor and selects the type of examination from a menu so that the image will be processed correctly. A small beam from a high-intensity laser in the processor converts the latent image to a visible one that is captured by a photomultiplier tube, similar to those used in fluoroscopic image intensifiers. The photomultiplier tube emits an electronic signal that is digitized and stored in a computer. The image can then be displayed on a high-resolution monitor. Hard copies can be produced using a laser film printer.

Digital radiography is another type of filmless imaging system. Special radiographic tables and upright cabinets contain digital receptors that react to the pattern of the remnant radiation and transmit a digital signal directly to the computer system. No cassettes and no processing are involved. While digital radiography has for some time been used for special applications such as fluoroscopy and angiography, technical limitations and cost factors have prevented widespread adoption of digital systems for general radiography.

Once stored in the computer system, digital images from either CR or digital radiography systems are organized and cataloged and can be accessed on screen from multiple locations connected to the system network. These digital images can be manipulated electronically to enhance visibility. Analog images (conventional radiographs) can be added to the system by scanning them with a laser device called a film digitizer.

The computer hardware and software technology used to manage digital images in hospitals and large health care systems is called a picture archiving and communication system (PACS). These systems provide archives for the storage of images, connect images with patient database information, facilitate laser printing of images, and display both images and information at work stations throughout the network as needed. PACS may include transmission equipment for teleradiology, allowing images to be viewed in remote locations such as a physician's home, and receiving images from remote locations such as outlying clinics. PACS technology can transmit images directly over telephone lines and via the Internet.

IMAGE QUALITY

The more exposure received by a specific portion of the film, the darker that portion of the image will be. The visibility of the radiographic image depends on two factors: the overall blackness of the film and the differences in blackness between the various portions of the image. The clarity and sharpness of the image are also important, as is the degree to which the image is a true representation of the subject. These features make up the four elements of radiographic quality.

Radiographic Density

The overall blackness of the image is referred to as the radiographic density. When the radiographic density is optimum, the film is both dark enough and light enough for you to see the image clearly on the viewbox. Fig. 1-28 shows radiographs of varying radiographic density. Density is influenced by many factors, but it is primarily controlled by the mAs. Since exposure darkens the film, an increase in mAs will result in a darker radiograph, while a decrease will make the film lighter.

Radiographic Contrast

The difference in the radiographic density of adjacent structures within the image is referred to as the radiographic contrast. Even when a radiograph has the proper radiographic density, it is possible that structures may be too similar in density to be easily distinguished from one another. Fig. 1-29 shows radiographs with high, low, and optimum contrast. You will note that the high-contrast image has a "black and white" appearance. Structures in the gray areas are easily distinguished, but no details can be seen in the very dark or the very light portions of the image. The low-contrast image has an overall gray appearance, and the structures tend to blend into one another. The optimum contrast radiograph shows details within all areas of the image, although the contrast in some areas is less pronounced.

Contrast is influenced by a number of factors, including the nature of the subject and the amount of scatter radiation affecting the film, but kilovoltage is the primary contrast control factor. High kilovoltage produces an x-ray beam that penetrates more completely, leaving no white areas in the image. The dark, easily penetrated portions of the subject are not quite as dark when the kVp is high because less mAs is needed to obtain the desired radiographic density. When more contrast is desired, the kVp is decreased. Since this will result in less penetration by the x-ray beam, a beam of greater intensity is needed and the mAs must be increased.

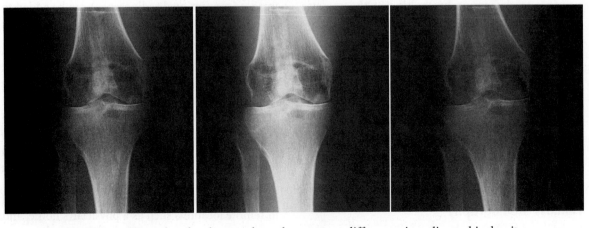

FIG. 1-28 Radiographs of a phantom knee demonstrate differences in radiographic density. **A,** Optimum density. **B,** Underexposed. **C,** Overexposed.

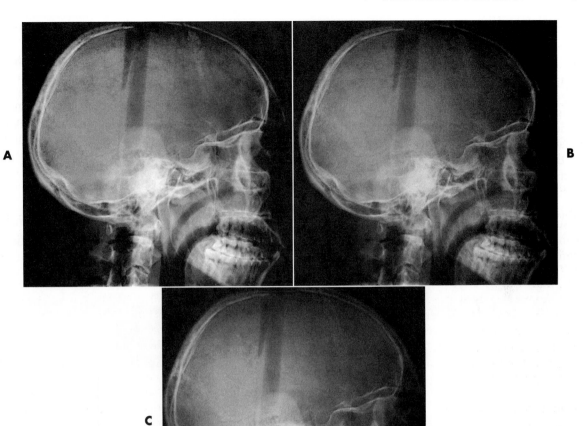

FIG. 1-29 Radiographs of a phantom skull demonstrate differences in radiographic contrast. **A,** High contrast. **B,** Low contrast. **C,** Optimum contrast.

Contrast is best evaluated when the overall radiographic density is optimum.

Radiographic Definition

The third element of image quality is radiographic definition. This refers to the sharpness of the image. When definition is high, the edges and lines that make up the image are crisp and precise; whereas with low definition, these lines and edges are less distinct and appear somewhat blurred or "out of focus." Among the factors that affect radiographic definition are the SID; the distance between the object and the film, referred to as *object-image distance (OID);* the size of the intensifying screen crystals and the thickness of the phosphor layer; and whether the patient is able to hold still during the exposure.

Radiographic Distortion

The fourth element of image quality is radiographic distortion. This refers to a variation in the size or shape of the image in comparison to the object it represents. Size distortion is always in the form of magnification, and all radiographic images are magnified to some degree. The factors that affect magnification are the OID and the SID. The angulation of the diverging x-rays that define the edges of a subject affects the degree of magnification (Fig. 1-30). When the x-ray tube is farther from the film, the central, more parallel rays will define the subject, resulting in less magnification. As the x-ray beam continues past the subject to the film, the rays continue to diverge, increasing the magnification.

The closer the object is to the film, the less magnification there will be.

Shape distortion is the result of unequal magnification of various parts of the subject. The least shape distortion occurs when the plane of the object is parallel to the plane of the film and the central ray is perpendicular to it. Angulation of the x-ray beam, the film, or the object in relation to the film will all cause some degree of distortion (Fig. 1-31).

RADIATION UNITS

Radiation measurements can be made in two different, but related, systems: the traditional (British) system, still most commonly used in the United

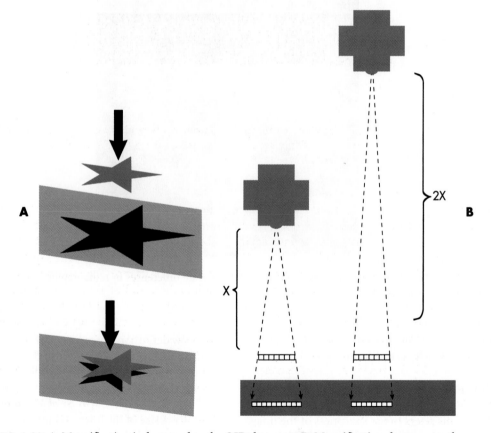

FIG. 1-30 **A,** Magnification is decreased as the OID decreases. **B,** Magnification decreases as the SID increases.

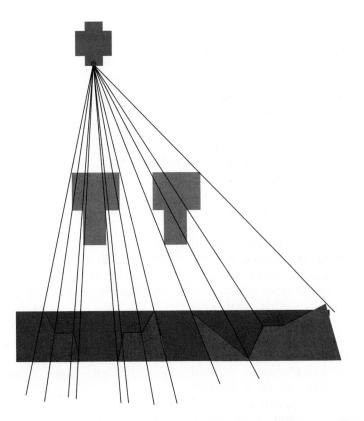

FIG. 1-31 Radiographic distortion. Distortion is minimized when subject is parallel to film and central ray is perpendicular to film. Shape distortion results when there is angulation of x-ray beam in relation to subject or film.

States, and the SI (*Systeme Internationale*) units established by the International Commission on Radiation Units in 1981. These units and their relationships are summarized in Table 1-2.

The traditional unit of radiation exposure is the **roentgen (R),** a measurement of radiation intensity in air. The roentgen is equal to the quantity of radiation that will produce 2.08×10^9 (over 2 billion) ion pairs in one cubic centimeter of dry air. The SI unit for measuring radiation intensity is coulombs per kilogram (C/kg), specifying the quantity of electrical charge in coulombs produced by the exposure of 1 kilogram of dry air. One roentgen equals 2.58×10^{-4} (.000258) C/kg.

The roentgen is useful for measuring the quantity of radiation present, but it is not a useful dose measurement. Dose varies with the depth of measurement and the quantity of radiation energy absorbed in the exposed tissue. To measure therapeutic radiation doses, as well as specific tissue doses received in diagnostic applications, the traditional unit is the **rad.** Rad stands for **r**adiation **a**bsorbed **d**ose and is equal to 100 ergs (an energy unit) per gram of tissue. One roentgen of exposure will result in approximately 1 rad of absorbed dose in muscle tissue. The SI unit for dose measurement is the Gray (Gy). One Gray equals 100 rad, and conversely, 1 rad equals 1 centigray.

The biological effect of radiation exposure varies according to the type of radiation involved and its energy. Equal doses of various types of radiation will not necessarily result in equal biological effects.

TABLE 1-2

RADIATION UNITS

	CONVENTIONAL UNITS	SI UNITS
Exposure units	Roentgen (R)	Coulombs per kilogram (C/kg)
	Quantity of radiation that will produce 2.08×10^9 ion pairs in 1 cc of air	$1 R = 2.58 \times 10^{-4}$ C/kg
Dose units	Rad (radiation absorbed dose)	Gray (Gy)
	100 ergs per gram of tissue	1 Gy = 100 rad
Dose equivalent units	Rem (roentgen equivalent in man)	Sievert (Sv)
	rem = rad $\times$ QF	Sv = Gy $\times$ QF
		1 Sv = 100 rem

Some radiation workers, such as engineers in nuclear power plants, nuclear submarine construction workers, or technologists in nuclear medicine laboratories, may be exposed to several types of radiation with unequal levels of biological effect. Neither the roentgen nor the rad is a useful unit for measuring the occupational dose of combined radiations with different levels of effects.

To simplify the process of measuring occupational dose, a **quality factor (QF)** number is assigned to each type of radiation based upon its relative biological effect as compared to x-rays. The quality factors for different types of ionizing radiation are listed in Table 1-3. For example, note that thermal neutrons have a QF of 5. This is because 1 rad of thermal neutrons causes biological effects that are approximately equal to those produced by 5 rads of x-ray energy. The absorbed dose is multiplied by the QF to obtain the

dose equivalent. The resulting unit is called the **rem,** which stands for **r**oentgen **e**quivalent in **m**an. Thus, the worker exposed to 1 rad of thermal neutrons would receive 5 rem of occupational exposure.

$$rad \times QF = rem$$

The SI unit used to measure dose equivalents is the Sievert (Sv). The Sievert is determined by multiplying the dose in Gy times the QF; thus,

$$Gy \times QF = Sv$$

and

$$1 Sv = 100 rem$$

Since the radiation quantities involved in diagnostic radiology are so small, radiographers commonly use units that are 1/1000 of the common unit (e.g., milliroentgens [mR], millirad [mrad], and millirem [mrem]). For example, a chest radiograph may result in a skin entrance dose of 15 mrad, or 0.015 rad.

Students often find it confusing to determine which dose units should be used in a given situation. This is made more difficult by the tendency of many radiographers to use the traditional roentgen, rad, and rem units interchangeably. This does not cause serious inaccuracy when speaking only of diagnostic x-rays, because exposure to 1 roentgen of x-ray energy will result in approximately 1 rad of absorbed dose in muscle. Since the QF of diagnostic x-rays equals one, 1 rad is also equal to 1 rem.

In general, the reason for the measurement determines which unit is most appropriate.

TABLE 1-3

QUALITY FACTORS* FOR DIFFERENT TYPES OF IONIZING RADIATION

TYPE OF RADIATION	QUALITY FACTOR
X-ray photons	1
Beta particles	1
Gamma photons	1
Thermal neutrons	5
Fast neutrons	20
Alpha particles	20

*Quality factor is derived from relative biological effectiveness measurement.

The roentgen and C/kg are used to measure the presence of x-radiation without any reference to its absorption or attenuation (i.e., the quantity of radiation present in air). The rad and the Gray are used to measure radiation dose. These units are used to prescribe radiation therapy. The amount absorbed by a specific tissue is what is being measured, so a statement indicating the part of the body involved usually modifies the rad dosage. For example, a radiation oncologist may prescribe a treatment involving 150 rad to the liver, or a research report might state that the average patient who has a routine chest radiograph receives a thyroid dose of 4 mrad. The laboratory that processes the personnel monitor badges will report occupational dose in dose equivalent units: rem, mrem, or mSv.

BIOLOGICAL EFFECTS OF X-RAY EXPOSURE

As mentioned earlier in this chapter, x-rays can ionize substances, removing electrons from their orbits. This process results in a free, negatively charged electron and leaves the remainder of the atom with a positive charge. When human beings are irradiated, ionization may occur to any part of a living cell, such as the material that makes up its membrane, the water within the membrane, or the DNA that makes up the cell's chromosomes and directs its activity. The initial ionization may produce a "domino effect," causing ionization in the surrounding area. Exposure also creates free radicals, temporary molecules and parts of molecules with electrical charges. Free radicals may interact directly with the DNA or may produce toxic substances that are injurious to DNA.

Most effects of exposure are extremely short-lived because electrons find new homes in the orbits of other atoms, and the balance of charges returns to normal. Free radicals combine to form more stable compounds. Occasionally, however, the damage is not resolved instantly. A cell may be so damaged that it cannot sustain itself and dies. Cell death is an insignificant injury unless the number of cells involved is massive. Cells may sustain damage that requires several days for the body to make repairs. The body produces special enzymes that

function to repair the DNA protein molecules. A cell may be damaged in such a way that its DNA "programming" is changed, and the cell no longer behaves normally. This type of injury may eventually result in the runaway production of new, abnormal cells, causing a tumor or malignant blood disease.

The relative sensitivity of different types of cells is summarized in the Laws of Bergonié and Tribondeau, which state that cell sensitivity to radiation exposure depends on four characteristics of the cell:

1. **Age.** Younger cells are more sensitive than older ones.
2. **Differentiation.** Simple cells are more sensitive than highly complex ones.
3. **Metabolic rate.** Cells that use energy rapidly are more sensitive than those with a slower metabolism.
4. **Mitotic rate.** Cells that divide and multiply rapidly are more sensitive than those that replicate slowly.

According to these laws, we see that blood cells and blood-producing cells are very sensitive. Cells in contact with the environment are quite simple, have relatively short lives, and are quite sensitive. These include the cells of the skin and the mucosal lining of the mouth, nose, and gastrointestinal tract. Some glandular tissue is also particularly sensitive, especially that of the thyroid gland and the female breast. The tissues of embryos, fetuses, infants, children, and adolescents tend to be more sensitive than adult tissues because of their younger age and their higher metabolic and mitotic rates. Nerve cells, which have a long life and are quite complex, are much less vulnerable to radiation injury. Cortical bone cells are also relatively insensitive.

Radiation effects are classified in various ways. Short-term effects are those observed within 3 months of the exposure. They are associated with relatively high radiation doses (greater than 50 rad). Short-term effects may be further categorized according to the body system affected: central nervous system (CNS), gastrointestinal, and hematological effects. Long-term effects, sometimes referred to as latent effects, may not be apparent for as long as

30 years. Somatic effects are those that affect the body of the irradiated individual directly, whereas genetic effects occur as a result of damage to the reproductive cells of the irradiated person and are observed as defects in the children or grandchildren of the irradiated individual.

Short-Term Somatic Effects

One observable short-term effect is a reddening of the skin, **erythema.** This phenomenon is sometimes called a "radiation burn." In the very early days of radiation use, the amount of radiation necessary to produce reddening of the skin was called the "erythema dose." It was the first unit used to measure radiation.

Other short-term effects from high doses in excess of 50 rad have been observed and studied in radiation therapy patients and in the victims of radiation accidents and atomic bomb blasts. This is vastly more exposure than is delivered by diagnostic x-ray machines. Extremely high doses produce CNS effects, seizures and coma that result in death in a short period of time. Lesser doses will result in "radiation sickness," a gastrointestinal effect in which the mucosal lining of the digestive tract is damaged, breaks down, and becomes infected by the bacteria that normally inhabit the bowel. These victims also have a compromised immune system, due to the death of white blood cells, and are unable to fight the infection. Radiation sickness is usually fatal, and suffering may be prolonged. A lesser dose, affecting primarily the blood, results in hematological effects: anemia and compromise of the immune system. These victims are prone to infectious diseases that may or may not be fatal, depending on the radiation dose and the severity of the disease process. The whole-body radiation dose fatal to 50% of the irradiated population within 30 days is approximately 300 rad for humans.

Long-Term Somatic Effects

"Long-term" here refers to the length of time between exposure and observation of the effect. The time required for long-term effects to manifest is generally considered to be 5 to 30 years, with the greatest percentage occurring between 10 and 15 years.

Short-term radiation effects are predictable, and the quantity of exposure required to produce them is well documented. Long-term effects, on the other hand, are apparently random. They may involve repeated small doses, such as those used in radiography. Certainly, the percentage of observable effects from the radiation involved in typical x-ray examinations is extremely low and the risk to any one patient is minimal. Most of us take greater risks when we drive a car or cross a busy street. Nevertheless, there is a risk of long-term effects that has been demonstrated by studying large populations over long periods of time. The incidence of certain conditions is greater when results for irradiated groups are compared to those of nonirradiated control groups.

Long-term radiation effects are not easily identified as such because they occur so long after exposure and because these same effects also occur in the absence of radiation exposure. Only extensive research with large populations and computer analysis can demonstrate the role of radiation in causing these effects. In other words, radiation causes increased *risk* of these effects, but the effects cannot be predicted with respect to any one individual. While the individual risk may be extremely small, increasing exposure to the entire population poses public health risks that require the attention and concern of everyone involved in applying ionizing radiation to human beings.

The documented latent effects of low doses of ionizing radiation include the following:

- **Cataractogenesis.** The formation of cataracts, clouding of the lens of the eye. This effect concerns radiologists and radiographers who work extensively in fluoroscopy and those who perform other work that involves repeated exposure to the eyes.
- **Carcinogenesis.** Increased risk of malignant disease; particularly cancer of the skin, thyroid, and breast; and leukemia, a malignant blood disease associated with radiation exposure.
- **Life span shortening.** A study of the life span of radiologists who died during a 3-year period before 1945 showed that they had shorter life spans than physicians who did not use

radiation in their practices. This group included radiologists who had used radiation since the early days of x-ray science. More recent studies show that occupational exposure no longer has a measurable effect on the life span of radiologists. Nevertheless, since radiation exposure has been linked to life span shortening, it is a public health concern and another reason to practice a high level of radiation safety.

Genetic Effects

Genetic effects, in the form of changes or mutations to the genes, may be caused when the ovaries or testes are exposed to ionizing radiation. In the female, all the ova cells that the individual will ever produce are present in an immature state at birth. Since no new egg cells are produced as the individual ages, the effect of radiation exposure to the ovaries is cumulative. The genetic effects of radiation to the testes also have a longer-term effect than may at first be presumed, because damage to the stem cells that produce the sperm may result in continued production of sperm with the genetic mutation. The majority of genetic mutations are considered negative, or less well suited to survival of the individual than nonmutated cells.

Since reproductive cells have only half the number of chromosomes in all other cells, each parent contributes one chromosome to each pair in the new individual, and nature makes the choice as to which gene of each pair will affect the characteristics of the offspring. Those genes that are "chosen" are said to be dominant, and those that are not selected are called recessive. Mutated genes are usually recessive and therefore do not manifest their characteristics in the offspring. Both dominant and recessive genes, however, occur in the reproductive cells of the offspring and may be passed on to future generations.

As an increasing percentage of the population is exposed to radiation from natural, occupational, and health care sources, the likelihood increases that an individual will be conceived with mutation of both genes in a strategic pair, resulting in some type of deformity or maladaption. Public health officials and governments are very concerned about preserving the integrity of the population's gene pool by minimizing harmful, defect-causing radiation. This concern should motivate those who apply ionizing radiation to humans to minimize gonad doses in every way possible. Gonad shielding for this purpose is addressed later in this chapter.

Genetic effects from mutations caused by x-ray exposure have long been demonstrated in animal research. Interestingly, very little genetic effect has been confirmed by the continuing research of the Japanese populations affected by the atomic bombs dropped on Hiroshima and Nagasaki during World War II or in other studies of human populations.

RADIATION SAFETY

Clearly, exposure to x-rays creates some risk for both patients and radiographers. It is therefore an essential part of your education and your ethical responsibility to be knowledgeable about radiation safety and to use this knowledge to avoid all unnecessary radiation exposure to your patients, your coworkers, and yourself. A comprehensive course on the subject of radiation biology and radiation safety will be a part of the curriculum in your radiography program.

Personnel Safety

Radiographers may be exposed to radiation either from the primary x-ray beam or from the scatter radiation that results from the interaction of the primary beam with the patient or other material in its path. Because radiographers are considered to be "occupationally exposed individuals," they are prohibited from activities that would result in direct exposure to the primary x-ray beam. This means that they are not allowed to hold patients or cassettes during x-ray exposures and must stand clear of the path of the primary x-ray beam during fluoroscopic and mobile radiographic examinations.

As explained earlier in this chapter, scatter radiation is ambient radiation in the x-ray room during an exposure. Radiographers are not exposed to any significant amount of this radiation in a typical radiographic room when standing well behind the protective lead barrier of the control booth.

The exposure increases when the radiographer assists with fluoroscopic procedures or uses mobile x-ray equipment.

The three principal methods used to protect x-ray equipment operators from unnecessary radiation exposure are time, distance, and shielding.

The amount of exposure received is directly proportional to the time spent in a scatter radiation field, so occupational dose is decreased when this time is minimized. For example, a radiographer might shorten the time of exposure by stepping into the control booth during fluoroscopic procedures when not required to be near the patient.

The second method involves using distance. Increasing the distance between yourself and a radiation source decreases your exposure in proportion to the square of the distance, so small increases in distance have a relatively large effect. Mobile x-ray units have long cords on the exposure switches, enabling the radiographer to get as far from the radiation source as possible while making an exposure.

The third method is shielding and is by far the most common method of dose reduction used by radiographers. The lead wall of the control booth provides the primary barrier and is the radiographer's primary defense. Other types of shielding include lead aprons, gloves, goggles, and thyroid shields (Fig. 1-32). These types of shielding are worn during fluoroscopic procedures and mobile radiographic examinations.

An essential part of your clinical education will be learning to protect yourself and your coworkers from unnecessary radiation exposure. This includes doing a "safety check" before each exposure—making certain that all personnel are properly protected and that the door is closed before initiating exposures.

Personnel Monitoring

Devices for monitoring radiation exposure to personnel are called **dosimeters.** They should be worn in the region of the collar and should be outside the lead apron when a lead apron is worn.

Film badges were once the principal type of dosimeter. They are still in use today, but are much

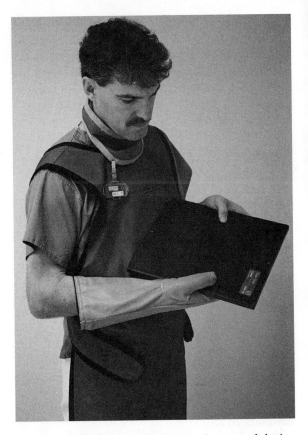

FIG. 1-32 Radiographer wears protective apparel during fluoroscopic and mobile radiographic examinations.

less common. They consist of one or two pieces of dental film, paper-wrapped and enclosed in a badge-like holder. Several filters are incorporated in the badge so that, if the unfiltered exposure exceeds the capacity of the film, additional exposure can be measured in the filtered area. The disadvantage of this type of personnel monitor is that the dental film is subject to fog when exposed to heat or fumes, and this exposure could result in a false reading. The film is also ruined if it is laundered! After a period of use, the film is returned to a laboratory that processes it and measures the film density. The exposure is calculated and reported based on this measurement. Many radiographers still refer to their dosimeters as "film badges," but today they are more likely to be TLDs or OSLs.

TLD stands for *thermoluminescent dosimeter.* The roots of this word mean, "dose-measuring device that gives off light when heated." The TLD is a type of personnel monitor commonly used by radiographers (Fig. 1-33). It consists of a plastic badge containing one or more lithium fluoride crystals. These crystals (and several others with similar characteristics) absorb x-ray energy and give off the energy again in the form of light when heated. The TLD is more durable than the film badge insert and responds only to ionizing radiation exposure. At the end of the measurement period the badge is sent to a laboratory where the crystals are placed in a special tray and inserted into the TLD analyzer. This instrument heats the crystals to the required temperature, measures the light emitted, and transmits the data to a computer.

OSL stands for *optically stimulated luminescence* and refers to the most recently developed monitoring dosimeter (Fig. 1-34). Aluminum oxide is the radiation detector in this device. The dosimeter is processed using a laser rather than heat as for TLDs. OSLs have several advantages over TLDs. They can measure very small doses more precisely and can be reanalyzed to confirm results. They are accurate over a wide dose range and have excellent long-term stability.

Radiation monitor badge service laboratories provide badges, processing service, and reports and

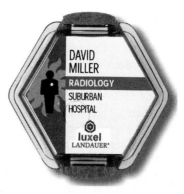

FIG. 1-34 Latest generation of personnel dosimeters is the optically stimulated luminescence (OSL) type.

keep permanent records of the radiation exposure of each person monitored. Service may be arranged on a weekly, monthly, or quarterly basis. Personnel who receive relatively high doses of occupational exposure change their badges most frequently. With the exception of OSL badges, dosimeters cannot accurately measure total exposures of less than 5 mrem (0.005 rem). For this reason, personnel who receive very small amounts of exposure will get more accurate measurements with less frequent badge changes. Personnel involved in diagnostic radiography who are always, or nearly always, in a control booth during exposures are usually best monitored with quarterly service. Monthly service is a better choice for those who work in fluoroscopy and perform bedside radiography.

Service companies provide an extra badge in every batch that is marked CONTROL. This badge's purpose is to measure any radiation exposure to the entire batch while in transit. Any amount of exposure measured from the control badge will be subtracted from the amounts measured from the other badges in the batch. The control badge should be kept in a safe place, away from any possibility of x-ray exposure. It should never be used to measure occupational dose or for any other purpose.

Radiation badge service companies will want to know the name, birth date, and Social Security Number of all persons to be monitored so that all records can be accurately identified. If there has been a history of previous occupational radiation

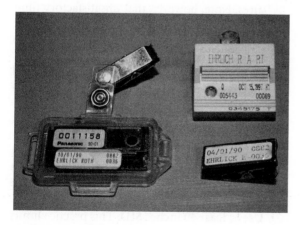

FIG. 1-33 An assortment of TLD radiation dosimeters as worn by radiographers.

exposure and the dose is known, this information should also be provided so that the record will be complete and accurate. Exposure reports are sent to the subscriber for each batch, and an annual summary of personnel exposure is also provided. Personnel should be advised of the radiation exposure reported from their badges and should be provided with copies of the annual reports for their own records. Personnel exposed to ionizing radiation should not leave their employment without a complete record of their radiation exposure history. Employers are required to provide this information.

Effective Dose Equivalent Limits

The ALARA principle is the guiding philosophy associated with all radiation use that involves exposure to humans, both patients and workers. It states that all radiation exposure to humans should be limited to levels that are **As Low As Reasonably Achievable.**

The effective dose equivalent–limiting (EDE) system is used to calculate the upper limits of occupational exposure that is permitted. For occupationally exposed personnel, the upper EDE limit is 5 rem (50 mSv) per year. This applies to workers over the age of 18 who are not pregnant and is assumed to be a whole-body dose. These limits apply to occupational exposure only and not to exposure that workers may receive as a result of imaging or tests related to their own health care.

The EDE system also states a retrospective or cumulative dose limit that is equal to 1 rem (10 mSv) times the worker's age. For example, a 30-year-old worker with no previous occupational exposure would have a cumulative EDE limit of 30 rem (300 mSv). This is referred to as the "rem bank." The worker is permitted to exceed the annual limits by small amounts as long as the rem bank is not depleted.

The EDE system specifies dose equivalents for specific body organs and tissues. For example, workers who receive exposure to their hands while their bodies are protected may wear ring or wrist dosimeters. A higher dose limit is established for this limited exposure.

The established EDE limits ensure that the safety of radiation workers is comparable to that of workers in other safe occupations. The risk from the allowable exposure is considered to be so low as to pose an insignificant risk. The occupational dose received by radiographers is usually well below the established limit.

The upper boundaries of occupational dose were formerly referred to as "maximum permissible dose" or MPD. This term is now out of favor because it implies that exposure in excess of the lowest achievable dose is permissible. The ALARA principle must be applied in conjunction with the use of EDE limits. It is important that radiographers not be complacent simply because their dose is below the limit. Radiation control agencies require that occupational dose be kept to the lowest levels that are reasonably achievable.

Patient Protection

This topic will be addressed repeatedly in various contexts throughout your education in radiography. You will be able to understand it far more completely at a later date. For now, you should be aware that the following methods are employed to minimize patient dose:

- **Avoid errors.** Double-check requisitions and patient identification so that the right patient gets the right examination.
- **Avoid repeat exposures.** Establish good routine procedures, and follow them strictly so that careless errors do not necessitate repeat exposures. Note, however, that unsatisfactory films *must* be repeated. Radiation safety cannot be used as a reason for failing to produce a satisfactory examination.
- **Collimate.** Use the smallest radiation field that will encompass the area of clinical interest. In no case should the size of the radiation field be greater than the size of the film.
- **Use the highest kVp that is consistent with acceptable film quality.** This permits using the lowest possible mAs to obtain an acceptable exposure.
- **Use at least 40 inches SID.** This practice limits patient exposure from tube housing leakage and collimator scatter.

- **Fast films and screens.** Use the fastest films and screens consistent with the necessary film quality.
- **Provide shielding** for gonads, eyes, breasts, and thyroid, as appropriate.

Gonad Shielding

Lead shields that prevent unnecessary radiation to the reproductive organs are required when the patient is of reproductive age or younger, whenever the gonads are within the primary radiation field, and when the shield will not interfere with the examination. Generally, this applies to most patients under the age of 55. A shield device consisting of at least a 0.5-mm lead equivalent is placed between the x-ray tube and the patient. Shields attached to the collimator (shadow shields) may be positioned by viewing their shadows within the collimator light field. Shields placed on or near the patient's body are referred to as contact shields and are somewhat more effective than shadow shields. Both types meet the legal requirements for gonad shielding. Fig. 1-35 demonstrates shield placement for both males and females. It is helpful to note that the pubic symphysis is at the same level as the greater trochanter of the femur, avoiding the necessity of palpating the pubic symphysis for proper shield placement.

RADIATION AND PREGNANCY

It has been recognized for some time that radiation exposure poses specific risks to the developing embryo or fetus. In general, we now know that radiation during pregnancy may result in spontaneous abortion, congenital defects in the child, increased risk of malignant disease in childhood, and an increase in significant genetic abnormalities in the children of parents who were exposed in utero.

Animal studies first alerted scientists that radiation could cause spontaneous abortion of the developing embryo and could increase the rate of congenital abnormalities seen in those that survived to birth. These findings have been confirmed in humans by studying the pregnancies of women who survived the atomic bomb blasts of Hiroshima and Nagasaki and the nuclear accident at Chernobyl. Studies of smaller groups of women exposed to radiation as a result of diagnostic and therapeutic procedures confirm that radiation in excess of 5 rad to the uterus is cause for some level of concern. In the 1950s, Alice Stewart, an English researcher, demonstrated a fourteenfold increase in the incidence of childhood leukemia among children who had been exposed to radiation in utero as a result of x-ray pelvimetry examinations in the third trimester of pregnancy.

The greatest risks for spontaneous abortion, fetal death, and significant birth defects exist when significant levels of exposure occur during the first trimester of pregnancy (i.e., the first 3 months). The embryo is most vulnerable to radiation insult while tissues are in the process of differentiation. Unfortunately, this creates the greatest hazard at a time when a woman may not yet be aware she is pregnant.

Radiation control agencies address the issue of radiation exposure to pregnant radiation workers. The EDE limit of whole-body radiation for the pregnant worker is 0.5 rem over the 9-month course of the pregnancy. When a worker declares that she is pregnant by submitting a written document to her employer, the employer is responsible for providing fetal radiation monitoring and for ensuring that the occupational dose does not exceed the EDE limit for pregnant workers. Here again, the ALARA principle is important. Every effort should be made to minimize exposure, keeping the dose as far below the limit as possible.

For a pregnant radiographer, the safest work assignment would be one in which a permanent lead barrier (control booth) always shields the worker during exposures (Fig. 1-36). Pregnant radiographers, or those of childbearing age who may be pregnant, should pay particular attention to personal safety measures when assisting with fluoroscopy or using mobile x-ray equipment.

The public is generally aware that x-radiation is to be avoided during pregnancy, and this may lead to irrational fears on the part of pregnant women or their families. The chance is extremely remote that a routine x-ray examination of the chest or an extremity would harm the developing child. On the other

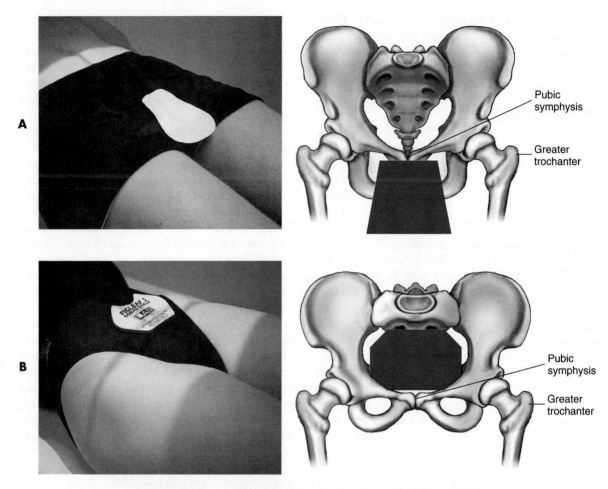

FIG. 1-35 Gonad shield placement. **A,** Male shield is placed in the midline with its top margin 1 inch inferior to pubic symphysis. **B,** Inferior margin of female shield is placed at or near the top of the pubic symphysis. It is centered in the midline, halfway between the level of the anterior superior iliac spine and the symphysis pubis. Note that in both males and females the pubic symphysis is at the level of the greater trochanters.

hand, examinations requiring direct radiation to the pelvis, especially relatively high-dose fluoroscopic studies or computed tomography scans of the abdomen or lumbar spine, may be cause for concern.

Radiation control regulations require that female patients of childbearing age be advised of potential radiation hazards before x-ray examination. This requirement is usually met by posting signs in the radiology department advising women to tell the radiographer before the examination if they may be pregnant (Fig. 1-37). Such signs should be written in all languages commonly used in the community.

The patient's physician is in the best position to be aware of an early pregnancy. The patient's history may indicate the possibility of pregnancy, and specific questions to rule out pregnancy should be a part of any medical history that precedes the ordering of pelvic x-ray examinations. If pregnancy is a

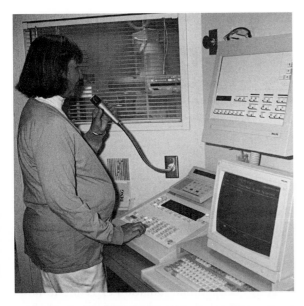

FIG. 1-36 Lead barrier of control booth protects pregnant radiographer.

possibility, an early pregnancy test, easily and quickly performed in the physician's office, may clarify the situation. If the patient is pregnant and the proposed x-ray examination involves direct pelvic radiation, the physician must weigh the potential risks and benefits of the examination and discuss them with

the patient before proceeding with the study. In the case of minor or chronic complaints, it is common to delay the examination until after the child is born.

In practice, however, the possibility of pregnancy may not even be considered. This is especially true with accident or injury where the emergency department or office visit is brief and the history is limited to the injury complaint. For this reason it is essential that the radiographer consider the possibility of pregnancy in any female of childbearing age. Ask specific questions to determine that the patient's physician has addressed the issue of pregnancy before ordering the examination.

Until the early 1980s, the American College of Radiology recommended the use of the "10-day rule" to limit the likelihood of accidentally irradiating an embryo. Reduced radiation dose for all radiography due to technology advances has caused this group to reverse this recommendation. Some radiology departments, however, still use the 10-day rule to screen potentially pregnant patients before radiography. The rule states that nonemergency x-ray examinations of the female abdomen and pelvis are done only during the first 10 days of the menstrual cycle, the onset of menstruation being considered as Day 1. Because menstruation usually indicates that the patient is not pregnant, and

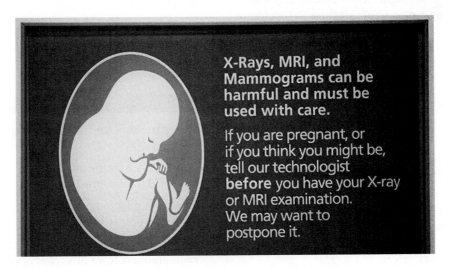

FIG. 1-37 Signs in dressing rooms and imaging suites alert patients to the potential hazard of examination when pregnant.

pregnancy cannot commence until 13 to 15 days later when the patient ovulates, the first 10 days of the cycle is the period when the patient is least likely to be pregnant. Where this rule is used, exceptions are usually made only after the radiologist has considered the case and spoken with the referring physician. Neither the 10-day rule nor an early pregnancy test can guarantee that the patient is not pregnant, but these methods can greatly decrease the likelihood of irradiating an otherwise unsuspected embryo.

If x-ray examinations of a pregnant patient must be done, modifications in procedure can help to minimize the dose to the embryo or fetus. If the part to be examined is not the abdomen or pelvis, this area can be shielded with a lead apron. If the abdomen or pelvis is to be evaluated, the number of views and/or the size of the radiation field may be minimized, resulting in less radiation exposure than that required for a routine procedure. The decision to do a limited study and the determination of the exact limitations to be imposed are prerogatives of the radiologist.

CONCLUSION

From the discovery of x-rays by Roentgen more than 100 years ago to the highly technical environment of today's imaging center, many arts and sciences have made contributions to radiography: physics, chemistry, mechanics, photography, anatomy, electronics, medicine, nursing, and social sciences, to name a few. The safe use of x-rays to aid in the diagnosis of illness and injury will now be the focus of your studies and the setting in which we will consider patient care in the chapters that follow.

REVIEW QUESTIONS

1. Of the following types of electromagnetic energy, which has the shortest wavelength?
   A. radio waves
   B. gamma rays
   C. microwaves
   D. green light
   E. ultraviolet light

2. Which of the following is **NOT** an accurate statement regarding the characteristics of x-rays?
   A. They can penetrate matter that is impenetrable to light.
   B. They cause certain crystals to fluoresce.
   C. They can be refracted by a lens.
   D. They have an exposure effect on photographic emulsions.
   E. They cannot be detected by the human senses.

3. The mAs value of an exposure is varied to provide control of:
   A. radiographic density
   B. radiographic contrast
   C. radiographic definition
   D. radiographic distortion
   E. all of the above

4. The effective dose equivalent limit for whole-body occupational radiation exposure to non-pregnant radiation workers over the age of 18 is:
   A. 1.25 rem per year
   B. 5.0 mrem per year
   C. 0.5 mrem per calendar quarter
   D. 0.5 rem per year
   E. 5.0 rem per year

5. Which of the following is a personnel radiation dosimeter?
   A. SID
   B. kVp
   C. TLD
   D. OID
   E. rem

CRITICAL THINKING EXERCISES

1. Compare and contrast radiography and fluoroscopy.

2. Explain the significance of x-ray wavelength in the radiographic process.

3. What should a radiographer do to prevent inadvertent exposure to an embryo or fetus?

4. List the three principal methods used to protect radiographers from unnecessary radiation exposure, and explain how each method is applied in practice.

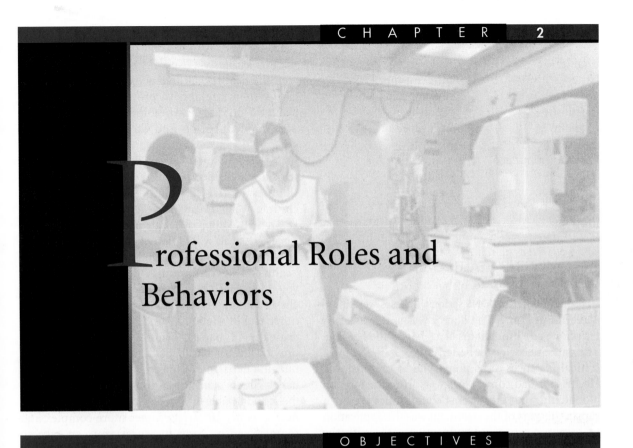

Professional Roles and Behaviors

At the conclusion of this chapter, the student will be able to:

- State three reasons why a study of professional behavior is important to the radiographer.
- Describe the radiographer's role in relation to the radiologist, referring physician, hospital administration, nursing personnel, and other hospital staff.
- List three aspects of self-care that demonstrate responsible behavior by the radiographer.
- List three ways that a radiographer can contribute to the advancement of radiologic technology.
- Define ethics.
- Explain the rationale for confidentiality of professional communications.

- List four patient rights that the radiographer is responsible for protecting.
- Define the terms *negligence* and *malpractice.*
- List three specific acts of intentional misconduct that may occur in radiology departments.
- Discuss the most frequent circumstances causing patients to initiate litigation.

assault	malpractice
battery	misdemeanor
defendant	mission statement
diagnostic	moral agent
empathy	negligence
ethics	plaintiff
false imprisonment	radiologist
fellow	resident
felony	slander
intern	therapeutic
libel	tort

THE CHANGING HEALTH CARE DELIVERY SYSTEM

IN EARLIER GENERATIONS serious illnesses were often cared for at home. The doctor was summoned by telephone and brought his black bag to the bedside. The patient usually got better, and only in the most critical instances did a patient go to the hospital. Health care had come a long way from leeches and bloodletting, but there were no antibiotics yet and a substantial part of the treatment was the application of common sense and supportive care. With the discovery of antibiotics and more sophisticated medical treatments, simple measures gave way to intensive treatment protocols. Now, after years of professional treatment for even the slightest discomfort, we have lost the incentive to take personal responsibility for prevention and self-care. Reluctance to rely on simple remedies, plus inappropriate and excessive use of medications, have reduced the efficacy of many of our "modern" treatments. The steadily increasing costs of this approach have placed health care at a crossroad, forcing us to adopt new ways to cope with disease and health maintenance. For these reasons, health care is returning to many of the preventive measures and natural treatments that once were part of the medical knowledge in most households. Prevention is an important part of the solution because it is demonstrated to be more affordable than the costs of treating disease.

Delivery of health care can be viewed in many ways. Crisis intervention is one approach in which the patient or client seeks help only when unable to manage alone. As soon as the emergency has passed, the former lifestyle is usually resumed. In comparison, the health maintenance or preventive health care system attempts to promote well-being and avoid the need for medical intervention. It encourages good nutrition and exercise and promotes self-care that avoids such habits as smoking and the use of "recreational" drugs. Potential health problems are identified before they manifest as illness. Illnesses are treated promptly before they become chronic or life threatening.

These two approaches are not mutually exclusive, since each deals with different points on a line drawn between optimum health and fatal illness called the health-illness continuum. On one end of this line you might find a healthy patient required to obtain a chest radiograph for employment purposes. On the other end of the spectrum you could encounter a critically ill patient whose examination might provide lifesaving information. Since patients in the imaging department may fall anywhere along this health-illness continuum, you must be both empathetic and flexible in your approach to widely varying needs. As health care becomes more complex and more expensive, any measures you can take to promote health will help reduce hospital stays and prevent duplication of services. This increases cost-effectiveness as well as patient satisfaction.

Health Care Insurance and Benefit Systems

Until 20 years ago, most health care was provided on a fee-for-service basis. Under this system insurance companies reimburse patients for the costs of their health care within the limits of the policy and the patient is responsible for any costs that are not covered. Patients can seek care from their choice of physicians and hospitals. Since private physicians may provide a more personal service and greater continuity of care under this system, many individuals find this kind of care reassuring and are willing to pay a high premium for this type of insurance coverage.

Medicare, a federal health insurance program in the United States, covers a portion of the medical care costs for those over age 65. The federal government also provides funds to aid the medically indigent through a program called Medicaid.

As health care and hospital services became more technical and more expensive, health insurance premiums and uninsured charges began to cost more than many individuals could afford. In an effort to deliver more affordable care, health maintenance organizations (HMOs) were formed. These organizations provide complete and comprehensive health care for the cost of the premium and a small fee called a co-payment for each visit. HMOs control costs by promoting good health and by providing care only in specified facilities. The physicians and other professionals who provide care may be salaried employees of the organization. Physician assistants and nurse practitioners may provide many aspects of care formerly provided only by physicians.

If you belong to an HMO and have a health concern, the first person you see is your primary health care provider. This might be a physician or perhaps a nurse practitioner (a nurse with advanced education and credentials for providing primary care). If your condition necessitates additional diagnostic attention or care, you will be referred to a secondary provider. This provider might be a specialist such as an ophthalmologist, a gynecologist, or a radiologist. At times your condition might be serious enough to demand care within the hospital setting, which is called tertiary (third level) care. Your primary care provider will coordinate your treatment and provide follow-up care after you are discharged from the hospital.

By promoting good health, the HMO tries to reduce the average cost of health care for all its members. Regular physical examinations, immunizations, weight control, treatment for hypertension, and other forms of preventive care, such as fitness programs and classes on health-related topics, are typically included among benefits of these organizations. This preventive care system is in direct contrast to crisis intervention or episodic care in which you see your physician only when you are ill. An inherent part of an HMO system is that patients are expected to become more involved in meeting their own health care needs. They seldom have the ongoing, one-to-one relationship with a primary care provider that was once common with a family doctor.

As HMOs have succeeded and become more popular, many private physicians and hospitals have cooperated to form managed care systems. These systems allow private hospitals and physicians to provide private services while also providing care through insurance plans similar to HMOs. Managed care systems save money by limiting access to expensive services when they are not needed. Their benefits vary from modified fee-for-service programs to comprehensive HMOs.

Unfortunately, even HMOs have had difficulty coping with the escalating cost of diagnostic procedures and hospital care. Health insurance rates have soared, and the number of families unable to afford health care has increased dramatically. One outcome is that many low-income families have turned to emergency departments to provide care for all kinds of illnesses. This crisis intervention model of care is expensive on a per patient basis, and since many of these patients are unable to pay, the cost is spread over the entire span of hospital care.

To relieve the pressure on hospital emergency departments and provide care on a more cost-effective basis, a system grew to meet the needs of patients who need urgent care or minor surgery for conditions that are not immediately life threatening. New facilities were established called immediate or urgent care clinics. Patients are seen without waiting several days for an appointment. These centers cope with acute but minor illnesses and accidents. Conditions such as broken fingers, middle ear infections, and severe upper respiratory infections can be seen quickly and treated effectively in such centers.

Outpatient surgical facilities are also becoming common. In these "surgicenters," patients are admitted in the early morning for minor procedures such as simple hernia repair and are released to home care the same evening. Once again, the impetus for such centers was the need to cut costs. In this case, the charges involved are less than those for the use of a major surgical suite and a subsequent overnight hospital stay.

Consumers need to know how to use the coverage available, since insurance programs vary greatly and are often subject to change. Must you be referred to an emergency department for a sudden illness, or is there an urgent care center? Does your policy cover x-rays and medications? If benefits are not used correctly, the insurance may not cover the care received and patients may be faced with large, unexpected bills. It definitely pays to be an informed and assertive consumer.

Health Care Facilities

Hospitals may be owned and operated as either public or private agencies. Public hospitals and health care facilities are operated by federal or local governments. Military hospitals and facilities for veterans operated by the Department of Veterans Affairs are examples of federal agencies. Counties, cities, and communities may provide public health care services, including hospital care. Many hospitals are privately owned. These may be not-for-profit institutions, such as those owned by religious or charitable groups, or proprietary hospitals, which are health care businesses run for profit. While there are still independent hospital institutions, many hospitals are members of a hospital system that cooperates to cut costs by sharing the use of highly technical equipment and by purchasing supplies in volume.

The role of the hospital in relation to the community it serves is reflected in its **mission statement,** a one- or two-paragraph declaration of the institution's basic philosophy and primary goals. This statement provides guidance for the decisions that govern the activities of the facility. An example of a mission statement for a hospital system belonging to a religious order is in Box 2-1.

Many patients today are cared for in outpatient clinics, when only a few years ago they would have been admitted to a "short stay" ward for minor surgical procedures or invasive diagnostic procedures such as colonoscopies. Hospitals often include outpatient clinics for certain services such as follow-up care for oncology patients and well-baby check-ups. Many public health departments also provide clinics, especially for prenatal and pediatric care.

Patients with chronic diseases may receive home health care provided by the health department or by an HMO or managed care system. Others may be

---

BOX 2-1

EXAMPLE OF A MISSION STATEMENT FOR A HOSPITAL BELONGING TO A RELIGIOUS ORDER

Our Mission
Providence Health System continues the healing ministry of Jesus in the world of today, with special concern for those who are poor and vulnerable. Working with others in a spirit of loving service, we strive to meet the health needs of people as they journey through life.

Our mission is carried out by employees, volunteers, physicians and others who work together in a spirit of service that reflects our core values.

---

cared for in long-term care facilities, often called "nursing homes," or in a foster care facility. Foster care is sometimes provided in private homes. Medicare and state health programs help defer the expenses of foster care or long-term residential facilities for the elderly and infirm.

THE HEALTH CARE TEAM

Despite changes in the health care delivery system, patients continue to be the most important people in the health care community. They come to us for help in preserving health and solving health-related problems and all the efforts of the health care team should be directed toward meeting these needs. You will be an important member of this team, so it will be helpful to become acquainted with other team members and their functions in the hospital. Although you may see patients in physicians' offices, outpatient clinics, and other health care settings, most of your clinical experience will occur in a hospital, the setting on which this book is focused.

Physicians

Patients may be brought directly to the hospital for emergency care. As noted above, some may seek primary care in the emergency department. Many patients are sent to the hospital by a doctor known as the referring physician. On admission the referring physician may also serve as the attending physician who continues to provide direction for care, or another physician may be assigned to the case. The attending physician is responsible for assessing the patient's needs and prescribing therapeutic procedures to promote health.

The attending physician may determine that the expertise of one or more specialists would be helpful in the patient's diagnosis or treatment and may refer the patient to a specialist for consultation. A list of specialty areas is found in Table 2-1. This list will assist you in learning the hospital language.

The physicians who practice in the hospital form the medical staff. Depending on the institution's size and organization, this group may also include **interns** (recent medical school graduates gaining practical experience), **fellows** (licensed physicians receiving advanced training), and **residents** (licensed physicians in an educational program to become certified in a specialty area).

Hospital Organization and Management

The hospital is governed by an executive board that establishes goals, policies, and financial plans and hires the director or administrator. One of the

TABLE 2-1	
ABBREVIATED TABLE OF MEDICAL SPECIALTIES	
SPECIALTY	**FUNCTIONS**
Anesthesiologist	Administers anesthetics and monitors the patient during surgery
Dermatologist	Diagnoses and treats conditions and diseases of the skin
Emergency department physician	Specializes in trauma and emergency situations; a triage expert in disaster situations
Family practice physician	Treats individuals and families in the context of daily life
Gastroenterologist	Diagnoses and treats diseases of the gastrointestinal tract
Geriatrician	Specializes in problems and diseases of elderly persons
Gynecologist	Treats problems and diseases of the female reproductive system
Internist	Specializes in diseases of the internal organs
Neurologist	Specializes in functions and disorders of the nervous system
Obstetrician	Specializes in pregnancy, labor, delivery, and immediate postpartum care
Oncologist	Specializes in tumor identification and treatment
Ophthalmologist	Diagnoses and treats problems and diseases of the eye
Otorhinolaryngologist	Specializes in conditions of the ear, nose, and throat
Pathologist	Specializes in the scientific study of the alterations in the body caused by disease and death
Pediatrician	Specializes in the care, diagnosis and treatment of diseases affecting children
Psychiatrist	Specializes in diagnosis, treatment, and prevention of mental illness
Radiologist	Specializes in diagnosis by means of medical imaging
Surgeons	
Abdominal	Specializes in surgery of the abdominal cavity
Plastic	Restores or improves the appearance and function of exposed body parts
Neurologic	Specializes in surgery of the brain, spinal cord, and peripheral nervous system
Orthopedic	Diagnoses and treats problems of the musculoskeletal system
Thoracic	Specializes in problems of the chest
Urologic	Diagnoses and treats problems of the urinary tract and the male reproductive system

responsibilities of the board is to extend the privilege of staff membership to qualified physician applicants and to organize the staff to cooperate in making the rules that govern professional activities. Many of these rules relate to standards of care and medical records.

The administration must see that suitable facilities and equipment are provided and that a staff of well-trained professional, technical, and support personnel is present. Fig. 2-1 shows a typical organizational structure for hospitals and the lines of authority and responsibility that form a chain of command for the health care team.

The hospital may have one or more assistant administrators who have clearly defined areas of responsibility for several departments. They do not need specific training and experience in the areas under their direction because their expertise is in health care management. They rely on department supervisors for decisions and communications at the level where specialization is required.

Each department has a chief or supervisor whose education and expertise relate directly to the area of responsibility. For example, the supervisor of the hospital pharmacy is a registered pharmacist, whereas the supervisor of the radiology department is usually a radiographer. Each supervisor leads a group of skilled employees who carry out the department's goals.

Some departments meet patient needs directly. Nursing service, for example, provides patient care by implementing nursing care decisions, carrying out physician orders within the framework of hospital policies, and communicating plans for patient care and physician orders to other departments. Some typical hospital departments are listed in Table 2-2. Note that some are categorized according to whether their functions are **diagnostic** (related to identification of patient problems) or **therapeutic** (devoted to treatment). Still other departments serve patients indirectly by providing support services such as purchasing, central supply, and laundry. Social service departments may support patients and their families by providing a hospital chaplain, a trained counselor, or a translator. These departments also coordinate with other agencies and services as needed when a patient is discharged or transferred. Many hospitals also have auxiliary groups consisting of volunteers who tend to special needs of patients and their families. Very large institutions often

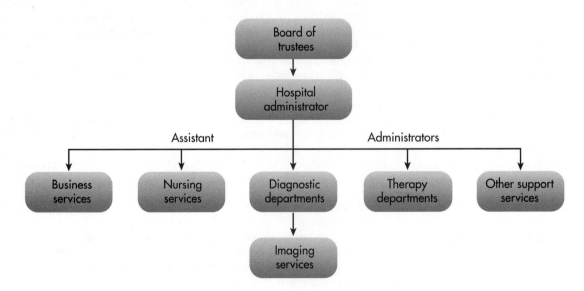

FIG. 2-1 Simplified example of hospital organizational chart.

SOME TYPICAL HOSPITAL DEPARTMENTS

| GENERAL | DIRECT PATIENT SERVICES | | SUPPORT SERVICES |
	DIAGNOSTIC	THERAPEUTIC	
Admissions	Computed tomography (CT)	Dietary	Accounting
Emergency	Electrocardiography (ECG)	Occupational therapy	Central/sterile supply
Nursing service	Electroencephalography (EEG)	Oncology	Human resources
Social services	Magnetic resonance imaging (MRI)	Physical therapy	Housekeeping
Chaplain/counseling services	Nuclear medicine	Respiratory therapy	Laundry
	Pathology (medical laboratories)	Surgery	Medical records
	Radiography		Purchasing
	Sonography		Security

include research and education departments as well as separate departments or clinics for providing outpatient services. The names of many departments and how they fit into the chain of command vary with the institution's size and its management philosophy. It is useful to study the organizational chart of the clinical facilities affiliated with your radiography program.

Few patients use the services of all departments, but the well-being of most patients requires the cooperative efforts of many team members. You may gain a better understanding of how the team functions by focusing your attention on one patient.

Judy Colton was admitted to the hospital with chronic back pain. Her family physician, Dr. Evans, requested a lumbar myelogram to aid in diagnosis and the planning of an effective course of treatment. The examination request was actually a referral to a specialist, the radiologist, for diagnostic consultation. As her attending physician, Dr. Evans wrote the order in Ms. Colton's chart, and a nurse made arrangements for the procedure.

A transportation orderly brought Judy and her chart to the radiology department, where the radiographer greeted her and checked the chart to confirm the orders. The radiologist explained the procedure, and the radiographer assisted the radiologist to perform the examination. Clean linen used during the examination

was provided by the hospital laundry. Several members of the radiology department staff assisted by handling her paperwork, processing the images, and helping to move the patient. A supervising radiographer checked the exam to see that they met the standards of the radiologist, the department, and the hospital. The orderly then returned Judy to the care of the nursing service.

Meanwhile, the radiologist studied the images and dictated a report of the findings. A medical transcriptionist typed the report, and a clerk filed the exam. A copy of the report was placed in the chart, and a second copy was sent to Dr. Evans, who was then able to confirm the diagnosis of a herniated intervertebral lumbar disk.

Dr. Evans contacted Dr. Ortiz, a neurosurgeon, who recommended a laminectomy.

Following this surgery, Judy received medication for pain from the hospital pharmacy. As soon as her condition permitted, physical therapy was implemented with the help of other team members.

Members of the business office staff used information from the various departments to prepare the billing, and copies were sent to Ms. Colton and to her insurance company. The payment received helped support the many services rendered by the hospital, including the purchase of imaging supplies and the radiographer's salary.

Ms. Colton's chart was reviewed by a medical staff committee in a random sampling to ensure that hospital regulations had been followed and to gather statistics about hospital services. Her chart was then stored for future reference, since it might be needed again to assist in her care. The images are part of Judy's medical record and were also kept on file.

This case is a simplified representation of a hospital stay. How many departments shared responsibility for Judy's care? What types of communication were required to coordinate the team's efforts? Were any of the team members unnecessary or unimportant?

SERVICES AND ROLES IN THE IMAGING DEPARTMENT

The department where you receive your clinical experience in radiography may be called the radiology department. Since the early use of x-rays in medicine, *radiology* has been the term applied to the science of medical imaging. As technology has added new imaging methods to the medical repertoire, radiologists have included these methods within their practices and within existing radiology departments. Since some of the new imaging modalities do not involve the use of x-rays, some radiology

departments have been renamed diagnostic imaging departments. This text uses the two terms interchangeably.

Whether it is called radiology or diagnostic imaging, this department provides various diagnostic services that relate directly to the patient. The administrative structure is diagrammed in Fig. 2-2. **Radiologists** are members of the medical staff and serve as consultants in one or more of the imaging modalities in radiology. The line of responsibility for radiologists goes through the medical staff organization. Radiologists play a major role in establishing standards of care and technical quality within the department in addition to performing many examinations with the assistance of radiographers (Fig. 2-3). Each examination must be interpreted by a radiologist and the information provided to the referring physician.

The radiology services in a modern hospital are divided among several departments under the supervision of a radiology manager, who works with radiologists and the hospital administration to establish policies and budgets for the various imaging departments. The radiology manager may also

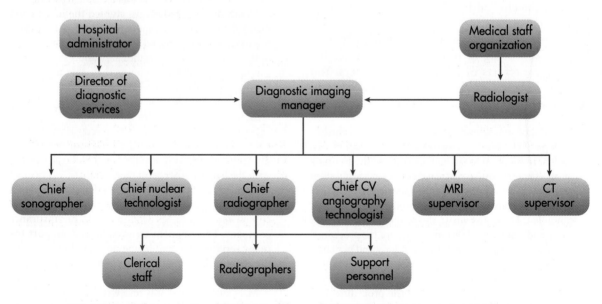

FIG. 2-2 Typical organizational structure of the medical imaging department. Actual titles may vary.

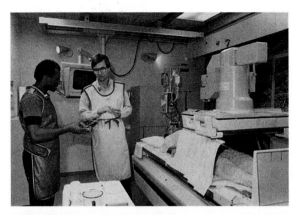

FIG. 2-3 Radiologists perform many examinations with radiographers' assistance.

supervise several groups of employees such as those in radiography, nuclear medicine, ultrasound, cardiovascular angiography, computed tomography (CT), and magnetic resonance imaging (MRI). Groups of employees under the manager's direction may be referred to as teams or "quality teams." The team approach to management is popular because it rewards cooperative effort and encourages team members to work together for the benefit of the patient. This book primarily focuses on the radiography department team. Chapter 12 provides an introduction to other imaging modalities and corresponding aspects of patient care.

The chief radiographer, sometimes called the department coordinator, manages the day-to-day activities in the radiography department. He or she also schedules the staff of radiographers and support personnel in this area and orders the necessary supplies. Division of responsibility between the chief radiographer and the radiology manager varies with the institution. The chief radiographer is often promoted from the ranks of staff radiographers because of both technical expertise and supervisory capability. Exact titles for these positions vary greatly among institutions.

Staff radiographers may report directly to the chief radiographer or to a lead radiographer or team leader responsible for a given area. In practice, they also work and communicate directly with

radiologists rather than along the established chain of command.

Imaging departments also require support staff. Depending on the size of the department and the organization of the hospital, support personnel may include administrative assistants, receptionists, a medical secretary, and transportation service personnel. There may also be an information systems manager with a staff to maintain patient files, image files, and the computerized images organized in the picture archiving and communication system (PACS).

Good communication systems depend on the ability of all team members to relay information systematically, preventing essential details from being overlooked. As you begin to understand each team member's responsibilities, you will appreciate the cooperation and communication lines that help the team function smoothly.

RADIOGRAPHY AS A PROFESSION
Professionalism

What is a profession? Many different definitions have been advanced. At one time, profession meant "calling." Knowledge of the profession was handed down from master to student, and students honored their teachers by upholding the traditions as they had been taught. This was called "professional behavior," and young persons received into a profession who failed to live up to its highest principles brought shame to themselves and their teachers. Classical professions included medicine, law, and the clergy. While these professions required scholarship and dedicated study, it was not necessarily the length of the education that separated the professions from other occupations. The nature of the work required professionals to place a high value on their service to others; the client and the community would suffer if high standards were not upheld. Commitment to truth and the highest good were hallmarks of the professional.

Today a profession might be defined somewhat differently, but the primary characteristics are similar. A profession is not only a field of study but also the application of specialized knowledge to benefit others. A profession is organized to govern itself—to effectively set standards of professional behavior, education, and qualification to practice, and to enforce those standards within its ranks. Having a peer review journal or publication is also expected of a profession, since this allows the profession to advance and to continually review and challenge the basis of knowledge on which it functions.

Clearly, radiographers and other radiologic technologists, working primarily through their principal professional organization, the American Society of Radiologic Technologists (ASRT), have brought medical imaging technology to the professional level. As a professional radiographer, your work must focus on your patients and your efforts must be devoted to providing quality service. One of this book's primary goals is to assist you in becoming a professional radiographer.

Professional Organizations

The oldest and largest national professional association for technologists in the radiologic sciences is the ASRT.* It was founded to advance the profession and to promote high standards of education and patient care. Fourteen visionary x-ray pioneers founded the original organization in 1920, calling it the American Association of Radiological Technicians. Since that time the organization has grown from a membership of 46 to 100,000 members, and ASRT is one of more than 70 national organizations of technologists around the world that are members of the International Society of Radiographers and Radiological Technologists (ISRRT). Other organizations of imaging technologists, some of which are affiliated with ASRT, serve those with specific professional interests. For example, American Healthcare Radiology Administrators (AHRA) provides a network and resources for technologists with administrative positions, while the Association of Collegiate Educators in Radiologic Technology (ACERT) and the Association of Educators in Radiological

Sciences (AERS) provide forums to meet the needs of technologists and others who teach in this field. Organizations also exist for those involved in imaging modalities other than general radiography, such as the Society of Diagnostic Medical Sonography (SDMS), the Society of Nuclear Medicine (SNM), and the Association of Vascular and Interventional Radiographers (AVIR). Some of these imaging specialty organizations, such as SNM, are international organizations with membership categories for physicians, technologists, and others.

ASRT is the only nationally recognized professional society representing all radiologic technologists in the United States today. It reaches radiographers on the local level through the affiliated state societies. These affiliates must conduct their business according to ASRT standards, and each state society elects a board of directors to conduct the society's business. State societies also sponsor continuing education programs and have roles similar to the national organization.

At the time of this writing, the ASRT is revising its governance structure. The proposed model for the new ASRT governance structure includes a House of Delegates, a Board of Directors, and a Commission. The House of Delegates is the legislative body of the organization. It may be downsized to include 54 affiliate delegates, elected or appointed by the state societies, and 28 chapter delegates, elected by the membership at large. Chapter delegates represent the different areas of practice in the radiologic sciences (including management and education) and imaging and therapeutic professionals in the military. The role of the House of Delegates is to debate and vote on issues that have a major impact on professional practice. The Board of Directors is the governing body and consists of the chairman, president, vice president, president-elect, and secretary-treasurer, plus the speaker and vice speaker of the House of Delegates. The first five members of the board are elected by the membership at large, and the remaining members are elected by the House of Delegates. The role of the Board is to consider and act on issues that relate to the business functions of the ASRT. The Commission comprises a seven-member panel with backgrounds in administration, education, and extensive professional practice. The Commission is

---

*Information about ASRT, including membership applications and copies of the ASRT documents mentioned in this chapter, are available directly from ASRT. Write to ASRT at 15000 Central Ave SE, Albuquerque, NM 87123-3917. Telephone: 800-444-2778 or 505-298-4500. Fax: 505-298-5063. Or visit the ASRT website: www.ASRT.org.

appointed by the Board of Directors, the speaker and vice speaker of the House of Delegates. The role of the Commission is to review issues relative to professional practice, business, and governance and to refer these issues to either the House or the Board for consideration and action.

ASRT serves its membership in many ways, including significant contributions to education, professional advancement, legislation, and public relations. ASRT also appoints technologist representatives to other organizations and committees whose work is significant to the profession.

With respect to education, ASRT provides guidelines for the organization, correct operation, and curriculum design for programs in the various imaging modalities. In addition, ASRT sponsors educational conferences and self-study materials for technologists. ASRT publishes a peer-reviewed scientific journal and a magazine that covers timely topics and key issues in the radiologic sciences. The organization also reviews and approves educational programs for continuing education and maintains education records for members, providing copies of these records to members annually.

ASRT actively supports legislation to protect the public from excess radiation exposure by inadequately trained workers. This includes efforts to mandate state licensure and to set minimum standards for both the accreditation of educational programs and granting credentials to individuals who administer radiation. *Voluntary* federal minimum educational standards for the practice of radiologic technology are part of the Consumer-Patient Radiation Health and Safety Act of 1981. ASRT has been instrumental in attempting to amend this act through the introduction of the Consumer Assurance of Radiologic Excellence (CARE) bill into Congress in 2001. If enacted, the CARE Act will require mandatory education and credentialing standards for *everyone* who uses ionizing radiation or magnetic resonance as well as for those who plan and deliver radiation therapy. States that fail to meet these standards will lose Medicare and Medicaid reimbursement for radiologic procedures.

Through its public relations program, ASRT promotes awareness of the profession and the duties of radiographers. To commemorate the anniversary of the discovery of x-rays, ASRT sponsors National Radiologic Technology Week each year during November. This observance honors the contributions of radiographers to the health care field.

Practice Standards

For many years the ASRT has worked to attain professional status for radiologic technologists. To meet this goal, ASRT has developed a written statement that describes the radiographer's duties and responsibilities. This document, entitled The Practice Standards for Medical Imaging and Radiation Therapy, defines the clinical practice, technical activities, and professional responsibilities of imaging and therapeutic professionals. The Practice Standards for Radiography are printed in Appendix A. These standards include desirable and achievable levels of performance against which actual performance can be assessed. Because of its general format, the standards can be adapted to any area of practice and region of the country. The practice standards may be used by radiology managers to develop job descriptions and performance appraisals, and in the case of medical malpractice or negligence claims, a lawyer may use this document to determine the accepted level of care and to show whether the professional standard has been met.

Education

Hospitals, community colleges, and universities offer approved education programs in radiography with a minimum program length of 2 years and some lasting as long as 5 years. All of these programs must meet the same rigorous standards for academic excellence and clinical experience.

Hospital-based programs provide a comprehensive academic and clinical curriculum under the sponsorship of one or more health care institutions. They usually require a time schedule of at least 40 hours per week divided between formal classses and clinical practice. Graduates receive a diploma or certificate of completion.

Community college programs provide a comprehensive academic curriculum and are affiliated with hospitals that provide the requisite clinical experience. Graduates are awarded an associate degree.

University programs may require at least a 4-year commitment with a greater portion of the student's work devoted to academic courses. These programs lead to a bachelor's degree and may also qualify the graduate for advanced postgraduate programs.

Credentials

In the field of radiologic technology such credentials as registration, permits, certificates, and licenses all refer to documents that attest to the qualifications of individuals.

The American Registry of Radiologic Technologists (ARRT) is a national organization of appointees from both ASRT and the American College of Radiology (ACR). The ACR is an organization of physician specialists in radiology that is affiliated with the American Medical Association (AMA). ARRT establishes minimum standards for certification in various imaging specialties and radiation therapy. Applicants must have high school diplomas or equivalent and must have completed an approved education program in radiologic technology. ARRT conducts qualifying examinations that entitle the applicants who pass to use the designation registered technologist (RT) in association with their names. ARRT conducts primary specialty examinations in radiography (R), nuclear medicine (N), and radiation therapy (T) and permits use of these abbreviations with the RT designation. Postprimary specialty examinations are offered in computed tomography (CT), magnetic resonance imaging (MR), mammography (M), cardiovascular-interventional technology (CV), quality management (QM), sonography (S), vascular sonography (VS), and bone densitometry (BD).

Certification by ARRT is recognized nationally, and to some degree internationally, as a standard qualification to practice radiologic technology and is a prerequisite for employment in this field by most accredited institutions in the United States. Once certified, you must renew your registration annually with the ARRT by paying a nominal fee. Prior to your birth month, you will be sent a renewal form and a questionnaire to complete, documenting current employment status and eligibility for renewal. Proof of 24 credits of continuing education is also required every 2 years. Certification by ARRT is an important goal for student radiographers.

Licensure refers to the granting of "official permission" and is a prerogative of state governments. All states have laws requiring drivers' licenses and licenses to practice medicine and nursing. State licensure of radiologic technologists began in the early 1970s when laws were enacted in New York, New Jersey, and California. Now many states and territories have a license requirement to practice radiologic technology, and several others have licensure bills pending. These laws vary greatly among states. If the CARE Act is implemented, all states will require licensure and licensure will be granted to any person certified by ARRT who applies and pays a fee.

Radiographers may also be required to have certification in other specific areas. For example, the State of Washington requires completion of an approved 7-hour course on human immunodeficiency virus (HIV) infection. Additional examples include the periodic cardiopulmonary resuscitation (CPR) certification that is required of all patient care personnel in most hospital settings and venipuncture certification that may be required for personnel who draw blood or administer intravenous fluids and medications. These certification requirements provide incentive to maintain competencies and document qualifications.

Some states issue permits to practice radiologic technology under limited circumstances or in limited scope. These permits do not require the same high standards necessary for ARRT certification or licensure. Limited permits may allow a public health nurse to take chest radiographs or an orthopedic assistant to take extremity radiographs while helping with application of a cast. To obtain a permit, an applicant must demonstrate knowledge of radiation safety and technical expertise in a limited area of radiography.

Continuing Education

In radiologic technology, as in any rapidly changing technological field, continuing education is essential to stay abreast of current trends and to maintain competencies. This also is an important professional responsibility.

Many opportunities for continuing education are available to the radiographer. Hospitals, colleges, and professional organizations all provide educational

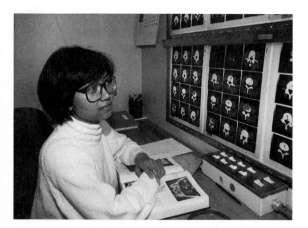

FIG. 2-4 A radiographer earns continuing education credits through independent study.

opportunities for radiographers to stay abreast of current developments and expand their skills. Education may take the form of courses, classes, workshops, seminars, and other group experiences, but there is also a variety of materials available for individual learning and self-study (Fig. 2-4). ASRT provides self-study materials for continuing education, which helps individuals who cannot attend classes or individuals who wish to study subjects that are not otherwise immediately available.

In addition to the continuing education requirements for renewal of ARRT certification, states may also require continuing education as a condition of license renewal. In some states (e.g., Texas) renewal of ARRT certification is accepted as proof of required continuing education for renewing a state license.

When you are required to provide evidence of continuing education, be sure to determine in advance whether the education you plan to receive is approved and accredited for this purpose. Keep an accurate record of your continuing education activities, including any documentation of participation that you receive. Documentation is valuable even if it is not immediately required, as it may help you later in qualifying for a promotion or a new position.

Failure to maintain competency, licensure, registration, or required additional certification places the employer and the employee at risk and may result in loss of employment and professional reputation. Knowing the credentials required in a given situation and maintaining current credentials are important professional responsibilities. Violation of state licensure laws may result in fines and imprisonment.

Employment Outlook

The employment outlook for graduates of radiography programs looks very promising. The Bureau of Labor Statistics predicts that by the year 2010, 75,000 more radiographers will be needed than in the year 2000. Historically the demand for radiographers has been cyclical and has changed with changes in the economy and in the health care industry. Although these cycles existed previously, it is predicted that the demand for radiographers will remain constant for the foreseeable future.

There are several reasons cited for the continued demand for radiographers. Aging baby boomers, a large segment of our society, will be making more hospital visits and using more diagnostic services, including medical imaging. In addition, aging radiographers will be retiring at a faster rate than new radiographers can enter the profession. Currently, most radiographers are age 30 years or older. In addition, continued improvements in equipment and technology will create more opportunities for radiographers to specialize in advanced imaging areas, and this will create openings in general radiography. Expanding health care facilities will also contribute to the continued need for radiographers. The anticipated passage of the CARE Act will also have an impact on the demand for qualified and registered radiographers. Employers will no longer be able to hire individuals who have no formal education and certification to take x-rays.

Radiographers entering the profession will have job security, geographic mobility, and salaries competitive with other health care professionals. Radiographers will have the freedom to work anywhere in the country and hold either a permanent or temporary position; working in a variety of settings from physicians' offices to major medical centers. Employers will continue to offer many fringe benefits to recruit and retain their staff.

Career Ladder

Many possibilities exist for radiographers to achieve promotion and advancement, depending on their interests, skills, experience, and education. At this point it may be fun to speculate how your career will develop into the professional life that is right for you. Giving some thought to the possibilities now may help you to begin setting professional goals and to recognize opportunities that may present themselves later.

As a staff radiographer gains experience and demonstrates ability, the first promotional step is likely to be the position of lead technologist or team leader. A lead technologist supervises the work in a specific area or on a given shift, helping to implement the directives of the chief technologist. Excellence in clinical performance and a demonstrated ability to relate well to other team members may qualify a radiographer for this position.

The position of chief radiographer, sometimes known as radiography department coordinator, varies significantly with the size of the institution and department. In small hospitals, the position of chief radiographer may be quite similar to that of the lead technologist in a large medical center. Chief radiographers need management skills and an understanding of the entire institution's operation so that they can relate the needs and contributions of the department to the mission of the institution. In most cases education and experience beyond those needed to practice radiography are required.

The title of radiology administrator designates the manager of a large diagnostic imaging department. This executive must have management ability and experience. The position usually requires a master's degree in health care administration or equivalent experience.

The position of educator in radiologic technology usually requires advanced education (a degree in a related field) plus at least 3 years of clinical experience. This position may involve classroom, laboratory, and/or clinical work. Experience and further study may lead to advanced positions in education such as program director or dean of health sciences.

Commercial positions in radiology also exist. A strong technical background and good interpersonal skills may qualify a radiographer as a representative of a company that sells x-ray equipment, supplies, or both. Commercially employed radiographers may perform technical services such as the repair and maintenance of film processors. They may provide education and problem-solving consultation to customers of companies that manufacture x-ray film and intensifying screens, or digital imaging systems. Alternatively, they may be involved in the direct marketing of x-ray equipment to the radiologists and administrators who make major purchasing decisions. Employers may provide specialized training for these positions to qualified radiographers.

Opportunities also exist for qualified radiographers to work in research and development positions as employees of either corporations or educational institutions.

Technologists who provide services in special imaging departments may be recruited from the ranks of radiographers. Skills in CT, MRI, mammography, and angiography may be learned on the job and through independent study. Specialty certification in these areas is granted by examination through ARRT.

The specialty areas of radiation therapy, nuclear medicine, and sonography may be entered directly through educational programs for these technologies or through formalized programs open to technologists with any of the primary certifications.

Current trends indicate changes in baccalaureate degree programs in radiologic technology that will provide advanced *clinical* career paths for technologists. Four-year degree programs in radiologic technology have traditionally offered a broad general education, often with curriculum options in health care management and/or education, but the clinical credentials conferred by these programs have been equal only to those received by community college graduates. Within the past decade, however, several colleges and universities have developed degree programs leading to advanced clinical competencies and credentials. Graduates of these programs are given various titles such as advanced practice technologist, RT clinical specialist, and radiology practitioner assistant. They may qualify to supervise the work of other technologists, make decisions about the quality of images, and perform procedures such as fluoroscopy, venography, and arthrography under the direct supervision of a radiologist. Recognizing the value and popularity of these programs, ASRT is in the process of developing a curriculum guide for a baccalaureate program leading to advanced clinical credentials in radiologic technology.

ACCREDITATION

Accreditation is a process that applies to institutions and results in documentation attesting to the attainment of certain minimum standards. Hospitals seek accreditation by the Joint Commission on Accreditation of Healthcare Organizations (JCAHO), which indicates that the institution meets criteria for equipment, staff, safety, funding, management, and patient care. This credential is required for the hospital to receive Medicare payments and insurance payments from many private carriers.

The Centers for Medicare and Medicaid Services (formerly Health Care Financing Administration [HCFA]) is the federal agency that administers Medicare and Medicaid. Hospitals and other health care providers that wish to receive reimbursement for services under these federal programs must submit applications and provide documentation of appropriate credentials and accreditation.

Accreditation of colleges and universities is the province of state and regional agencies and attests to certain standards of education in accredited institutions. It is the basis for determining the value of the diplomas granted as well as the value of credits transferred from one institution to another.

The independent agency responsible for program accreditation in radiologic technology and radiation therapy technology is the Joint Review Committee on Education in Radiologic Technology (JRCERT). It is made up of members appointed by ASRT, ACR, and AERS. JRCERT establishes minimum educational standards, conducts inspections, and grants accreditation to programs that comply with the standards.

The accreditation processes for both hospitals and schools involve periodic self-assessment in which the institution evaluates its objectives, outcomes, resources, strengths, and weaknesses, and documents how it meets the established criteria for quality in its field. This activity is followed by an on-site visit by accrediting agency representatives during which interviews, physical surveys, and document reviews are used to assess the institution. The accreditation process provides insight that allows the institution to strive for improvement while assuring quality service for the consumer.

JOB SATISFACTION

Most students choose to study radiography because it is a caring, helping profession, but the desire to help is not enough. The stressful demands of clinical practice often tend to overshadow humanitarian considerations. The patient's needs may be overlooked while you are coping with highly technical material unless you make an effort to learn from the beginning to handle both at once.

Your work will be the most satisfying when your contributions and the personal contacts they involve are genuine and sincere. Performing tasks because you enjoy them will make your work more productive and much less stressful.

Self-Care

Health is a state of physical, mental, and social well-being, and being healthy implies that you are capable of promoting health. Health professionals are responsible for their own well-being and are also expected to serve as health role models for their patients and members of the community. Take care not to project an attitude that announces, "Do as I say, not as I do." This attitude undermines credibility in the eyes of the very people we most want to help.

An unhealthy radiographer is not a good health role model and cannot function effectively for both physical and psychological reasons. To help others, we must first meet our own physical and mental needs. Certain needs are universal and can be listed and ranked in importance (Fig. 2-5). Any unmet need causes stress and prevents an optimum state of well-being.

Our most basic needs are foremost until they are adequately satisfied. As we achieve satisfaction on

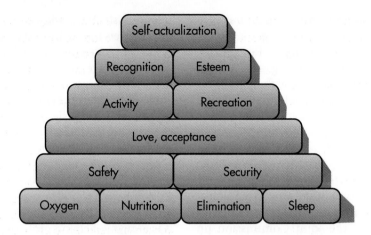

FIG. 2-5 Hierarchy of human needs.

one level, the needs of the next level occupy our attention. Self-actualization is the state in which a person welcomes tension and effort as a stimulus to creativity and self-expression. Your need for esteem and self-actualization may be the reason you are a student in this program. Constructively meeting our needs for well-being, knowledge, and self-esteem enables us to function more fully, free from self-preoccupation at those times when the patient requires full attention.

Since many patients have a lowered resistance that makes them especially vulnerable to infection, the radiographer who is ill should stay at home. However, since the team is counting on full attendance, it is better to prevent illness. Everyone experiences grief and acute anxiety occasionally, and such stresses can make you susceptible to illness. Whenever possible, you should stay at home to deal with such problems until some resolution is reached because anxiety and stress can prevent you from properly fulfilling your responsibilities.

Recommendations for the practice of good nutrition and exercise habits may sound trite, but these practices are rewarded with less time lost from work and an increased sense of well-being. In addition, knowledge and practice of the principles of body mechanics (see Chapter 4) will help you avoid the types of injuries that can result from lifting and moving patients or equipment.

Preventive health measures are equally important. For example, hospitals are required to offer employees the hepatitis B vaccine, but you are responsible for taking advantage of this important protection. The precautions discussed in Chapter 5 have been developed to help prevent disease transmission from patient to patient and from patient to you. Such precautions are completely useless unless you understand and use the principles involved. Minimizing the risk of disease in a health care setting depends on your willingness to learn and use the information offered to you.

Radiation exposure over the course of a career can have serious health consequences for you if proper precautions are not observed. Chapter 1 provides an introduction to safe practice, and your curriculum will include an extensive study of radiation protection. Adherence to radiation safety practices is another important aspect of self-care.

Empathetic Care

Job satisfaction depends on your ability to deal effectively with clinical situations and involves several attributes. One such attribute is **empathy,** a sensitivity to the needs of others that allows you to meet those needs constructively rather than merely sympathizing or reacting to a patient's distress. Understanding and compassion are accompanied by an objective detachment that enables you to respond appropriately. For example, you could express sympathy for the victim of a tragic accident by crying or by smothering him with pity. A more productive expression of empathy would show concern and care while quickly and accurately providing the films that could aid in rapid diagnosis and treatment.

Beginning students often express concerns such as, "What will I do if the patient vomits? I just know I'll get sick too!" or "I faint at the sight of blood." As you gain confidence and experience, you will learn to deal with an emergency first and let your knees shake later. Focusing on the patient while projecting a calm, reassuring attitude will be your best reinforcement.

By focusing on patient needs, you will be able to respond calmly and assertively if a patient acts inappropriately. It may seem strange or frightening when an individual responds to stress and anxiety by becoming hostile or even threatening. These actions are often coping mechanisms patients use to feel in control of a situation. Maintaining a calm, objective attitude is most effective in dealing with such patients. Overt sexual expressions by patients are encountered infrequently and usually indicate anxiety by patients who no longer feel sexually functional because of their current physical state. With this in mind, you can be less judgmental while setting limits on patient behaviors. In other words, you can refuse to accept the behavior while continuing to reassure and care for the patient.

Burnout

Health care workers are particularly susceptible to the condition known as "burnout." Burnout is a response to the chronic strain of dealing with the constant demands and problems of people under our care. This emotional overload can be exacerbated by personal problems as well as by unreasonable demands in the workplace. Burnout typically causes exhaustion, dissatisfaction, anxiety, and eventually apathy. Burned-out workers often experience depersonalization and may tend to withdraw. When required to relate to others, their attitude may be hostile. The decline in job performance may be severe enough to jeopardize employment. Victims of burnout are also subject to health problems and are likely to abuse substances such as tobacco, caffeine, and alcohol.

If you are working long hours and work seems to be the entire focus of your life, it is wise to examine your motivation. Positive motivation characterizes the individual who works for positive results. Even when this person works very hard, enthusiasm is maintained. Hard workers with a positive attitude might be called "work enthusiasts." Those with a negative motivation, however, work to avoid negative consequences such as losing their jobs or dealing with unpleasant aspects of their personal lives. Such workers are referred to as "workaholics."

The likelihood of burnout is decreased by attention to the aspects of self-care discussed earlier in this chapter. Stress relief is also important. It helps to "lighten up." Humor is a stress reliever that helps us connect with others, and difficult situations have less power to defeat us when we can laugh at them. Humor also increases creativity and has health benefits. Stress is diminished when we remember that occasional mistakes are bound to happen and that no one is perfect.

Care of Supplies and Equipment

Hospitals must stock tremendous quantities of supplies to function effectively. In such an environment, one can easily assume that free access implies free use, but in truth someone must pay the bill. Added to the purchase price of each item is an overhead factor that may be two or three times the item's basic value. For example, when a film is accidentally exposed, the loss includes not only the price of the film but also the proportional cost in work hours of the stock clerk, receiving clerk, purchasing agent, and accountant, as well as the administrators who supervise these employees, plus the overhead costs for shipping and storage.

Medical equipment is expensive, and proper care is required to ensure that its value is preserved and that it is available when needed. The misuse of equipment or supplies, or their diversion for personal use, wastes money and increases health care costs. The radiographer who avoids such waste is demonstrating a high standard of ethical behavior.

Participation in Professional Activities

Health care professionals value the acquisition of additional skills and regularly expand their knowledge. Those who are content with the status quo quickly find that the profession marches on without them. Standard practice changes rapidly, and today's knowledge will soon be out of date. Textbooks often contain information that is valid when the manuscript is completed but is outdated by the time the book is published. Formal and informal continuing education also helps us to maintain interest in our work and to avoid the boredom and routine that are detrimental to emotional health.

In the area of professional growth, cooperation is often more productive than individual effort. ASRT has 54 affiliate societies, one in each state and one each in the District of Columbia, the city of Philadelphia, and the territories of Guam and Puerto Rico. There are also many district groups within the state societies. These groups provide an opportunity for radiographers to become acquainted, share problems and ideas, hear speakers, present papers, and exhibit their work.

Professional associations provide opportunities to advance the profession while helping their members. Members may further a profession's goals while developing leadership skills through chairing committees, holding office, and participating in business and educational sessions.

The importance of scientific contribution should be emphasized. Professionals often respond to problems or new situations by developing new methods of performing their work, and many of these ideas can assist others. We owe a large debt to those who have advanced the art and science of our profession. We can acknowledge these gifts and receive recognition and a sense of belonging through our own contributions.

PROFESSIONAL BEHAVIOR

Litigation has become all too common in our society today. For this reason, it is important that health care workers become familiar with the moral, ethical, and legal implications of their behavior and performance. For many of us, these terms seem almost interchangeable. In practice, however, they have somewhat different applications.

Morals and Ethics

Personal morality is based on lessons of right and wrong that were taught to us at an early age. As we grow older, we expand our understanding of these principles and apply them in a general way to other circumstances. The customs, beliefs, and rules of our formative years play an important part in our decision making. Morals provide an internal motive that governs our relationships with others and permits us to live together in harmony.

Lawrence Kohlberg studied and wrote on the subject of moral development in the 1970s, and his description of the stages of moral development is called Kohlberg's theory. Kohlberg's work describes how individuals learn morality at first through experience with obedience and punishment. In time, they learn to behave morally to gain acceptance and approval. An advanced state of moral development is characterized by a principled conscience that recognizes the value of morality to society and to the human condition. More recent moral development research by Carol Gilligan using female subjects indicates that there is more emphasis on the significance of caring in the moral development of women, as compared with a greater emphasis on justice in the moral development of men.

The beliefs that we share with our community about values and duties constitute societal morality that influences the laws, customs, and moral components of our culture. As stated in the Declaration of Independence, our founding fathers believed that "all men are created equal" and that they were entitled to "life, liberty and the pursuit of happiness." These concepts form a central part of our societal morality as a nation.

Group morality refers to moral principles that apply specifically to certain groups of people. For example, professionals have certain duties to clients and to the public that do not apply to the population in general. The moral duties of physicians were defined in ancient Greece in the Hippocratic oath. Examples of group morality for today's health professionals include the duties to provide due care, to maintain professional competence, and to maintain confidentiality of patient information.

Ethics is a branch of philosophy and may be defined as a systematic reflection on morality. This application of moral principles to specific human activities might be thought of as "applied morality." Ethical actions are behavior that is within the accepted principles of right and wrong. There are a number of different analytical approaches to answering ethical questions. If you are fortunate to have a course in ethics as part of your education program, you will have an opportunity to explore the thought processes used by ethicists to arrive at conclusions. Basically, these approaches consider the proper response to any situation, measured against the standard of a deep respect for the dignity of all life and of the environment.

Group ethical behavior includes duties and obligations placed on us by our profession. Ethical questions that arise in the practice of professions have been considered and addressed by most professions and their organizations. The essential principles of ethical behavior for the group are stated in a document called a code of ethics. Because professionals have important moral duties, they are responsible for knowing and honoring the principles of ethics that govern their professional activities.

While the application of moral, ethical, and legal standards may be confusing, there are a few clear differences. Our moral principles instill a sense of right and wrong and a desire to do the right thing. Professional ethics define correct moral behavior in the context of performing professional duties. Laws are the means used by government to enforce commonly accepted moral standards in the interests of society. When injured individuals believe that we have caused them harm by failing to fulfill our moral or professional responsibilities, laws exist to provide remedies. They ensure that the rights of carelessly or unjustly injured parties will be protected by the courts.

Standards of Ethics

A code of ethics is a hallmark of a profession because it signifies high principles of professional behavior and a willingness by the profession to control its own conduct. As stated earlier in this chapter, most professions have their own codes of ethics that govern behavior. The ASRT Code of Ethics, printed in Box 2-2, is developed and jointly adopted by ASRT and ARRT. It establishes broad principles of professional conduct. Specific behaviors to achieve these ends are detailed in the Standards of Practice. Some principles of the ASRT Code of Ethics are self-explanatory, and some are expanded in other sections of this chapter. Four of them (the third, fifth, seventh, and ninth principles) are not discussed elsewhere in this chapter and deserve additional attention.

The third principle requires radiographers to put aside all personal prejudice and emotional bias when rendering professional services. This is more difficult than it may first appear. Most of us can easily identify prejudice in others, but our own biases or judgments are beyond our awareness and are justified as "only common sense." We all have natural preferences that may result in discriminatory treatment if we are not fully aware of them. With what patients do you feel most comfortable? Men? Women? Those of your own race? Those over 16? Under 65? Middle class? Do you feel greater compassion for a patient with a heart problem than for one with a sexually transmitted disease? Once we identify areas in human relationships where we are most at ease, it becomes apparent that we are less at ease in other situations and would prefer to avoid them altogether. It is instructive to pay attention to how we deal with patients who are outside our "comfort zone." Sometimes we tend to act more friendly or solicitous to cover up feelings, while at other times we may remain aloof, appearing to be preoccupied. Lack of interest and concern is unacceptable; feigned concern is never the same as the real thing. Faithfulness to the spirit of the third principle requires a high degree of self-awareness and presents a serious professional challenge to the radiographer.

The fifth principle deals with the issue of professional responsibility, implying that radiographers are truly professional because they are sufficiently educated and experienced to be capable of independent discretion and judgment. Within the scope

BOX 2-2

AMERICAN SOCIETY OF RADIOLOGIC TECHNOLOGISTS CODE OF ETHICS

- The radiologic technologist conducts himself or herself in a professional manner, responds to patient needs and supports colleagues and associates in providing quality patient care.
- The radiologic technologist acts to advance the principal objective of the profession to provide services to humanity with full respect for the dignity of mankind.
- The radiologic technologist delivers patient care and service unrestricted by concerns of personal attributes or the nature of the disease or illness, and without discrimination on the basis of sex, race, creed, religion or socio-economic status.
- The radiologic technologist practices technology founded upon theoretical knowledge and concepts, uses equipment and accessories consistent with the purpose for which they were designed and employs procedures and techniques appropriately.
- The radiologic technologist assesses situations; exercises care, discretion and judgment; assumes responsibility for professional decisions; and acts in the best interest of the patient.
- The radiologic technologist acts as an agent through observation and communication to obtain pertinent information for the physician to aid in the diagnosis and treatment of the patient and recognizes that interpretation and diagnosis are outside the scope of practice for the profession.
- The radiologic technologist uses equipment and accessories, employs techniques and procedures, performs services in accordance with an accepted standard of practice and demonstrates expertise in minimizing radiation exposure to the patient, self and other members of the health care team.
- The radiologic technologist practices ethical conduct appropriate to the profession and protects the patient's right to quality radiologic technology care.
- The radiologic technologist respects confidences entrusted in the course of professional practice, respects the patient's right to privacy and reveals confidential information only as required by law or to protect the welfare of the individual or the community.
- The radiologic technologist continually strives to improve knowledge and skills by participating in continuing education and professional activities, sharing knowledge with colleagues and investigating new aspects of professional practice.

Revised and adopted by The American Society of Radiologic Technologists and The American Registry of Radiologic Technologists, July, 1998.

of our professional activity, we are expected to make decisions and to be accountable for our decisions. A very important aspect of this responsibility is awareness and acceptance of our limitations. Although responsibilities may vary with the working environment, regular duties should be specified in written job descriptions and should be consistent with the scope of practice authorized by one's credentials as permitted by law and institutional policy. The Standards of Practice provide guidance with respect to these duties and responsibilities. It is in no one's best interest to perform tasks without adequate knowledge or to undertake a responsibility without adequate qualification. This principle also holds the

radiographer accountable for errors committed under the orders of another person if the radiographer knew, or should have known, that the order was in error.

The seventh principle requires that radiographers adhere to accepted practices and make every effort to protect themselves and all patients and staff from exposure to unnecessary radiation. The ethical implications of this issue are very important. When a radiographer violates this principle, there is no telltale evidence. The negative consequences of other breaches of ethics might be immediate, but the latent and genetic effects of unnecessary radiation may not be apparent for 10 to 30 years, or even for several generations. Making every effort to minimize radiation exposure—even when the patient is difficult to handle, you have been awakened for an emergency in the middle of the night, you are really in a hurry, and no one is watching—requires both good habits and a strong ethical commitment to radiation protection.

The ninth principle relates to confidentiality in a health care setting, one of the cardinal concepts in all codes of ethics relating to health care. The confidentiality of conversations between patients and their physicians is considered so important that, along with communications to lawyers and the clergy, it is protected by "legal privilege." This means that the professional cannot be required to divulge such information, even when it is of material value in a court of law. Although the information provided to a radiographer is not legally privileged, radiographers often hear conversations between patients and their physicians and have access to confidential information contained in patient charts. You may witness circumstances in which patients are unable to preserve their dignity and behave in ways that would embarrass or shame them if known to friends or family members. Many patients do not want it known that they are ill or have been hospitalized, and others may wish to keep their diagnosis confidential. Information that may seem of no consequence to you may constitute a very sensitive issue for the patient.

Any breach of confidence, even if no names are mentioned, may rightly be interpreted by others as an indication that you do not respect professional confidence. Betrayals of confidence cause mistrust of the health care team and may prevent patients from revealing facts essential to their care.

The patient's right to confidentiality is not violated by appropriate communications among health care workers when the information is pertinent to the patient's care. It is justifiably assumed in such a case that the transfer of information is for the patient's benefit and that all personnel involved are bound by the ethics regarding confidentiality. Appropriate communications are those directed privately to those who need the information. Conversations about patients must never be held in public areas such as waiting rooms, elevators, or cafeterias.

The ethics of patient-staff communication also require sound judgment and restraint to avoid exposing patients to the radiographer's personal concerns or the problems of the hospital staff. Using the patient as a sounding board for complaints or gossip is inexcusable.

Rules of Ethics

In addition to the Code of Ethics, which is an aspirational document, the standards of ethics for the profession as published by ARRT also include Rules of Ethics. These are mandatory specific standards of minimally acceptable professional conduct for all registered technologists and applicants for certification by ARRT, and they are enforceable by ARRT. The Ethics Committee and the Board of Trustees of ARRT handle challenges to the Rules of Ethics through established administrative procedures. These rules are published in their entirety by ARRT. They prohibit the practices summarized below:

- Use of fraud or deceit to obtain employment or credentials
- Dishonest conduct with regard to the ARRT examination
- Conviction or no-contest plea with respect to a felony, gross misdemeanor, or misdemeanor (except speeding or parking infractions)
- Failure to report to ARRT that legal or ethical charges are pending against the person in any jurisdiction
- Failure or inability to practice the profession with reasonable skill and safety
- Any professional practice that is illegal, contrary to prevailing standards, or that creates an unnecessary danger to the patient
- Delegation, or acceptance of delegation, of professional functions that might create an unnecessary danger to a patient
- Actual or potential inability to practice radiologic technology safely by reason of illness, use of alcohol or drugs, or any physical or mental condition; adjudication of mental incompetence, mental illness, chemical dependency, or posing a danger to the public
- Revealing privileged communication except as permitted by law

- Knowingly engaging in or participating in abusive or fraudulent billing practices
- Improper management of patient records, such as failure to maintain records, or actions that may result in a false or misleading record
- Assisting a person to engage in the practice of radiologic technology without current and appropriate credentials
- Violating an administrative rule of a state board, or violating any state or federal law governing the practice of radiologic technology or the use of controlled substances
- Providing false or misleading information directly related to the care of a patient
- Practicing outside the scope of practice authorized by one's credentials
- Making a false statement to ARRT or failing to cooperate with an investigation conducted by ARRT or the Ethics Committee
- Engaging in dishonest or misleading communication regarding one's education, experience, or credentials
- Failing to report to ARRT any violation or probable violation of any Rule of Ethics by any registered technologist or applicant for certification by ARRT

Ethical Judgments and Conflicts

The process of ethical analysis is helpful in any situation where the correct action is in question. The first step is to be sure you have all the pertinent information. Measure possible actions against the standard of deep respect for the dignity of life. If there is a conflict, consider which value, duty, or guideline is most important and why. In a new situation, consider which aspects of existing moral principles provide the most reliable guide. Finally, consider what new thinking is needed to deal with a novel situation.

Ethical analysis is being used increasingly to solve institutional problems. When several individuals have analyzed the situation, the next step may be to seek resolution through discussion that leads to consensus. Once the question is resolved, action can be taken. The one responsible for implementing the ethical decision is called the **moral agent**.

Ethical conflicts may trouble us when the ethics of the group are not compatible with our personal beliefs. For example, there are health professionals who find that caring for some patients with acquired immunodeficiency syndrome (AIDS) offends their personal sense of morality because they disapprove of the homosexual lifestyle. For others, the conflict between their religious beliefs and the legal right of a patient to receive an abortion may be a problem. Professionals must not permit issues of personal morality to supersede the group moral duty to provide quality patient care. While ethical standards might pose personal moral challenges, these standards assure us that professional moral judgments can be made that will hold true for everyone in similar circumstances. They test whether a specific behavior will support the values and duties of our profession. If you experience frequent ethical conflicts that cannot be resolved, you may need to find a new position or career that conforms more closely to your own moral standards.

Patient Rights

A major ethical concern for radiographers is to protect patient rights at all times. Considerable emphasis is placed on consumer advocacy in our society, and this value is especially significant in health care. There are many different statements of patient rights, and patient rights legislation is currently pending in the U.S. Congress. The patient rights statement of the American Hospital Association is printed in Box 2-3. This statement was developed prior to the introduction of recent patient rights legislation and may be subject to change, but the key concepts that are especially pertinent to the work of radiographers are the same in all statements of patient rights.

Foremost is the right to considerate and respectful care. This statement is self-explanatory and is essentially the same professional behavior prescribed by the second and third principles of the Code of Ethics for Radiologic Technologists. It applies to all patients, regardless of status.

The patient also has a right to information, but this does not obligate the radiographer to provide any and all information that may be requested.

```
BOX 2-3
```

AHA PATIENTS' RIGHTS STATEMENT

The Patient Care Partnership: Understanding Expectations, Rights and Responsibilities

When you need hospital care, your doctor and the nurses and other professionals at our hospital are committed to working with you and your family to meet your health care needs. Our dedicated doctors and staff serve the community in all its ethnic, religious and economic diversity. Our goal is for you and your family to have the same care and attention we would want for our families and ourselves.

The sections explain some of the basics about how you can expect to be treated during your hospital stay. They also cover what we will need from you to care for you better. If you have questions at any time, please ask them. Unasked or unanswered questions can add to the stress of being in the hospital. Your comfort and confidence in your care are very important to us.

What to Expect During Your Hospital Stay

- **High quality hospital care.** Our first priority is to provide you the care you need, when you need it, with skill, compassion, and respect. Tell your caregivers if you have concerns about your care or if you have pain. You have the right to know the identity of doctors, nurses and others involved in your care, and you have the right to know when they are students, residents or other trainees.
- **A clean and safe environment.** Our hospital works hard to keep you safe. We use special policies and procedures to avoid mistakes in your care and keep you free from abuse or neglect. If anything unexpected and significant happens during your hospital stay, you will be told what happened, and any resulting changes in your care will be discussed with you.
- **Involvement in your care.** You and your doctor often make decisions about your care before you go to the hospital. Other times, especially in emergencies, those decisions are made during your hospital stay. When decision-making takes place, it should include:

Discussing your medical condition and information about medically appropriate treatment choices. To make informed decisions with your doctor, you need to understand:
- The benefits and risks of each treatment.
- Whether your treatment is experimental or part of a research study.
- What you can reasonably expect from your treatment and any long-term effects it might have on your quality of life.
- What you and your family will need to do after you leave the hospital.
- The financial consequences of using uncovered services or out-of-network providers.
Please tell your caregivers if you need more information about treatment choices.

Discussing your treatment plan. When you enter the hospital, you sign a general consent to treatment. In some cases, such as surgery or experimental treatment, you may be asked to confirm in writing that you understand what is planned and agree to it. This process protects your right to consent to or refuse a treatment. Your doctor will explain the medical consequences of refusing recommended treatment. It also protects your right to decide if you want to participate in a research study.

Getting information from you. Your caregivers need complete and correct information about your health and coverage so that they can make good decisions about your care. That includes:
- Past illnesses, surgeries or hospital stays.
- Past allergic reactions.
- Any medicines or dietary supplements (such as vitamins and herbs) that you are taking.
- Any network or admission requirements under your health plan.

Continued

BOX 2-3

AHA PATIENTS' RIGHTS STATEMENT—cont'd

Understanding your health care goals and values. You may have health care goals and values or spiritual beliefs that are important to your well-being. They will be taken into account as much as possible throughout your hospital stay. Make sure your doctor, your family and your care team know your wishes.

Understanding who should make decisions when you cannot. If you have signed a health care power of attorney stating who should speak for you if you become unable to make health care decisions for yourself, or a "living will" or "advance directive" that states your wishes about end-of-life care; give copies to your doctor, your family and your care team. If you or your family need help making difficult decisions, counselors, chaplains and others are available to help.

- **Protection of your privacy**. We respect the confidentiality of your relationship with your doctor and other care-givers, and the sensitive information about your health and health care that are part of that relationship. State and federal laws and hospital operating policies protect the privacy of your medical information. You will receive a Notice of Privacy Practices that describes the ways that we use, disclose and safeguard patient information and that explains how you can obtain a copy of information from our records about your care.
- **Preparing you and your family for when you leave the hospital.** Your doctor works with hospital staff and pro-fessionals in your community. You and your family also play an important role in your care. The success of your treatment often depends on your efforts to follow medication, diet and therapy plans. Your family may need to help care for you at home.

You can expect us to help you identify sources of follow-up care and to let you know if our hospital has a finan-cial interest in any referrals. As long as you agree that we can share information about your care with them, we will coordinate our activities with your caregivers outside the hospital. You can also expect to receive information and, where possible, training about the self-care you will need when you go home.

- **Help with your bill and filing insurance claims.** Our staff will file claims for you with health care insurers or other programs such as Medicare and Medicaid. They also will help your doctor with needed documentation. Hospital bills and insurance coverage are often confusing. If you have questions about your bill, contact our business office. If you need help understanding your insurance coverage or health plan, start with your insurance company or health benefits manager. If you do not have health coverage, we will try to help you and your family find financial help or make other arrangements. We need your help with collecting needed information and other requirements to obtain coverage or assistance.

While you are here, you will receive more detailed notices about some of the rights you have as a hospital patient and how to exercise them. We are always interested in improving. If you have questions, comments, or concerns, please contact _____.

A Patient's Bill of Rights was first adopted by the American Hospital Association (AHA) in 1973. The Patient Care Partnership was copyrighted by the AHA in 2003.

Radiographers must be prepared to explain radiographic procedures and to identify themselves and the radiologists. Patients have the right to copies of their billing records, medical records, and radiographs. When these records are requested, they should be provided according to the established policies of the institution. *Questions regarding diagnosis, treatment, and other aspects of care should be referred to the physician.*

The right to privacy implies that the patient's modesty will be respected and that every effort will be made to maintain the patient's sense of personal dignity. The radiographer must remember that many common procedures (enemas, for example) threaten the patient's modesty and dignity. Patients are likely to be much more sensitive in these situations than health care workers who perform these procedures daily. Physicians or health care workers should not be left alone with patients of the opposite sex in a physical examination setting that requires undraping the patient or examining the genitalia or female breasts. A "chaperone," preferably of the same sex as the patient, should be present. The main reason for this practice is to ease the patient's mind if he or she fears such an encounter and to provide a witness in case the patient later claims to have been assaulted or touched in an unprofessional manner. Many institutions have policies for these situations, and physicians usually prefer to be chaperoned even when no such policy exists. The radiographer should be aware of the institution's policies and sensitive to others' needs in this regard. Students and others not required for a procedure must have the patient's permission to be present. Taking photographs other than for the sole purpose of the patient's care also requires consent.

The right of privacy also includes the expectation of confidentiality introduced earlier in this chapter. The Health Insurance Portability and Accountability Act (HIPAA) was enacted under the U.S. Department of Health and Human Services (HHS) to protect the privacy rights of patients. In April 2003, hospitals were required to provide protection for patients concerning the release of individual financial and medical information without the written consent of the patient. No information may be released to employers, financial institutions, or other medical facilities without specific permission by the patient. In brief, this law requires the following:

1. The patient must receive a clear written explanation of how the health provider may use the disclosed information.
2. The patient will be able to see and copy records and request amendments.
3. A history of routine disclosures must be available to the patient.
4. Health care providers must obtain consent before sharing routine information on treatment, payment, and health care operations. Separate authorization is needed for nonroutine disclosures and nonhealth purposes.
5. Patients have the right to request restrictions on uses and disclosures of their information.
6. Patients may file complaints with a covered provider or with HHS about violations of these rules.

Patients have the right to refuse treatment, which also implies the right to refuse examination. If a patient chooses to exercise this right, the radiographer *must not* proceed with the study. *Note that signing an informed consent does not invalidate the patient's right to refuse treatment once the procedure has begun.* Consent may be revoked at any time during the procedure. If this occurs, take time to find out why the patient is unwilling to continue, since this may be a response to a temporary discomfort and not an objection to the procedure itself. If the patient still refuses to complete the procedure, comply gracefully and allow the patient to leave or return to the nursing service. Notify the attending physician.

Informed consent

Although patient consent for routine procedures is given on admission and is implied by the continued acceptance of hospital care, informed consent is necessary for any procedure that is considered experimental or that involves substantial risk. Certain imaging procedures such as myelograms require that you explain the procedure and its potential risks and benefits to the patient and witness that the patient signs a consent form. For some procedures, providing information and obtaining consent is the physician's duty, but for patients undergoing most routine procedures, a staff member provides the necessary form and explanation on the physician's behalf.

When it is your duty to obtain informed consent, be sure that you fully understand the procedure and its risks and benefits so that you can adequately explain them to the patient and answer any questions. If the patient asks a question you cannot answer, seek the correct answer before continuing, because an improper response may invalidate the consent. The legal implications of informed consent cannot be overemphasized. Successful litigation has been based on lack of compliance with the following guidelines:

- Patients must receive a full explanation of the procedure and its risks and benefits and sign the consent form before being sedated or anesthetized.
- A patient must be competent in order to sign an informed consent.
- Only parents or legal guardians may sign for a minor.
- Only a legal guardian may sign for a mentally incompetent patient.
- Consent forms must be completed before being signed. Patients should never be asked to sign a blank form or a form with blank spaces "to be filled in later."
- Only the physician named on the consent form may perform the procedure. Consent is not transferable from one physician to another, not even to an associate.
- Any condition stated on the form must be met. For example, if the form states that a family member will be present during the procedure, the consent is not valid if the family member is not there.
- Informed consent may be revoked by the patient at any time after signing. This is an invocation of the patient's right to refuse examination.

A typical consent form is reproduced in Appendix B. The radiographer is responsible for knowing which procedures require written consent and for checking the chart to be certain that these forms are in order before beginning the examination.

Genetic information

In the near future, matters of who has access to the information contained in an individual's genetic code will pose questions that relate to confidentiality and patient rights. In June of 2000, the Human Genome Project reported that, for the first time, human beings are able to read their own recipe! The human genome is essentially the instruction for how to build and operate a human being. This almost incredible achievement brings us closer to identifying and potentially altering the genes responsible for the transmission of genetic-based diseases. For example, research in cancer-suppressing genes offers a new approach in the treatment of many kinds of tumors.

While these discoveries open an entire new world of research and potential treatment, they also open the door to new ethical dilemmas. Many of the genetic-based diseases are relatively rare but present long-term care problems with extremely high medical costs. Should everyone be screened for these diseases? Should families with a history of these diseases be compelled to undergo screening? What should be considered if a fetus is tested and found to have inherited a severe familial disease? Should prenatal genetic screening be as much a part of prenatal care as blood pressure screening?

These questions will continue to pose ethical problems as genetic counseling becomes a more frequent component of health care. Physicians, social workers, and others with training in this sensitive field will be used with increasing frequency to help patients make informed decisions about genetic questions.

Death with dignity

Although the right to die is not specifically mentioned in the Patient Bill of Rights, it has received considerable public attention in recent years. This can present important ethical questions about health care workers' commitment to do everything possible to preserve and prolong life and the responsibility to relieve suffering, respect patient choice, and honor the patient's right to die with dignity. Recently the news media have focused attention on physician-assisted suicide for qualified terminally ill patients. There is a wide array of definitions and beliefs within this debate.

As a separate issue, resuscitation of patients for whom there is a reasonable expectation of recovery is considered to be medically and ethically correct, but sometimes heroic measures may only serve to prolong the patient's suffering at great cost to the family and the public. This has become an important issue because modern technology has made it possible to sustain life indefinitely by providing artificial life support to individuals who would otherwise not survive.

When the patient's condition is terminal or when chronic illness or suffering has resulted in a substantial decrease in quality of life, the physician and the patient (or the patient's family, if the patient is incompetent) may agree to a "no-code" or "do not resuscitate" (DNR) order. This means that if death is imminent, no effort at resuscitation is to be attempted. When a DNR order is instituted, a notation is placed in the patient's chart so that everyone involved in the patient's care will be aware of the order.

Many patients have "advance directives." An advance directive is an outline of specific wishes about medical care in the event that an individual loses the ability to make or communicate decisions. Copies of these directives are usually given to the family physician and an attorney or family member and should be part of the medical record.

Another way for individuals to influence decision making about their health care is to appoint a personal representative (durable power of attorney for health care). This action enables a trusted person to act on the patient's behalf if and when the patient is unable to communicate his or her wishes. The designated person is empowered to sign a valid informed consent form and should be aware of the patient's wishes, values, and beliefs about life-sustaining treatments in a wide array of situations.

To avoid confusion or contention at critical times, all members of the immediate family should be informed when an advance directive is executed or when a health care representative is appointed.

Laws are legal requirements for behavior. Laws govern the practice of health care delivery, the practice of radiography, and certain interpersonal interactions. In general, laws may be divided into two categories: criminal law and civil law.

Criminal law deals with offenses against the state or against society at large. Crimes may be further distinguished according to gravity or importance. Serious crimes are called **felonies** and may be punished by imprisonment. Less significant crimes are called **misdemeanors** and are usually punishable by fines.

Civil law deals with the rights and duties of individuals with respect to one another. A civil wrong committed by one individual against the person or property of another is called a **tort.** Lawsuits pursued under tort law claim that the **plaintiff,** the suing party, has been injured in some way by the **defendant,** the party being sued. Civil lawsuits seek "damages" rather than punishment; they are satisfied by court-ordered payment to the injured party by the defendant. In other words, civil law allows compensation to individuals who have been injured by a noncriminal act.

Crimes: Felonies and Misdemeanors

Criminal acts committed by radiographers could include either felonies or misdemeanors. Thefts and some drug-related crimes, for example, are felonies. Violations of laws that regulate practice, such as licensure requirements or scope of practice limitations, are usually classified as misdemeanors. Violations of criminal law could make it impossible for you to obtain professional standing and/or employment as a radiographer in the future.

Intentional Misconduct

Civil lawsuits alleging personal injury are becoming increasingly common in the health care field. The torts involved may fall into one of two categories: intentional misconduct or negligence. The intentional torts that occur in a hospital setting include assault, battery, false imprisonment, invasion of privacy, libel, and slander (defamation of character).

False imprisonment is the unjustifiable detention of a person against his or her will. This becomes an issue when the patient wishes to leave and is not allowed to do so. It is acceptable to use physical restraints when appropriately applied for safety reasons with the patient's permission. For example, hospitals have policies requiring use of safety belts on stretchers and of side rails on hospital beds at night. The least restrictive restraints that provide adequate safety should be used. Inappropriate use of physical restraints, however, may constitute false imprisonment. Reasonable judgment must be used to decide whether restraints are necessary. Hand or leg restraints are used only when the patient's physician orders them (see Chapter 4).

Invasion of privacy charges may result when confidentiality has not been maintained or when the patient's body has been improperly and unnecessarily exposed or touched. The significance of confidentiality is reemphasized here. Hospitals and their employees may be liable if they disclose confidential information obtained from a patient or contained in the medical record. If the information disclosed reflects negatively on the patient's reputation, one may also be liable for defamation of character. Protection of the patient's modesty is vitally important and is noted throughout this text as it pertains to specific procedures. Liability can also result if photographs are published without a patient's permission.

Libel and **slander** refer to the malicious spreading of information that causes defamation of character or loss of reputation. Libel usually refers to written information, and slander is more often applied to verbal information. It should be clear that a breach of confidentiality is not only unethical but sufficient grounds for a slander suit against the radiographer.

Assault is defined as the threat of touching in an injurious way. Note that the person need not be touched in any way for assault to occur. If the patient feels threatened and is made to believe that he or she will be touched in a harmful manner, justification may exist for an assault charge. To avoid this, the radiographer must explain what is to occur and reassure the patient in any situation where the threat of harm may be an issue. Never use threats to force a patient's cooperation; this also applies to both adults and pediatric patients.

Battery is defined as unlawful touching of a person without consent. If the patient refuses to be touched, that wish must be respected. Even the most well-intentioned touch may fall into this category if the patient has expressly forbidden it. This should not prevent the radiographer from placing a reassuring hand on the patient's shoulder as long as the patient has not forbidden it and when there is no intent to harm or to invade the patient's privacy. On the other hand, a radiograph taken against the patient's will or on the wrong patient could be construed as battery. This emphasizes the need for consistently double-checking patient identification and being certain that proper informed consent has been obtained for procedures that require it.

Unintentional Misconduct

Unintentional torts include negligence and malpractice. **Negligence** refers to the neglect or omission of reasonable care or caution. The standard of reasonable care is based on the doctrine of the reasonably prudent person. This standard requires that a person perform as any reasonable person would perform under similar circumstances. In the relationship between a professional person and a patient or client, the professional has a duty to provide reasonable care. An act of negligence in the context of such a relationship is defined as professional negligence or **malpractice.** The radiographer is held to the standard of care and skill of the "reasonable radiographer" in similar circumstances.

You may also hear the terms *gross negligence, contributory negligence,* and *corporate negligence.* Gross negligence refers to negligent acts that involve "reckless disregard for life or limb." It denotes a higher degree of negligence than ordinary negligence and results in more serious penalties. Contributory negligence refers to an act of negligence in which the behavior of the injured party contributed to the injury. Corporate negligence applies when the hospital as an entity is negligent.

To legally establish a claim of malpractice, a claimant must prove to the court's satisfaction that four conditions are true:

- The defendant (person or institution being sued) had a duty to provide reasonable care to the patient.

- The patient sustained some loss or injury.
- The defendant is the party responsible for the loss.
- The loss is attributable to negligence or improper practice.

The doctrine of *res ipsa loquitur* means literally, "the thing speaks for itself." This doctrine is sometimes applied when negligence and loss are so apparent that they would be obvious to anyone. For example, if a patient who has had surgery is demonstrated to have a surgical instrument inside his body at the surgical site, the fact of the instrument's presence establishes the negligence of the surgeon.

Although a patient may sustain some loss, the court must be convinced that the loss is a result of negligent care or treatment before the patient can collect damages. Usually a determination of negligence is based on whether the usual standards and procedures were followed. In another case, a patient may prove that someone was negligent, but the patient is not entitled to damages unless it can be demonstrated that a loss occurred as a result. Nonetheless, it is inexcusable to be complacent about negligence simply because there was "no harm done," or to be callous about loss just because accepted and established procedures were followed.

Because malpractice lawsuits against physicians and hospitals are becoming increasingly common, rates for malpractice insurance coverage have soared. This topic is a serious concern to all health professionals. There has been much discussion concerning whether radiographers should carry malpractice insurance. Hospitals carry liability insurance that covers negligence of employees acting in the course of their employment. Radiographers must learn the extent of malpractice coverage in their institutions.

Traditionally, there has been a tendency to place legal responsibility on the highest authority possible. For instance, according to the legal doctrine of *respondeat superior* ("let the master respond"), the employer is liable for employees' negligent acts that occur in the course of their work. This liability by one person or agency for the actions of another is called vicarious liability. According to the doctrine of the "borrowed servant," a physician may be liable for wrongful acts committed by hospital employees under the physician's orders. Under these doctrines, actions of radiographers may result in lawsuits against their employers or against the physicians with whom they work.

In recent years, however, the "rule of personal responsibility" has been increasingly applied. This means that each person is liable for his or her own negligent conduct. Under this rule, the law does not allow the wrongdoer to escape responsibility even though someone else may be legally liable as well. Although radiographers themselves are seldom named specifically in malpractice lawsuits, the rule of personal responsibility has resulted in some unfavorable judgments against radiographers as individuals.

Some believe that the increasing application of the rule of personal responsibility places radiographers in legal jeopardy, and for this reason they should be protected by their own liability insurance policies. Others argue that the potential for a large insurance settlement is an incentive to sue and that if the radiographer has no means of paying a large claim, no suit will be filed. ASRT sponsors the offering of professional liability coverage on a group basis, indicating that this organization thinks such coverage is important. The possibility of losing personal assets such as one's home may provide motivation for joining such a plan.

Lawsuits can result in conflict, expense, professional embarrassment, and loss of public confidence, even when the plaintiff is denied any award. Thus a great need for caution exists, both in the interest of patient care and in the avoidance of possible malpractice claims. Research indicates that lawsuits are most likely when patients feel alienated from the people providing their care. When a trusting professional relationship is established, suits are less likely to occur. With this in mind, you can minimize the risk of medicolegal problems by remembering and applying The Seven Cs of Malpractice Prevention listed in Box 2-4.

Proper patient identification (see Chapter 4), accuracy in medication administration (see Chapter 7), and compliance with patient safety requirements (see Chapter 4) are other positive steps the radiographer can take to avoid malpractice suits.

BOX 2-4

THE SEVEN Cs OF MALPRACTICE PREVENTION*

- **Competence.** Knowing and adhering to professional standards and maintaining professional competence reduce liability exposure.
- **Compliance.** The compliance by health professionals with policies and procedures in the medical office and hospital avoids patient injuries and litigation.
- **Charting.** Charting completely, consistently, and objectively can be the best defense against a malpractice claim.
- **Communication.** Patient injuries and resulting malpractice cases can be avoided by improving communications among health care professionals.
- **Confidentiality.** Protecting the confidentiality of medical information is a legal and ethical responsibility of health professionals.
- **Courtesy.** A courteous attitude and demeanor can improve patient rapport and lessen the likelihood of lawsuits.
- **Carefulness.** Personal injuries can occur unexpectedly on the premises and may lead to lawsuits. [See Chapter 4.]

*The Seven Cs are printed here with the permission of David Karp, loss prevention manager for the Medical Insurance Exchange of California.

Harm may result from contrast media administered without proper precautions (see Chapter 10) or when reactions are not immediately identified and appropriately treated (see Chapter 8). Poor radiographs pose a potential for misdiagnosis that may have serious consequences for the patient and the radiographer. Since the possibility of harmful error is often greatest in stressful situations, appropriate responses in an emergency ensure the least risk. You must understand and accept that an appropriate response depends on your level of experience and education, so do not hesitate to ask questions and receive help when needed.

The radiographer can also help to protect the patient and the institution by reporting illegal or unethical professional activities to the proper authorities. In such a situation, the radiographer must be neither too zealous nor too hesitant. A simple, written statement that includes the facts (dates, times, names, places), but avoids judgments or conclusions, should be prepared as soon as possible after the occurrence. This statement should be submitted to the appropriate person, probably your immediate supervisor unless he or she was involved in the incident. The supervisor receiving such a report is responsible for seeing that it is given to the proper authority, who must then follow up with an investigation. A single report may not produce change, but it may add strength to other reports or lead to increased supervision where needed.

CONCLUSION

As health care and health insurance have become more expensive, many individuals have been forced to assume the role of health advocates and to take more responsibility for their own health. This is true of radiographers as well. In addition to their participation as health care providers, they also have a responsibility to serve as healthy role models.

The health care team is a large group of people with varied skills and responsibilities. It is organized to form an effective chain of command that provides the best possible patient care. The radiographer is an important member of this team with significant responsibilities to patients and to the team.

Professional groups offer opportunities for continuing education and professional growth and also establish standards for ethical behavior. Ethical and professional behavior is essential to good patient care. Such conduct safeguards patient rights and reduces the likelihood of medicolegal difficulties.

REVIEW QUESTIONS

1. The only recognized professional society open to all radiologic technologists in the United States today is:
   A. AVIR
   B. NRA

C. AHRA

D. ASRT

E. AARP

2. Arm and leg restraints applied without either the patient's permission or a physician's order could result in charges of:

A. slander

B. false imprisonment

C. negligence

D. invasion of privacy

E. battery

3. The nationwide increase in patient visits to the emergency department is due to:

A. convenient hours

B. lack of doctors who make house calls

C. lower costs per visit than doctors' offices

D. inability of patients to obtain low-cost health insurance

4. Standards of correct behavior by professional groups are called:

A. morals

B. laws

C. codes of ethics

D. torts

E. regulations

5. The day-to-day scheduling of staff in the radiography department is the responsibility of the:

A. radiologist

B. chief radiographer

C. department secretary

D. admitting clerk

E. cashier

CRITICAL THINKING EXERCISES

1. Jon Russell, age 64, was brought to the hospital emergency department on Sunday afternoon for problems with his right ankle. Several days prior to admission he had stepped in a hole while carrying a heavy box, and the swelling had not gone down with frequent applications of cold and the use of a firm ankle support bandage. Carol, the radiographer on duty, was very reassuring, even though a busy schedule caused her to delay her lunch break once more. After positioning the ankle and completing and processing the films, she left them with the emergency department physician on call and went to lunch. Dr. Coal, the emergency department physician, looked at the films and said to Jon, "Well, these films are a little dark, but I don't see a fracture. You should stay off the ankle as much as possible, continue to use ice and your support bandage, and elevate your leg as often as you can." On Monday, the radiologist decided that the films were too dark to be diagnostic and Jon was asked to return for additional films. The final diagnosis was that Jon had suffered an avulsion fracture of the distal tibia. While Jon only suffered some inconvenience and no litigation was ever involved, do you think Carol was guilty of negligence? What do you think she should have done?

2. At lunchtime the cafeteria was full of employees and visitors. Sandy, a new radiographer, saw her friend, Janet, and sat down to eat and chat. "Wow, did we have a mouthy patient just before lunch!" she related. "Do you remember that Laura Moss who runs the dress shop downtown? She was so drunk she apparently fell down and broke her leg! I could hear her in the next room; and when I looked in at them, they were giving her some kind of stuff to calm her down." A chair at the next table was pushed back abruptly. "That is completely untrue! My wife was not drunk. She tripped and fell on the stairs. The medication was glucose because she was having an insulin reaction." A formal complaint was subsequently filed with the hospital administration. Were Sandy's comments wrong? If so, what was her offense? Was she merely rude, or is there possible cause for litigation?

Professional Attitudes and Communications

At the conclusion of this chapter, the student will be able to:

- List examples of how members of diverse groups may approach health care.
- List examples of how cultural diversity may influence or affect the communication process.
- Demonstrate five examples of nonverbal communication.
- Compare assertive and aggressive behavior.
- Discriminate between assumed and validated statements.
- Define the term *valid choice* and give an example that might be typical of a patient care situation in radiology.
- Describe three approaches used when dealing with children in the radiology department.

- Compare approaches for dealing with deaf patients to those that apply to patients with moderate hearing loss.
- List the two most important points to be remembered when dealing with patients in an altered state of consciousness.
- Locate the portions of a chart containing information relevant to diagnosis, history, current status, laboratory reports, radiology reports, allergies, and medications.
- List five reasons for keeping accurate medical records.

VOCABULARY

aggressiveness	diagnosis
aphasia	electrolarynx
ambulatory	ethnic
assertiveness	hospice
autonomy	oncology
chart	palliative
charting	prognosis
chronic	regimen
dermatitis	valid choice

WE OFTEN HEAR COMPLAINTS about poor communication skills, poor manners, and unprofessional attitudes. Perhaps it would be wise, then, to address some ways in which these terms apply to your work as a radiographer. In this context, to communicate means to convey information accurately, to express oneself clearly, and to have an interchange of ideas and information with others. Attitude, on the other hand, is a state of mind, an opinion, or a feeling, often revealed by body position, tone of voice, or other nonverbal signals. Manners are customs that express respect and are sometimes referred to as the oil that makes daily contacts run smoothly.

Accurate communication is essential for both immediate and ongoing patient care. The ability to give instructions depends on the speaker being clear and precise. The listener, on the other hand, is equally responsible for attentive and receptive behavior. The rapport we establish with both patients and coworkers by listening attentively and responding in a meaningful way can easily be overlooked under the pressures of a busy schedule. Stress in the workplace can accelerate rapidly when interpersonal communication breaks down and good manners are neglected.

Because culture has profound effects on our attitudes and on the ways in which we communicate and perceive others, this chapter addresses issues of cultural diversity before discussing the communication process. When cultural differences are not recognized and respected, relationships suffer and communication is much less effective. Until quite recently, much of the direct health care in the United States was administered by providers of Anglo-European descent.

There was little sensitivity to the importance of differences between cultures. Now businesses and industries, especially the health care industry, have begun to appreciate the advantages of cultural diversity in the workforce and of cultural awareness in providing the best possible service to clients.

ISSUES OF CULTURAL DIVERSITY

Our grandparents' generation was raised in communities that might be described as culturally homogeneous. The culture of the majority prevailed, and those who were "different" were expected to "fit in." This was especially true in rural areas and small towns. In cities, immigrants gathered into neighborhoods where their own languages and cultures prevailed and did their best to conform to the majority culture in the workplace. American society today, both urban and rural, is far more culturally diverse than in our grandparents' day. While this diversity poses certain social problems, it also creates a vast richness and creative potential.

The Scope of Diversity

The subject of ethnic and cultural diversity is complex and fills numerous textbooks. It is impossible within the scope of this book to anticipate the many diverse ethnic and cultural situations you will encounter as a radiographer. We hope that the limited examples in the discussion that follows will help to raise your awareness of those situations in which sensitivity is needed. The racial and **ethnic** (national) characteristics of individuals originally were identified with specific areas of the globe. Africans came from Africa, Chinese from China, and so forth. In many cases, racial characteristics such as skin color, hair texture, and the shapes of facial features were identified with specific cultures as well as with ethnic origins. As opportunities for emigration and travel increased, it became more difficult to identify the national origin of a specific individual. For example, not all patients with Asian features speak an Asian language.

Culture is determined by language and by the customs commonly observed. It can be misleading to generalize about the cultural attitudes and practices of any ethnic group, since individual variations within a group depend on so many factors. In addition, the physical appearance of an individual may have no relationship to how extensively he or she has integrated culturally into the mainstream of American life. A person who has recently arrived from Eastern Europe wearing the latest athletic shoes, a baseball cap, and blue jeans may speak little or no English, while a patient wearing a turban or a dashiki may have been born in Chicago of ancestors who have lived there for generations.

The relationship between culture and communication is an integral part of our everyday life. Our reactions and habits are learned from our parents, are passed down to our children, and largely govern the way we conduct our daily activities. Each society develops unwritten rules regarding such ordinary things as how close we stand when talking to another, where we touch another person in public, and other reflections of courtesy to those around us. For example, it is important in many Asian societies to avoid placing another person in an embarrassing position. Harmony is to be promoted, and loud or aggressive behavior is considered a sign of poor manners. Such patients may respond more positively to a soft, quiet tone of voice than to the brisk, assertive commands so easily adopted by many Americans when in a hurry. When apprehensive or nervous, Asian patients may become reticent and unsociable, which can hinder effective communication. The cultural differences in nonverbal behaviors are also highly significant. For example, a Vietnamese patient may smile to cover up disturbed feelings. Repeated head nods may indicate respect for the individual speaking rather than agreement with the subject being discussed.

The best way to understand people of another culture is to learn to know them personally. If your geographical area has a significant number of individuals from another culture, you can enrich your life and provide better care by learning as much as possible about ethnic groups with which you come in frequent contact. We hope that this discussion will heighten your awareness, not only of differences in ethnic backgrounds, but also of diversity within your own cultural group. The more sensitive you become to the reactions of all your patients, the more comfortable your interpersonal contacts will be.

When cultural diversity is mentioned, customs relating to nationality may be the first things that come to mind. Our society consists of many different groups in addition to ethnic groups, however, and each has unique characteristics that can affect the values and perceptions of individuals within the group. Historically, certain groups have been subjected to discriminatory treatment, causing some individuals to have a high level of sensitivity about their group identity. Examples of such cultural groups include the following:

- Gender groups: male/female
- Racial groups: distinguished by skin color and other physical characteristics
- Generational groups: the very young, generation X, baby boomers, and the elderly
- Geographic groups: North/South; East Coast/West Coast; native cultures in Hawaii, Alaska, and on and around reservations, plus areas where ethnic culture endures because large numbers of immigrants from a certain country have settled there (Mexican influences along the southern borders of Texas and California, and Scandinavian heritage in Minnesota, for example)
- Sexual preference groups: heterosexual, gay, lesbian, bisexual, and transgender
- Religious groups
- Groups based on nonracial physical characteristics: the blind, the deaf, the disabled, the obese
- Socioeconomic groups: low income (unemployed, welfare recipients, uninsured, underinsured), middle income, affluent
- Groups with various types of family structure: singles, unmarried couples with and without children, traditional nuclear families, single mother/single father heads of households, parents with children and grandchildren, and large, close-knit extended families

Culturally Significant Attitudes Toward Health Care

This section provides some examples of how various cultural groups approach health care and how their cultural status may affect the outcome. Although this discussion is limited in scope, it should help to increase your awareness of the diversity of needs, expectations, and fears that may influence your patients in the health care setting.

Some ethnic cultures have a high level of sensitivity surrounding modesty and physical contact in health care. This may apply to any situation but is most often an issue when the patient and the health care provider are not of the same gender, especially if the patient is female and the health care professional is male. These attitudes are particularly prevalent in both Hispanic and Islamic cultures, but are certainly not limited to these groups.

Research shows that women perceive health care more favorably than men do. In general, women are better informed about health care issues and more willing to talk about their health problems. Since men are less aware of health issues, they may fail to seek health care promptly when needed, hoping to avoid confronting that which they do not understand. They may perceive the need for treatment as a sign of weakness or vulnerability. Touching while providing health care is also perceived more positively by women than by men. Women find it reassuring and comforting, while men find personal touch less positive.

Our elders can remember lives lost to infections, polio, whooping cough, and diphtheria, before the days of antibiotics and vaccines. Having observed these advances in medicine, the majority of those over age 75 came to think of medicine as miraculous and doctors as all-powerful. This generation has faith in the medical establishment and is unlikely to question the need for any test, prescription, or intervention that doctors may recommend. On the other hand, members of the baby boom generation were at a formative stage in the late 1960s or in the 1970s. One of the catch phrases of that time was, "Don't trust anyone over thirty!" This attitude is reflected in a more conservative and questioning approach to the medical establishment. Generation X has taken this approach even farther, as demonstrated by an increased willingness to seek alternative health care options.

Geographic differences in population size also affect health care. The availability of sophisticated health care services in cities has generally resulted in a higher level of expectation in urban areas. Even those in lower socioeconomic strata are likely to receive adequate health care through publicly funded facilities. In a rural setting, on the other hand, patients are less likely to have access to subsidized health care. In addition, the limited selection of available services and the constraints of distance often limit options and contribute to health care problems. Consider the plight of a middle-aged woman with rheumatoid arthritis who lives on a remote ranch. The nearest rheumatologist may be many miles away, and traveling to visit this specialist will be time-consuming, costly, and painful.

While it cannot be said that there is universal tolerance for gay, lesbian, bisexual, and transgender groups, there is more public discussion and acceptance today than was apparent during the twentieth century. Patients who do not conform to a heterosexual way of life need to feel confident that disclosing their sexual preference will not compromise their health care or their insurability.

Some religious groups dictate or prohibit specific health care practices. For example, some religions do not condone blood transfusions, some prohibit any practice that punctures the skin, and others oppose the practice of vaccination. Prayer and other religious healing practices may need to be accommodated in combination with medical treatments. Religious dietary requirements, such as kosher meals for orthodox Jews, may affect a patient's choice of medical facilities and may affect compliance with the medical **regimen** (system designed to provide benefit).

For patients with physical disabilities or with conditions such as sexually transmitted diseases or obesity, the major deterrent in seeking health care may have little to do with their condition, but may be powerfully influenced by the attitudes of insensitive health care providers. The young woman with cerebral palsy who is frowned on when seeking birth control, the deaf patient who feels ignored, the acquired immunodeficiency syndrome (AIDS) patient who is shunned, and the obese patient who is scolded rather than advised—all feel diminished and are likely to develop negative attitudes toward health care providers.

Inability to pay for health insurance prevents many people of lower socioeconomic status from planning and implementing a health care program. Even when these patients have access to a physician, they may be unable to purchase the prescriptions, foods, or medical supplies that are prescribed. Low-income employees often have less flexibility in their work schedules, so the ability to keep health care appointments may be affected by the need to keep a job. Limited financial resources may also prompt a patient to work when it would be a better health decision to take time off for rest and healing.

Until fairly recently, the term "family" referred to father, mother, and children. Grandparents, aunts, or uncles were sometimes also included. The dictionary now defines a family as "a group of individuals residing under one roof." As divorce has become more common, many single parents have been forced to cope alone with a multitude of parental responsibilities. Teaching children good health habits may fade under the pressures of work, laundry, shopping, and child care. Single parents may neglect their own health because of time and financial constraints. Homosexual families and families in which grandparents are primary providers are among the nontraditional families that you are likely to encounter as they seek health care for themselves and for dependent children.

Professional Responsibility and Ethics in Relation to Diversity

You will recall from Chapter 2 that issues of cultural diversity have significant ethical dimensions. The American Society of Radiologic Technologists Code of Ethics requires radiographers to put aside all personal prejudice and emotional bias, rendering services to humanity with full respect for the dignity of mankind. Specifically, they are to conduct themselves in a professional manner, support their colleagues and associates, respond to patient needs, and deliver patient care and service unrestricted by concerns of personal attributes or the nature of the disease or illness and without discrimination on the basis of sex, race, creed, religion, or socioeconomic status.

According to Kohlberg's theory (see Chapter 2), the development of these high moral and ethical standards does not come naturally to most people and is unlikely to be attained by simply reading a code of ethics or a chapter in this or any textbook. It is a process that begins with a commitment and continues with each encounter that presents an opportunity to listen, reflect, and learn. We must open our minds to the possibility that our own perceptions are not universal and that the differing perceptions and values of others have validity and importance.

COMMUNICATION SKILLS
Nonverbal Communication

Although we perceive verbal language as our primary means of communication, nonverbal behaviors reveal a great deal about how we feel. How nonverbal communication is interpreted is largely based on cultural background. Most of us learn to respond to common cues in childhood. We perceive frowns or pursed lips as disapproval. Refusal to look directly into an individual's face while speaking conveys avoidance, submission, or rejection, while clenched teeth or fists suggest angry feelings under rigid control. Patients in pain may present a tight and rigid protective posture. Leaning forward while listening to another gives the appearance of intense interest in the subject being discussed. What other nonverbal behaviors do you commonly see around you (Fig. 3-1)?

Eye contact

In the United States, eye contact is considered a positive behavior. Making direct eye contact with an individual while speaking is usually perceived as an expression of interest, concern, or honesty. Many Asian societies, however, use no eye contact during verbal communication and may resent direct eye contact, if perceiving as being impolite and an invasion of personal space. In countries with a high-density population, eye contact and touch are less acceptable among adults than in the United States.

Many Native Americans avoid direct eye contact, considering it a mark of disrespect. Pointing directly at an individual can also be considered insulting.

An old superstition of Mediterranean origin is occasionally seen among Hispanic clients. The "evil eye" or *mal ojo* is thought to bring bad luck or illness

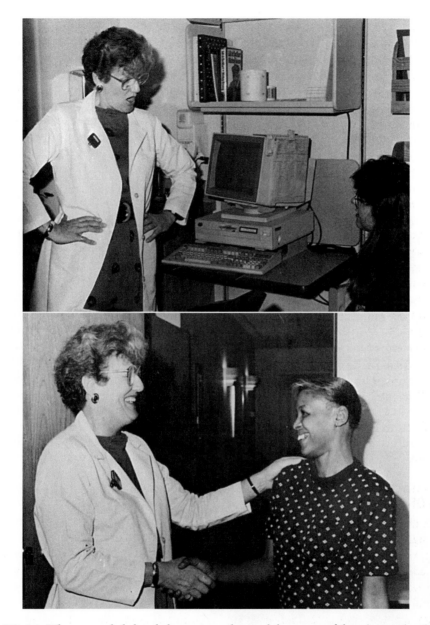

FIG. 3-1 What nonverbal clues help you to understand the nature of these interactions?

if children are praised or admired without also being touched. Eye contact with adults is perfectly acceptable, but when praising a child, it is wise to give a touch or pat while expressing admiration. While the parents may no longer express belief in the "evil eye," the ability of individuals to cause illness in a child by looking admiringly without touching is a very strong superstition.

Touching

Touch is a means of communication too. An abrupt or tentative touch may be perceived as distaste or reluctance to care for the individual. A positive touch is firm but gentle (Fig. 3-2) and reassures the patient that you are both capable and caring. People touch one another for a variety of reasons, for example:

- To provide reassurance, support, encouragement
- To imply domination, anger, frustration
- To form a positive connection, as in a handshake or shoulder pat
- To perform professional services, such as those provided by a doctor, hairdresser, or masseuse

The brief hug around the shoulder that is so reassuring to many Americans may be an upsetting invasion of personal space and privacy to those whose culture does not include a casual embrace. In Hispanic culture, for example, embracing, touching, and close proximity are easily accepted from familiar people. This may seem to contrast with a strong sense of modesty that can be demonstrated during physical examinations, so it is important to provide both men and women with ample gowns and covering during examinations in the imaging department. To Native Americans, personal space is very important, and while patients may embrace or touch others with whom they feel close, touching should be confined to that needed to provide health care. In some cultures and religions, touch by a stranger or a member of the opposite sex is unacceptable or strongly frowned upon.

When you must touch a patient, you are much less likely to unintentionally offend if you tell the patient in advance what you are about to do and then use a firm, appropriate touch. It is important that your touch have a professional purpose that is clear to the patient. As discussed in Chapter 2, touch is never forced on a patient.

Appearance

Patients tend to place their confidence in health care workers to the degree that they feel their expectations of a professional person are being met. Everyone we meet forms an impression of us from our appearance, and whether we realize it or not, appearance is another way we communicate how we feel about our work and our patients. What does your appearance tell patients about you? Uniforms are intended to present a simple, neat appearance and are washable and plain to make them easy to keep clean. They should fit comfortably and be worn with simple, appropriate accessories. Although fads and fashions change over time, a professional image will continue to be conservative.

The appearance of the examining room is equally important. An untidy, cluttered room is difficult to keep clean, and it shows a lack of respect for patients. It sends a nonverbal message that personnel may be too pressured or too uncaring to answer questions or provide reassurance (Fig. 3-3).

Listening Skills

How do you feel when you are interrupted, or when the listener looks out the window while you attempt to make your point? Are you irritated when others "put words in your mouth" or change the subject without responding to what you have just said? Good communication is a two-way street, and a good listener does more than await his or her turn

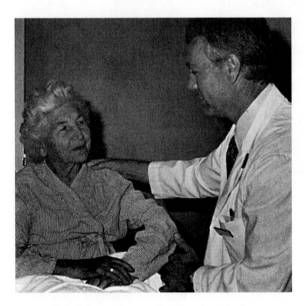

FIG. 3-2 Positive touch is firm but gentle.

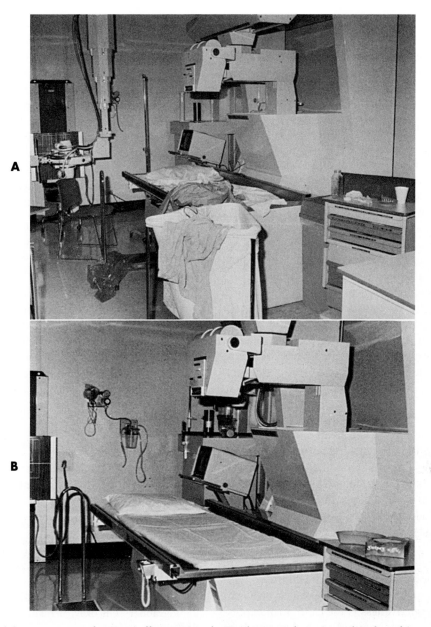

FIG. 3-3 Appearance of a room affects patients' attitudes toward care. **A,** What does this room communicate to you? **B,** A clean room inspires confidence.

to speak. Listening skill involves the ability to give full attention to the speaker. When you focus on the speaker, you can respond to what has been said rather than making a quick switch to the next item on your mental list. In conversation, patients often give us clues about a physical problem that could be easily missed if we rush to get to the next question. This approach may seem impractical in a busy imaging department, but it can become automatic with practice. Don't you have more confidence in people who really listen to what you have to say?

Verbal Skills

Clear, distinct speech habits are always preferable, regardless of the communication circumstances. Being a good communicator also implies the ability to use language and content appropriate to your listener. This is not meant to be patronizing or demeaning. After all, you would explain a procedure quite differently to a retired nurse than to a certified public accountant with little knowledge of anatomy. Use good eye contact, and make it a habit to speak face to face. This encourages others to feel that they have your full attention and concern. Be alert to the way your listener responds to your communication, and try to modify your approach if it does not seem to elicit the desired result. Cultural and individual expectations of social and health care interactions may affect the way you are perceived. These variations are discussed earlier in this chapter.

Attitude

Our attitudes are revealed by our nonverbal behaviors and also by our tone of voice and choice of words. Listeners receive more powerful messages from our attitudes than from what we actually say. Consider the difference between the following statements. The content is similar, but the message is very different:

"No! Don't do it that way!"

"Look, Martha, I think this way might work better."

Assertiveness can be a valuable strategy in communication and should not be confused with aggression. **Aggressiveness** involves anger or hostility, whereas **assertiveness** is the calm, firm expression of feelings or opinions. As a student you have the right to be assertive when you require assistance in a patient care situation that is beyond your ability. Employers may be assertive when requiring employees to meet the requirements outlined in their job descriptions. When dealing with uncooperative patients, pleasant assertiveness is the most effective attitude.

Validation of communication

Another important aspect of good communication is to validate whether you have been understood. An informal response such as a smile, nod, or brief "okay" may be a satisfactory acknowledgment in a social situation, but when essential information is being presented, the response must be one that reflects clear understanding. This is particularly true with all instructions that involve your professional activities. As a listener, you can be sure that you have understood the message by reflecting the elements of the speaker's statement in your response:

Radiologist: "Give Mrs. Johnson 50 ml of Isovue 300, and take the first film at 60 seconds."
Radiographer: "Mrs. Johnson gets 50 ml of Isovue 300, and I'll take the first film at 60 seconds."
Radiologist: "Right."

In the communication above, the speaker's instruction is complete. The listener's response reflects complete understanding, and the instructions are validated.

When the speaker receives an incomplete response, the situation changes:

Radiologist: "Give Mrs. Kirkland 50 ml Isovue 100, and take the first film at 3 minutes."
Radiographer: "Okay." (Turns to leave.)

At this point the speaker cannot be certain of having been understood, so the conversation must be continued:

Radiologist: "Wait. Tell me what you're going to do."
Radiographer: "I'll give Mrs. Kirkland 50 ml of Isovue and take the first film at 3 minutes."
Radiologist: "What strength Isovue?"
Radiographer: "Isovue 300."
Radiologist: "No. Isovue 100 this time."
Radiographer: "Oh, okay; 50 ml of Isovue 100."
Radiologist: "Right."

When presented with an incomplete message, the listener's responsibility is to obtain clarification:

Radiologist: "Give her 50 ml of Isovue."
Radiographer: "That's 50 ml of Isovue 300 for Mrs. Kirkland and the first film at 60 seconds, as usual?"
Radiologist: "Right."

If the listener's assumption was incorrect, the speaker must then state the intended message more accurately:

Radiologist: "No, no. Mrs. Kirkland should have 50 ml of Isovue 100 because of her decreased renal function, then start the filming at 3 minutes for the same reason."
Radiographer: "Okay; 50 ml of Isovue 100 and film at 3 minutes."
Radiologist: "Right."

When the speaker did not provide some essential information, both parties might have assumed that they were referring to the same patient and that the usual dose of Isovue and routine time would be used for the examination. When these points are not clear, the potential for error is greater. The lesson for both speakers and listeners is that messages must be clear and complete and that understanding must be validated or confirmed. Without validation, neither party can be certain that all elements of the message have been understood.

Communication Under Stress

Any situation that disturbs our everyday activities imposes stress. The hospital environment often proves stressful to patients and families, as well as to the health care workers responsible for their care. This is especially true in crisis situations when speed is a factor or when a complex situation causes disagreement about priorities.

Stress interferes with our ability to process information accurately and appropriately. We have all read newspaper accounts about victims of a house fire who fled with an object close at hand, such as a rubber plant, rather than important papers or treasured family possessions. In a stressful situation, accurate communication can be difficult. The principles of communication already discussed are always important, but these additional suggestions can improve your effectiveness in a crisis situation:

- Lower your voice, and speak slowly and clearly when a situation is very emotional.
- Be nonjudgmental in both verbal and nonverbal communication.

- Do not allow an upset individual's inappropriate actions or speech to goad you into a similar response.
- When you are uncertain whether the listener has understood you, request an answer. For example, "Did you read the consent form? What did it say?"

Extremely stressful situations may evoke hostile or even violent responses. If you express distaste or hostility, this can escalate the level of tension. Occasionally a patient who is recovering consciousness will become combative, or an elderly patient who is disoriented may threaten violent action. Most potentially violent situations occur in the emergency department. Hostile individuals, such as an inebriated patient involved in a motor vehicle accident or a group brought in following an unresolved gang fight, can be very threatening. The essential points to remember in such situations are the following:

- Do not attempt to handle the situation alone. Get help before the problem escalates, and leave the room if physical violence is threatened.
- Be pleasantly firm while explaining that your role is to provide health care only.
- Never let a combative individual get between you and the door.
- Review such situations with your supervisor and coworkers, and learn how to handle threatening events before they arise.

COMMUNICATION WITH PATIENTS
Addressing the Patient

The first contact with a patient is usually an introduction. In many social situations today, given names are used as soon as introductions are made. Although this may seem to project an air of friendliness and informality, it also poses certain problems. For many people, the stress of hospitalization is reflected in a strong feeling of helplessness or loss of **autonomy** (self-determination). Patients are told where and when to lie down, what to eat, when to take medications, and so on. This, in combination with anxiety over the need to seek treatment and the inability to comprehend much of the hospital jargon, magnifies the individual's need to maintain a sense of identity.

"Good morning, Mr. Torres. I'm Lynn Smith, the radiographer," is more than an example of good manners. It shows respect and concern and allows the patient to choose how he or she wishes to be addressed. In an effort to show friendliness, some staff may address adults as "honey" or "sweetie" instead of calling them by name. Others, who are focused on the work routine, may refer to "the gallbladder in room 2" or "that barium enema in the hall." Talking down to adults or treating them impersonally diminishes their self-esteem and raises feelings of resentment. Such feelings diminish patients' ability to understand and follow directions, prevent retention of information, and may hinder recovery.

Valid Choices

Another way to minimize these problems is to involve patients in their own care by giving them opportunities to make choices. Avoid the false sort of choice expressed by such statements as, "Would you like to come down for your x-ray now?" When the patient is scheduled for 10 AM, little choice is involved. **Valid choices** are alternatives, all of which are acceptable to you. Valid choices require a little more thought, but the rewards in terms of patient satisfaction are well worth the effort. Effective valid choices may be very simple. Questions such as, "Would you like a blanket over your knees?" and "Would you prefer to sit where you can see down the hall or over by the window?" reassure the patient who would like to feel capable of making decisions and having a share in his or her own care. Treating patients as individuals, allowing them to make valid choices, and using good nonverbal communication can help to alleviate fear while encouraging cooperation and self-care on the part of our patients.

Avoiding Assumptions

In determining why patients fail to follow instructions, a factor frequently encountered is the assumption that the patient has understood the procedure. To make an assumption is to make a guess. For example, we could assume that since you are reading this text, you are a student in a radiologic technology program. This may be true, or you may be an instructor, a nurse, or the proofreader for this book. Making assumptions about patients implies that you might also guess about their physical status and abilities, as well as their willingness to cooperate. Can you assume that Mr. White, who may have broken his ankle, can be positioned flat on the radiographic table? No. He may also have emphysema, which would interfere with his ability to breathe in a supine position.

Avoiding assumptions becomes critical when **ambulatory** patients (those capable of walking) come in for procedures that demand advance preparation. If, for example, Ms. Elwood is scheduled for a barium enema examination, an inquiry such as, "Did you follow the prep?" may not be a very effective way to find out what Ms. Elwood actually did. It implies that she was given a preparation kit, received clear instructions, and was able to comply. If you rephrase the question and ask her to explain exactly how she complied with the preparation instructions, you will get a more complete picture of how well she was able to cooperate. Reviewing the printed instructions with the patient may be helpful.

Assessment

Conversing with patients allows you to use your powers of observation. Is the patient alert or confused? How well does the patient hear? Is English comprehension a problem? From observation, you can often make a tentative assessment of the patient's ability to get on and off the examination table, walk unassisted to the bathroom, and so forth. In Chapter 6 we discuss patient assessment in depth, but you should learn from this chapter that good communication with patients can help you establish a spirit of trust and cooperation that will assist in patient care.

Older Adults

In this country, the health care field continues to be challenged by the increasing age of our population. Older patients may require special attention because of the many physical problems that often accompany aging. The visual and hearing problems discussed later in this chapter may have direct application to many of these patients. Good lighting and checking to ensure the patient has glasses or a hearing aid available will help both of you feel more comfortable. A typical attribute of aging is a tendency to proceed at one's own pace, both mentally and physically. Most older patients do not respond well to feeling pushed or hurried.

Occasionally, you will see older people who have lost varying degrees of the ability to understand why they find themselves in unfamiliar surroundings. This may be caused by Alzheimer's disease or organic brain syndrome or may occur as a direct result of medication, illness, or injury. Older patients who appear confused respond best to familiar situations. In these cases especially, use an individual's full name. During conversation, it helps to ask where the person was born, whether from a large family, and other questions about the past. Distant memory is often quite clear to those who cannot remember what was served for breakfast. Keep instructions simple, and give them one at a time. Using valid choices and treating older patients with the respect due any adult helps them maintain their sense of identity. We emphasize that relatively few older patients have these conditions, and it is important to evaluate the needs and abilities of each older patient on an individual basis.

Children and Adolescents

The fear and lack of comprehension that we often see in adults can be greatly magnified in children. Small children, who may have difficulty expressing themselves, respond to a friendly smile and a consistently firm, gentle, and reassuring touch. Try to find out what the child is called at home, and use the familiar name. If you are calm, cheerful, and unhurried, the child is much less likely to respond negatively to the strange surroundings and machines. Allowing the small child to take a favorite blanket or toy to the radiology department may help promote a feeling of security (Fig. 3-4). Talk to small children. Even if they do not understand all you say, a cheerful voice is reassuring. Strange adults are often intimidating to children because of their stature, so try to speak to children at their own eye level. You will find that this is very effective, especially when you

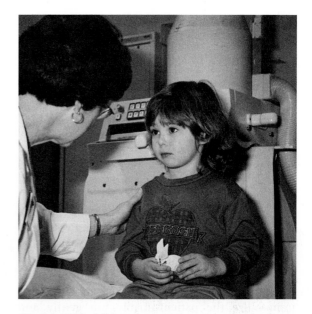

FIG. 3-4 With children, keep explanations simple, direct, and honest.

approach the child to "make friends" before entering the x-ray room.

Children over the age of 4 or 5 years require somewhat different approaches to communication. They are able to share information with you and cooperate more fully, but they also fear a loss of self-control and need to make valid choices even more than do adults. "Would you like to climb up on the table by yourself, or would you like me to help you?" is an example. Although children have no choice about submitting to the examination, they should be encouraged to cooperate as much as possible. Apprehensive children are not reassured by such statements as, "This won't hurt a bit." All too frequently the only word they assimilate is "hurt," and they become even more frightened. "Have you ever had your picture taken by x-ray?" allows you to add whatever simple explanation is necessary. "We're going to take a picture of your leg with this special big camera" is understandable to most children. Since children love to imitate adult behaviors, a demonstration is often more effective than verbal instruction. Show the child how to position the hand for a finger examination or how to hold a deep breath for a chest radiograph. If questions are asked, try to answer them simply. Never force information on children, since they may become more apprehensive if they do not understand everything that is said. It is better to treat the entire procedure in a matter-of-fact manner. Keep directions and explanations simple, direct, and honest. "We need to take five or six pictures, Johnny. We'll be as fast as we can."

How do you cope with the child who appears determined to be disruptive or refuses to follow directions? You set limits in clear terms, saying, "You must lie still," or "You may not get down." Above all, use praise for any attempt to cooperate. If after a patient and reasonable attempt the child continues to resist the examination, you should assume that cooperation is not possible. Do not hesitate to ask for more experienced help in dealing with a difficult situation. If the policy of your institution permits, immobilize the patient firmly but gently and complete the examination as quickly as you can. (See Chapter 4 for immobilization techniques.)

Remember that muscular activity is a natural response to anxiety in a small child. When the situation seems unbearable, kicking and squirming are quite normal. Crying also is normal for a frightened child. An order to stop crying only increases the anxiety, and trying to raise your voice over a child's screams is almost never effective. Sometimes, however, a whisper will capture a distressed child's curiosity and attention.

Special sensitivity is also required to deal with the emotional needs of younger adolescents (Fig. 3-5). Although they may act quite adult under normal circumstances, they become frightened and confused and may revert to childlike behavior when ill or in stressful situations. At this age, modesty and privacy are of paramount importance and x-rays may be feared as the "all-seeing eye," ready to unveil the patient's innermost secrets.

A professional approach, coupled with warm reassurance, promotes a more positive attitude in both children and adolescents. Many of the poor attitudes toward health care displayed by adults can be traced to a lack of sensitivity in the care given by health professionals during their formative years.

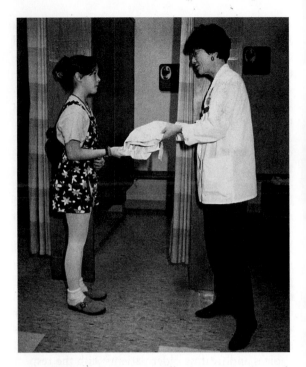

FIG. 3-5 Modesty is especially important in early adolescence.

SPECIAL CIRCUMSTANCES IN COMMUNICATIONS
Patients Who Do Not Speak English

Language barriers are not handled very effectively in the United States. Recent federal legislation has addressed the patient's right to communicate effectively in health care situations, regardless of language barriers. Most large hospitals now have a service that will arrange for an interpreter when necessary. In areas where languages other than English are typically used, the admitting and emergency areas must post signs in the most common languages advising patients of the availability of interpreters. In many cases, certified interpreters are "on call" and come immediately when needed. When a large percentage of the population speaks a single foreign language, full-time interpreters may be part of the hospital staff. If an outpatient procedure is scheduled in advance, an interpreter may be scheduled at the same time.

The difference between a certified interpreter and a friend or family member who assumes this role may be significant. The interpreter is trained to translate only what has been said, both by the patient and to the patient, and not to explain what is implied. Family and friends may tend to add extraneous information or to edit the conversation in an effort to be cooperative or to save time. For example, a complete explanation of positioning and breathing instructions may be abbreviated in translation to, "It's okay, Mama. Just hold still." Family members may hesitate to reveal information about the patient that they believe is private or embarrassing, and the patient may hesitate to reveal personal information through family or friends. Family members whose command of English is limited may have good intentions but may be unable to provide adequate translation of complex information.

The services of a trained interpreter provide a professional bridge in difficult communication situations. Certified interpreters must be used when:

- Obtaining the patient's medical history
- Obtaining informed consent or permission for treatment
- Giving a diagnosis
- The patient is conscious during treatment or surgery
- Confronting an emergency
- Explaining medication instructions, side effects, and dosages
- Physicians or medical staff are giving instructions
- The patient is being discharged

Your duty may be to arrange for an interpreter when appropriate, even though a "family translator" may be present. While this may result in a delay of routine procedures, the benefits may outweigh the disruption of your schedule. With professional translation, interpersonal relationships will not interfere, and the parties to the conversation can be certain that the translations are accurate. The interpreter will explain to the patient that all information is confidential and that interpretation is a part of the medical service that is provided at no charge.

When using an interpreter, look directly at the patient and speak as though the patient were able to understand you. The interpreter will translate as you speak or as soon as you have finished a sentence. Speaking to the interpreter directly tends to make the patient feel left out or talked about rather than involved in the process.

Telephone translation services are available, including unusual languages and obscure dialects. One such service called "Language Line" is provided by AT&T. Telephone translation is usually most efficient when a conference call format is used, but translators are patient if the telephone must be transferred from client to health care worker in the course of the conversation. If your hospital subscribes to a translation service, you will receive specific instructions about its use. This method may be very effective for obtaining a medical history or informed consent when translation is otherwise not available.

One hospital emergency department near a seaport maintains a file in six languages with phrases such as, "Please hold your breath," "Point to where it hurts," and other statements or questions that may be helpful in a health care setting. If a translator is unavailable, use demonstrations or pencil sketches to validate whether the individual understands, and make extensive use of nonverbal encouragement. A friendly smile and a warm touch may be worth many words. Appendix C provides a list of Spanish phrases with guides for pronunciation that may help you to greet Spanish-speaking patients and assist them in situations where only the simplest communication is required. Be cautious, however, about communicating in the patient's language if your language skills are limited. Even though you can express simple ideas clearly, you may be unable to interpret patient responses accurately. After all, even when we speak the same language, we don't always mean the same thing. In England, when a young lady is shopping for new "pants," she will be in the underwear section. If you ask, "Where can I find a lift?" while in London, you will be directed to the elevator, not to the cabstand. Since misunderstandings are common, even without a language barrier, it is especially important to clarify and validate instructions when our patients speak limited English.

The Hearing Impaired

In the past, many health care providers have treated deaf patients and those with some hearing loss essentially the same. In reality, the problems of communication are very different. Patients with a hearing loss may display levels of impairment that vary from the need to use a high-intensity hearing aid to only a mild difficulty hearing voices in a high or low register.

Certain rules are helpful in communicating with individuals who have hearing loss:

- Talk to, not about, these persons.
- Get the patient's attention before starting to speak.
- Face the person, preferably with light on your face.
- Hearing loss is frequently in the upper register, so speak lower as well as louder.
- Speak clearly and at a moderate pace. Do not shout.
- Avoid noisy background situations.
- Rephrase when you are not understood.
- Be patient.

When in doubt, ask the person for suggestions to improve communication. Avoid potential misunderstandings by using open-ended questions and asking patients to repeat instructions. Allow the patient who wears a hearing aid to retain it as long as possible, and give all instructions before the aid is placed in a safe location. Since visual clues become much more essential when hearing is impaired, try not to remove the patient's glasses until necessary.

Deafness

The deaf patient presents a challenge unlike that of one with a hearing loss. Many totally deaf individuals live in a cultural setting that has its own social structure, language, and even "inside" jokes. Certain cues help in differentiating between the patient with a hearing loss and the deaf patient, especially in an emergency. You may become aware that a seemingly alert patient is totally deaf when he or she:

- Does not respond to noises or words spoken out of the range of vision
- Uses lip movements without making a sound or speaks in a flat monotone
- Points to the ears and mouth while shaking the head in a negative motion
- Uses gestures or writing motions to express the need for paper and pencil

Some deaf people are adept at lip reading and are able to speak, at least to a limited degree. More often the deaf are educated in American Sign Language (ASL), which is the most common sign language. It is distinctly different from English and has unique grammar, syntax, and rules. Learning a few basic signs may aid in establishing rapport with deaf patients. A card showing the alphabet and some common useful signs in ASL should be available through your nursing service department.

As with patients who do not speak English, a certified interpreter is essential in any situation that requires complex instruction or an exchange of important information. Interpreters for deaf clients use the same ethical guidelines as foreign language translators, and the process of interpretation is essentially the same for all involved. Friends and relatives of a deaf patient should not ordinarily be used to interpret medical or treatment information, since they may add their own interpretation to the translation, changing its meaning. This could also compromise patient confidentiality and may cause the patient to delete or edit information that could have a direct bearing on diagnosis and treatment.

When a totally deaf patient is admitted for care, the chart should be flagged with this information. The deaf person has the right to request a specific interpreter, if available, and to have an interpreter replaced if communication is not proceeding well. Patients also have the right to choose the most preferred method of communication, which might be pencil and paper. Be sure that writing materials are available and that the patient's writing arm is free.

The medical setting can seem especially overwhelming to a deaf child. If possible, allow the child and parents to tour the area before the examination begins. Take time to fully explain the procedures and activities to the parents so they can help the child understand what to expect. If the child is distressed, you might consider allowing a parent to stay in sight or near the child, while following radiation safety precautions.

Impaired Vision

Most of us depend greatly on our eyes to sense our surroundings and ensure our safety as we move about. Vision enables us to recognize individuals and perform the activities of daily living. The ability of blind persons to accomplish these same tasks without vision can seem astounding. They rely on hearing, touch, and memory to a much greater extent than sighted persons. With the aid of a cane or guide dog, many blind persons lead very independent lives. Having learned to work outside the home, use public transportation, and maintain their own households, these patients may be insulted by attitudes that are too solicitous. On the other hand, they may welcome some special help in a strange environment. Some patients prefer to follow you by listening to your footsteps and using a cane, while others may wish to place a hand on your shoulder or elbow. Those who are more infirm may prefer your arm around their waist while you reassure and direct them verbally. None of these approaches applies to all blind persons. Good communication is the key to determining which form of help is acceptable and appropriate.

The person with recently failing vision and good hearing may need much verbal explanation and reassurance. Other visually impaired individuals are quite capable of proceeding confidently after a quick description of a room and the obstacles in it. You might say, "This is a square room, Mrs. Daley. The x-ray table is about 5 feet in front of you and a chair is at 7 o'clock. After you're on the table, I'll be in a booth to your left."

Patients with failing vision often see better in bright light. They may be able to recognize faces, but you should offer to read written material to them without waiting for a request for assistance.

Inability to Speak

Aphasia is defined as a defect or loss of language function in which comprehension or expression of words is impaired as a result of injury to language centers in the brain. Brain lesions large enough to damage language function will often produce multiple effects. The stroke patient who is unable to speak may also be unable to write. For this reason it is often helpful to ask the nursing staff how they have been able to communicate with the patient. Some patients are able to write. Many can indicate by a nod or shake of the head whether they understand your directions.

Many patients who have suffered the loss of speech due to throat cancer or an accident may choose to communicate using one of several different types of artificial speech. For some time, a handheld **electrolarynx** has been available. This device is placed on the external throat wall and operates by vibrations transmitted through the wall of the neck. While this certainly is an aid to communication, it has an extremely metallic tone and is not always easy to understand. Esophageal speech, in which the patient swallows air and then regurgitates it, is easily understandable but is low in volume and requires extensive practice as well as a fair amount of physical effort. Patients with aphasia may now take advantage of recent advances in artificial speech aids involving transesophageal puncture (TEP), in which a prosthesis is placed within the neck through a stoma. There are several variations. One is a semipermanent installation in which the prosthetic device remains within the stoma and is cleaned in place by the patient. Another is a removable aid that is inserted and removed by the patient for cleaning and maintenance. TEP devices also operate on a vibratory principle but are more easily understood than the external handheld electrolarynx.

Remember that the loss of the ability to see, hear, or speak is a communication impairment and not a reflection of the individual's ability to think. Patients with sensory deprivation or impaired ability to communicate challenge us to be more flexible and innovative in the ways we offer explanations, reassurance, and care.

Impaired Mental Function

Special sensitivity is needed when dealing with adult patients who are mentally or emotionally handicapped. Such patients may include those with congenital defects such as trisomy 21 (Down's syndrome), accident victims, those with illnesses affecting the brain, and those with severe emotional disorders that affect comprehension. As with children, you must assess the patient's ability to understand and follow instructions, since this ability may vary from a near infantile response to a functional capability close to normal. In general, the same clear, simple, and direct instructions offered to children are appropriate. You may need to repeat instructions if the attention span is short. It is not appropriate to talk to these patients as if they were toddlers. Use the adult form of address, and treat them with the respect and dignity due anyone their age.

Altered States of Consciousness

Another challenge to communication may arise with patients who have an altered state of consciousness. This change in the ability to respond, react, and cooperate may result from injury, illness, drugs, or medication. The impairment may range from a state of drowsiness, in which the individual can cooperate when aroused, to total unconsciousness. You must remember two points in communicating with patients who are drowsy or stuporous:

- They cannot be relied upon to remember instructions.
- They are not responsible for their actions or answers.

The individual who has loss of consciousness may seem to respond appropriately when regaining consciousness but may also attempt to sit up and get down from the table. Any patient with decreased level of consciousness (LOC) must be kept under close observation.

An important factor frequently overlooked in hospitals is the ability of many patients to hear and remember conversations that occurred while they were apparently unconscious. Patients who are unconscious because of anesthesia, trauma, or illness may be completely unable to respond while still retaining the ability to hear and remember what is said. A safe rule to follow is not to make any statements within hearing range of unconscious patients that you would not make if they were conscious. As a corollary to this, it is important to refer to unconscious patients by name and to reassure them about your actions. Medical literature gives many examples of patients who have regained consciousness after

prolonged periods and who have credited their recovery to health professionals who continued to call them by name and treat them as human beings with an identity uniquely their own.

PATIENT EDUCATION

Radiographers have a great deal of knowledge about health promotion and the treatment and diagnosis of disease. In the best of all worlds, this information would be directly applicable to patient education as well as to competent performance in the radiology department. The opportunities for health teaching in a radiology department are limited by the busy schedules of both the patients and the department. Under these circumstances, the most important opportunities for patient teaching include the following:

- During the explanation of procedures
- While responding to patient concerns
- As part of the instructions needed to prepare for a procedure
- During instruction for follow-up care

When you are responsible for direct patient teaching, include the patient in the plan whenever possible. After the teaching period, set aside a question-and-answer session and ask the patient to explain or demonstrate the principles to you. This validation of instructions makes patients feel involved in their care, promotes their sense of autonomy, and increases compliance with the medical regimen.

Explanation of the current procedure is essential for all patients. Patients will relax and cooperate much more readily when they know what to expect. Try to keep such explanations simple, and avoid technical details unless the patient expresses an interest. Use good listening skills to respond effectively to patient concerns. Patients frequently express apprehension about exposure to radiation. Reassure them that the risk is extremely small and is far outweighed by the benefits of the procedure. When the patient expresses any concerns, try to focus your response on both the subject and the level of anxiety. Avoid standard explanations that sound as though they were prerecorded. Such "canned" responses are impersonal and make the patient feel as though the question was unimportant. If you are unsure about the answer to a question, refer the patient to a knowledgeable coworker or physician.

When patient teaching involves preparation for a procedure:

- Use prepared written materials.
- Review each step with the patient.
- Validate that the patient understands by using open-ended questions and having the patient explain the preparation back to you.
- Use your best communication skills, even in these brief patient contacts. Listen carefully, be patient, and avoid a hurried appearance, which could discourage patients from asking questions.

COMMUNICATION WITH PATIENTS' FAMILIES

When we are sick or injured, the presence of those who care about us is very reassuring and may be essential to our ability to cope. It is natural that family members accompany patients to their appointments, rush to the emergency department after an accident, and visit patients during hospital admissions. You will often have to deal with family members who want to hold the patient's hand during a radiographic examination or who eagerly await the results of a diagnostic procedure. When you are busy and the patient is your primary concern, family members may appear as obstacles to your work. Dealing sensitively with families is often necessary and helps your patient in ways that may not be apparent.

Your communication with families often involves the transfer of practical information. Those waiting for a patient want to know how long the procedure will take, and they appreciate an update from you when a delay occurs. When the wait is prolonged, your attention to the waiting family's comfort might include directions to needed services such as the restrooms, cafeteria, or telephone.

If the patient is a minor, is incompetent, or is sedated, you may need to provide instructions to a family member regarding preparations or follow-up care. Be sure you are speaking to the person who will actually assist the patient, since information can be lost when it is passed from person to person.

Questions often arise regarding the immediate presence of family members during a procedure. The family must usually stay outside the room, preferably in a waiting area or lobby that is out of hearing range. This is done for reasons of radiation safety, but also because it allows the staff to proceed without interruptions from concerned family members who may not understand what is happening and may require excessive explanation and reassurance. Procedures that involve patient discomfort or some blood loss may be very unsettling to loved ones. If families are waiting near the procedure room, you should be aware of this and avoid making statements within hearing range that might alarm them or betray a professional confidence.

Occasionally a family member may need to stay with the patient in the procedure room, as with the deaf child mentioned earlier. In these situations, only one family member should be selected, and this person should receive a clear explanation before the procedure. You should answer questions at this point and clarify the role of the selected family member. A lead apron or other radiation shielding can be provided as necessary.

Sometimes dealing with families can be especially difficult. In an emotionally charged situation, we all use different means to cope with our anxiety. Some of us become dependent and wait for others to make decisions and give us instructions. Others maintain self-control by withdrawing or denying the importance of the situation. Anxiety can cause some individuals to be quite aggressive when asking personnel for information about patients dear to them. Families of patients in emergency situations naturally experience fear and anxiety, which may result in behaviors directed toward the closest professional person, possibly you! "Watch what you're doing." "You can't move him, he's hurt." "Are you in charge?" "Do you know what you're doing?" Such statements can elicit a negative reaction unless you recognize their hidden message. Fear frequently engenders anger. If you can understand aggressive demands for service and attention as an expression of fear, you can concentrate on providing reassurance rather than reacting to such comments as personal attacks.

Necessary activities, such as filling out forms and calling other family members, may serve to bridge the waiting period. Let families know when the patient will be moved and where the patient will be going. Although you should always refer inquiries about **diagnosis** (identification of condition) or **prognosis** (prediction of outcome) directly to the physician in charge, an expression of concern can demonstrate empathy. "I know you are worried about Barbara, Mr. Rudd. I've let the doctor know you're waiting for the results."

If families do not respond to your attempts to calm them and are preventing you from doing your work, you need help from someone who is in a better position to provide assistance. The social services department may send a counselor or chaplain to assist those who are grief stricken or in a state of panic. As a last resort, or if you feel at risk, security personnel may be summoned to intervene with hostile or belligerent relatives.

DEALING WITH DEATH AND LOSS

There may be an occasion in the future when you are present during a disaster involving fatal injuries, or even a situation involving sudden death within the imaging department. In an acute care hospital, despite the most sophisticated care, patients sometimes die. The medical and nursing staffs have developed specific procedures to follow in the case of death, and these responsibilities do not normally include the radiographer. The physician notifies the family while the nursing staff prepares the body for transport to the morgue.

Your role might be to provide support for the family while awaiting word from the physician. If so, do not volunteer information or discuss the staff's actions. Your observations and opinions must not be discussed at this time. When the family reaches the anger phase of their grieving process, they may want to place blame on someone for an unavoidable death. Spontaneous comments made by caregivers under stress are sometimes quoted by families in court actions to support accusations of malpractice.

If you have any question about the appropriateness of the staff's actions surrounding a patient death, this should be discussed later in private with your supervisor.

Once death has been pronounced on a candidate for organ donation, x-rays may be needed to determine correct placement of the various lines needed to support the integrity of the organs to be donated. You may hear the term *brain dead* used, but the determination of death is based on more than a flat brain wave recorded on an electroencephalogram. The criteria may vary slightly from state to state, but when organ donation is involved, there must be agreement among several physicians that death has occurred. The need to take radiographs of a dead body that is being maintained on oxygen and that does not appear deceased can be emotionally upsetting. Try to keep in mind that the organ donor is providing an opportunity for several other individuals to achieve a normal or improved quality of life.

Victims of some forms of abuse and certain types of homicide are also sometimes subjects for postmortem x-ray examinations. It can be difficult to maintain your professional composure under such circumstances. On these occasions, or when a patient dies unexpectedly during a procedure, the tension and the immediate activity may carry you through the actual event. How you cope with your feelings during the period that follows is important to your mental health, so talk about the events with a supportive person. Health professionals often see themselves as rescuers and may have unrealistic expectations that can lead to feelings of inadequacy and depression when nothing can be done for a patient. Do not be afraid to express emotion. All human beings are unique, and the death of any one of us diminishes humankind.

At some time in your professional or your private life, you will need to deal with someone who is grief stricken. The grieving process is experienced by anyone who suffers serious loss, and this includes patients who become disabled or disfigured. Terminally ill patients and their families often experience anticipatory grief. A great deal has been written on this subject. Early work written by Dr. Elisabeth

Kübler-Ross has greatly changed the way members of the helping professions view the dying process. Both terminally ill patients and their families are now perceived to need time to work through the grief process and achieve some measure of healing. Kübler-Ross points out that grief is an emotional readjustment to a new way of experiencing life and cannot be accomplished all at once. She identifies five phases of the grieving process. They may occur in any order, and not all people experience all five stages:

- **Denial.** At this stage the grieving person refuses to accept the truth and may refuse to discuss the possibility of loss or death.
- **Anger.** As denial is overcome, the person experiences the frustration of helplessness and a feeling of outrage at the apparent injustice of the loss. Rage may be vented on family, friends, and health care workers. This may be beyond the individual's control.
- **Bargaining.** At this stage the person seems to be attempting to earn forgiveness or mitigation of the loss by being "very good." Patients in this phase of grief are conscientious about following physicians' orders, are considerate of others, and seldom complain, even when suffering.
- **Depression.** The depressed person is often acquiescent, quiet, and withdrawn and may cry easily.
- **Acceptance.** At the conclusion of the grieving process, the person accepts the loss or impending death and deals with life and relationships on a more realistic, day-to-day basis. Those who accept their loss are often comfortable talking about it and generally display attitudes that are appropriate to their immediate circumstances.

Although the grieving process is facilitated by supportive acceptance at each stage of grief, the time required to pass from one phase to the next varies with individuals and cannot be hurried.

In dealing with the grieving patient, the radiographer may be presented with statements or questions that require a sensitive response. The patient may say, "I wish it was all over," "How long do you think I have to live?" or "Don't you think I'm much better today?" when there has been no change. In such circumstances you may feel a strong tendency to respond with the language of denial. A typical denial statement might be, "Don't talk like that! You're going to be fine." Such responses tend to block communication and may be insulting to patients who have long since passed the denial phase. Remember that the patient is not necessarily seeking a direct response. What is needed is a friendly, supportive listener.

Rephrasing the patient's remark encourages the patient to talk and conveys a message of acceptance. Examples of such responses to the previous remarks might be, "I'm sorry you're feeling tired of living," "You think it would help to know how long you have to live," or "You're feeling better today?" Don't be afraid to be involved or to show that you care. Be lavish with touch and comfort measures if the patient seems responsive to this type of attention.

Terminally ill patients have the right to be cared for in the facility of their choice. While some prefer the acute care setting, an increasing number choose to die at home. In the 1970s, a movement gained acceptance that emphasized home care for terminal patients. Instead of an emphasis on cure, care is focused on the pain relief and comfort measures that allow patients to die with dignity in familiar surroundings. This movement is called Hospice from the Greek term *hos,* meaning a place of shelter. Today **hospice** is a service rather than a place. When the physician determines that the patient is unlikely to live more than 6 months and a decision is made with the patient not to pursue further treatment of the underlying disease, a conference with the hospice staff determines whether the family is able to assume the responsibility of providing the major portion of care. The team of physicians, nurses, home health aides, psychologists, and social workers helps provide the patient with as much quality of life as possible during the short time that remains. Some communities have inpatient hospice facilities, but care is often given in the patient's home. The patient's home may be with family or in an assisted living or skilled nursing facility. Comfort measures and other **palliative** treatments (care that provides relief but is not intended to cure) are provided on call 24 hours a day. Respite care may be offered to permit the family caregiver time to rest and regroup. After the death of the patient, the hospice team may provide counseling to the bereaved that can help them with grief and healing.

This subject is often not included in the curriculum or texts on patient care. Few professionals are totally comfortable in the presence of death, and most of us find it difficult to objectively face our own mortality and eventual death. Those who work in an acute care setting need to learn to accept death as yet one more aspect of life. We strongly urge you to expand your awareness by reading and discussing this sensitive subject. Seek support and counseling for situations that are personally difficult to handle. Familiarize yourself with facility policies and protocols. Further education is advised for those working in situations such as radiation **oncology** (cancer treatment) where death is a likely occurrence. (See Chapter 2 regarding the patient's right to die and "do not resuscitate" [DNR] orders.)

COMMUNICATION WITH COWORKERS

Teamwork is defined as the cooperative effort by the members of a group to achieve a common goal. The pressures in a busy imaging department may sometimes make this concept hard to apply. Our goal is the best patient care possible, and it becomes easier to accomplish when we work cooperatively with others on the health care team.

The ability to relay information to other health professionals is essential in the multidisciplinary situation existing in modern hospitals. Many problems we encounter when dealing with patients are also met when communicating with professional workers. The pressures of time and patient load may cause or compound the personality conflicts encountered in any group. Good interpersonal relationships are built on the ability to make others feel good about themselves. The nonverbal behaviors that we use with patients, such as touch and appearance, are equally effective with coworkers. Use praise and appreciation as positive reinforcements when work is well done or when others go out of their way to offer assistance. Be a good listener, and

demonstrate your respect for your coworkers as individuals by avoiding cliques and gossip. Teamwork is a two-way street, so if you appreciate help when your workload is heavy, you should also assist your coworkers in similar situations. Being patient and considerate, avoiding assumptions, validating communication, and maintaining a positive attitude are all habits that will generally result in a positive response. Because good communication with your coworkers is important no matter where you work, we urge you to review the principles presented earlier in this chapter and to practice them in all your professional encounters.

One aspect of your interpersonal relationships with coworkers can have legal implications. The pressure of work within the department often makes it difficult to take the time to exchange general information. For this reason, break periods or lunchtimes are often used to catch up on recent developments and share information about difficult situations. *Never discuss patients in a public setting.* It is quite acceptable to talk about changes in schedules, the hospital picnic, or the new computer system, but discussions of interesting cases, important personages, or possible treatment errors could result in damaging litigation, since such conversations are invasions of the personal rights and privacy of patients.

In today's world, a great amount of technical information is exchanged. Although much of this is conveyed using charts and forms, informal messages may be equally important. Attention to details, such as adding your name and the date to telephone message forms, keeps information retrieval more accurate.

Here are some guidelines for avoiding problems with telephone communications:

- Be familiar with your telephone system, including forwarding and "hold" functions.
- Identify yourself and your department when calling or answering a call.
- Keep paper handy, and make notes during the call to avoid losing details.
- Use a pleasant, receptive tone of voice.
- Validate the message before concluding the call.
- Be sure the message is relayed to the proper person or department.

Any written communication is valuable only if the recipient receives it in good time. Whether this is a telephone message, a personal note, or a change in schedule, be sure that important messages are placed directly in the individual's hand, or posted in plain sight in a predetermined spot. Be sure to identify yourself, your department, the time sent or received, and if a reply is needed, include the address.

Fax transmissions and voice mail also facilitate transmission of information and instructions between hospitals and other health care facilities. Confidential information should not be communicated in a voice mail message, as there is no way of controlling who will receive the message. Extensive voice mail messages, even when not confidential, are usually not effective. It is better to simply leave your name and number and a general statement of the purpose of the call.

If you are responsible for faxing information to another institution, remember to fill out the cover sheet first. Confusion about where the information is needed or who is to receive it can cause needless delays in patient care. When sensitive, confidential information regarding a patient is to be sent by fax, it should be preceded by a phone call to alert the recipient. Confidentiality is difficult to preserve at best, and such information should be treated in a responsible manner. Fax transmission can be more convenient and efficient for a physician as well. Immediate, direct written communication of orders and scheduling requests may help prevent errors and improve service. The ability to print multiple copies of new orders makes fax transmission an especially useful tool.

Unlike the business world, where each individual in an office has a personal computer, it is more common in the radiology suite for a few computers to be used by the entire staff. Under these circumstances, using the computer system for personal communications is inappropriate.

Many troublesome situations can be avoided by maintaining a pleasant working relationship that allows you to solve small problems before they grow. Before recurring problems become monumental, follow the chain of command discussed in Chapter 2 to seek a solution.

MEDICAL INFORMATION AND RECORDS

Effective documentation of information about patients and their care marks the professional who recognizes efficient record keeping as a way to meet ongoing patient needs. Attention to clerical details may seem to be a nonprofessional function, but dates, account numbers, chart numbers, Social Security numbers, and similar data are necessary to your institution and the patients it serves. While different forms and types of data are used to meet the needs of various departments, certain terms are commonly used. **Charting** refers to any records you are expected to add to a document. In most imaging departments, the majority of the record keeping is done on requisition forms that usually have a limited area for charting. A **chart** usually refers to a more extensive compilation of information, such as an emergency department record or the chart brought with a patient who is hospitalized.

The forms may vary with your institution or department, but *any written records you initiate must be accurate, pertinent, and legible.* These medical records include not only written information on the condition of the patient, medications, and treatments, but also laboratory results, radiographs, and any other information that pertains to the health and welfare of the patient.

Health care providers today use computers extensively for clerical functions (Fig. 3-6). The storage of computer data on patients creates an individual file for each patient. Access to these files supplies not only basic information about the patient, such as room number, birth date, medical record number, and next of kin, but also diagnosis, treatment, and other observations pertinent to patient care.

Computer files can be used for scheduling, generating requisitions, or entering charges when procedures have been completed. However, computers are only capable of using the information provided them. If a date is incomplete or a name misspelled, the computer is unable to right the error and may reject the entire entry. Most hospitals provide in-service instruction applicable to their computer systems.

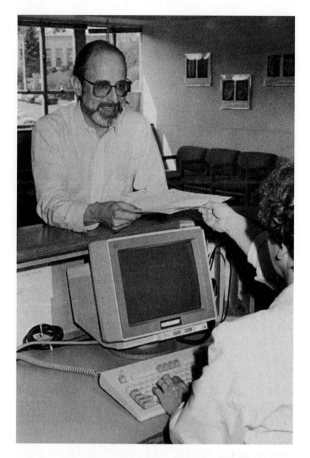

FIG. 3-6 Computers simplify clerical functions in imaging departments.

Responsibilities for Record Keeping

Health care agencies are also businesses. Proper record keeping is required to ensure that patients are billed accurately, that new supplies are ordered, and that insurance companies receive verification of the care given to their clients. Failure to process information accurately and promptly may inconvenience your coworkers and pose serious problems for patients.

The chief reason for keeping accurate, pertinent medical records is to provide data about the patient's progress and current status for other health team members. Not only does this prevent the need for repetitious diagnostic examinations by various professionals, it also encourages a systematic approach to therapeutic care, allowing for longitudinal comparisons that aid in a more comprehensive approach to extended health care. Well-kept records also serve as a resource for research investigations.

Accountability is an essential term when referring to the medicolegal aspects of patient care. We cannot overemphasize the importance of correct record keeping. Above all, medical records should be objective. For example, do not chart "patient is confused," because this does not demonstrate how you came to this conclusion. "Patient appears unable to relate why he is in hospital and who or what brought him here" is a clearer statement. Objectivity is particularly important when dealing with situations that have a strong potential for legal action, such as motor vehicle accidents. "Too drunk to climb on x-ray table" is an unvalidated clinical judgment. "Appeared uncoordinated, staggered severely, and was unable to climb on x-ray table without assistance; strong odor of alcohol on breath and clothing," is an objective statement.

Poorly kept medical records are often a major contributing factor when a defensible court case is lost. Charting should be complete, objective, consistent, legible, and accurate. The following list alerts you to some rules for avoiding mistakes frequently found when charts are audited:

- To delete an entry, simply draw a line through it; do not erase or use correction fluid.
- Always initial and date corrections.
- Never leave blanks on forms. Insert "NA" or "0."
- Never insert loose or gummed slips of paper.
- Always include all four digits of the year when dating written materials.
- Date and sign entries that you make, and include your title.

Remember that all information in patient records is considered confidential. The chart is a legal document that can substantiate or refute charges of negligence or malpractice and can also serve as a record of behavior, which may set a precedent. The course of treatment and quality of care are reflected in the chart.

The Chart as a Resource

Earlier in this chapter we discussed the need to validate impressions in assessing the status of patients in the radiology department. The chart is frequently your most accessible resource. Although the organization of charts may vary, certain elements are consistent. The diagnosis or "impression" is found at the conclusion of the history sheet. The patient's current status is found in the physicians' progress notes and in the nurses' notes. Allergic sensitivities are usually indicated in red on the chart cover and are also stated in the history sheet. Laboratory reports, radiology reports, and results of other studies are found in a separate section, whereas the medication record may be in the nurses' notes or on a separate record near the temperature sheet. The recording of pulse, blood pressure, and temperature on a graph form allows for a longitudinal comparison.

To reduce the time involved in the charting process, as well as the volume of hospital records, charting is a somewhat streamlined form of written communication. Many frequently used words are abbreviated, and comments are made in the form of brief phrases rather than complete sentences. Some practice is needed for beginners to translate this jargon accurately. The lists of abbreviations and terms in Appendix D are helpful to students learning to use medical charts.

Problem-Oriented Medical Recording

Problem-oriented medical recording (POMR) is a system of problem identification that started with systems analysis and is now used for medical, social, psychiatric, and demographic investigations. This system has been adapted to provide faster and more accurate medical information retrieval. To use this system, one must collect data, evaluate them and form a problem list, determine what intervention is appropriate, carry out the plan, and evaluate the results.

Traditional charts include a running commentary on the patient's total condition. Since most patients have several problems, retrieval of information on a specific point is rather cumbersome. Suppose Mr. Clark has been admitted with hypertension, but he also has **dermatitis** (skin inflammation) and mild diarrhea. In traditional charts, you would need to comb through the nurses' notes, progress record, graph sheet, or all three, to see if diarrhea is an immediate problem that will complicate today's radiographic examination. Using POMR, you may look at the list of problems in the front of the chart, find the number assigned to the problem that concerns you, and then look for that number in the joint progress notes kept by all medical staff providing care (Fig. 3-7).

When you look for information on a specific problem, you will find the letters S, O, A, and P in the margin with a narrative next to each letter. These initials stand for the words *subjective, objective, assessment,* and *plan.* Subjective observations are symptoms and personal reactions related by the patient. Objective observations are the signs and measurements that can be substantiated by the observer, such as weight, temperature, laboratory results, and emesis. Assessment is the definition of the problem, such as "obese—50 pounds overweight" or "diarrhea secondary to medication reaction." Plan is what the health provider intends to do to deal with the problem.

In essence, this charting system allows identification of each of the patient's problems. It permits differentiation between long-term and short-term problems, enabling you to focus on the immediate situation without ignoring long-term goals. (Reducing obesity, increasing exercise tolerance, or giving up smoking would be examples of long-term goals for the hypertensive patient.) POMR also permits ease of retrieval for specific information, such as cost analysis, quality control, and research. It remains the legal record of the course and quality of care.

Medical Recording by Radiographers

Requisitions and reports are forms of particular importance to radiographers. An x-ray requisition serves as the formal order for a diagnostic procedure. It includes patient data, a brief medical history, and specific instructions. In some situations it may be part of a multicopy form that eventually may include the radiologist's report. Both the requisition and the report are medicolegal records and may be filed with the films or separately. The original copies of inpatient reports become part of the patient's chart. Copies of reports are also supplied directly to physicians.

Although radiographers are not responsible for initiating these records, they rely on requisitions for information about each examination they perform. They may also refer to previous reports for information about the patient's problem or the radiologist's recommendations for further studies.

Medical recording by radiographers varies greatly from one institution to another, and you must become familiar with your facility's requirements. Documenting certain information about patients is an essential part of the medicolegal record. This includes administration of contrast media or medications, changes in patient status, and reactions to contrast or medications, as well as any treatment received in the radiology department. Examples of such treatment include oxygen given to a patient who becomes short of breath or cold packs applied to the site when an intravenous line has infiltrated.

Inpatient charts usually accompany patients to the imaging department. The chart is usually where you record changes in status, medications, and treatments. In your hospital, the information to be recorded might be placed in chart pages titled "Nurses' Notes," "Progress Notes," or "Medication Records." In some hospitals, completion of the procedure is routinely charted by the radiographer in the nurses' notes. The information you chart should include the date, the time (using the 24-hour clock; e.g., 2:15 PM is charted as 1415), a specific statement of what occurred, and your signature. When charting observations or treatments on behalf of the radiologist, include the radiologist's name followed by a slash mark and your signature. Although nurses often use only initials to identify their entries, they are part of a small group repeatedly using the chart, and their initials with their full name are recorded elsewhere in the chart for legal verification. When radiographers chart, they should use a full signature and a designation of their department or position so that identification is clear.

An increasing proportion of the patients seen in imaging departments are outpatients who do not have an actual chart, but accurate medical records are important for these patients as well. Your observations must be recorded on the proper form, which will be filed with either the report or the films. Initials may be adequate identification for routine notes on records generated in your own department.

PROBLEM LIST				
Date identified	Date of onset	Problem number	Problem title	Date inactive Resolved
9/27/02	9/27/02	1	Persistant nausea and diarrhea	
9/28/02	9/27/02	2	RUQ Pain	
9/28/02	9/28/02	3	Mild dehydration Fluid deficit	
4/23/98	1998	4	Adult-onset diabetes	7/1998

FIG. 3-7 Problem-oriented medical recording (POMR). **A,** Problem list used with POMR.

	REDLAND VALLEY COMMUNITY HOSPITAL		Kate E. Doble 573-82-6823 DOB-4/21/27
Date	Time	Problem #	Progress notes
9/28/02	1600	2	S. C/O RUQ pain, radiating to rt scapular area
			O. T.101, P. 96, R. 18, pain level 7
			A. Poss. acute cholecystitis; admitted for workup
			P. Dr. Erbele notified; will order meds p PE
	1630	1	S. C/O of constant nausea
			O. Emesis x 3 of clear green liquid approx 150 cc
			A. Unable to keep food down
			P. Hold evening insulin until M.D. visit
		4	S. Hx of adult-onset diabetes; held insulin this AM
			O. Alert and oriented
			A./P. Discuss diabetic orders with Dr. Erbele
	1725	3	S. C/O dry mouth and headache, nausea
			O. Further emesis x 3; approx 50 cc frothy green
			A. Dehydration
			P. Consult Dr. for parenteral fluid replacement order
			D. McCloskey, A.N.P. DMG

S, Subjective (symptoms)
O, Objective data (measurable signs)
A, Assessments (conclusions)
P, Plan (intervention or action)
E, Evaluation (effect of intervention)

FIG. 3-7—cont'd **B,** Example of joint progress notes using POMR.

Complete signatures, however, are needed for witnessing documents such as informed consents, consents to treatment, and incident reports.

Radiographs as Records

When medical images are recorded on film, the radiographs are legally considered to be a part of the medical record and belong to the institution in which they are made. Patients often assume that, because they have paid for the examination, the films belong to them. Tact is required when explaining that the charges cover the expense of the procedure and that every effort will be made to ensure the films are available when and where they may be needed to assist in the patient's care. Film copies of digitized images can be made when records must be transferred. These images can also be sent electronically to facilities equipped to receive them.

State laws vary with respect to the length of time images must legally be kept on file. Usually the retention period is 5 to 7 years, with the additional requirement that films on minors be kept 5 to 7 years after the patient reaches majority or legal age (18 to 21 years, depending on the state).

Since charts can easily be photocopied, the original is never allowed to leave the health facility.

Radiographs are more difficult to duplicate, however, and the quality of a duplicate is never equal to that of the original. For this reason, it is often helpful for original films to be made available for comparison or consultation outside the institution of origin. Digital images from computed radiography (CR), direct digital imaging systems, or computer-assisted modalities can be sent electronically to other providers or printed using laser cameras to produce hard copies of excellent quality when needed.

Since rules governing confidentiality also apply to all medical images, the patient must sign a release form when films are needed by another provider. A written record of the date and the borrower's name and address meets the legal obligation to keep original radiographs on file. Usually, follow-up procedures exist to ensure return of films that have been loaned, but radiographs are sometimes checked out for indefinite periods, as when a patient with a **chronic** (long-standing or slowly progressing) condition moves to another state.

It is usually recommended that films be sent directly to a consulting physician rather than allowing the patient to transport them. Sometimes, however, it is more convenient for the patient to carry the films. In this case, a physician should view the films with the patient and answer any questions in advance, since the patient's curiosity may result in an attempt to interpret the films. This can lead to unnecessary confusion and anxiety. For example, patients have been known to assume that a heart shadow is a lung tumor or that a gas bubble in the stomach indicates a serious disease.

CONCLUSION

The progress of humankind has depended on our ability to communicate with one another. In the hospital setting, many factors cause patient anxiety and fear. When we take time to empathize, we find greater personal satisfaction in our work and improve the quality of care. Sensitivity to cultural issues, good listening skills, positive attitudes, avoidance of assumptions, and validation of communication enhance the quality of our interactions. The same principles of communication that improve relationships with patients and their families will aid in our relationships with coworkers as well.

Charts serve as a valuable resource to the radiographer who needs to validate information on a patient's current status and record appropriate observations and procedures done in the radiology department. The ability to communicate well with patients and other health professionals is the mark of an effective professional.

REVIEW QUESTIONS

1. Which of the following terms best describes assertive behavior?
   A. forceful
   B. hostile
   C. persuasive
   D. firm
   E. argumentative
2. When instructions are given to a non-English-speaking patient, it is best to:
   A. speak English slowly and firmly
   B. use a sympathetic family member who speaks English
   C. draw detailed pictures
   D. use a trained interpreter
   E. send written instruction home with the patient
3. Deaf patients and hearing impaired patients differ in that the deaf patients:
   A. will not respond to sounds outside their field of vision
   B. may use ASL as their primary means of communication
   C. often move socially within a deaf community
   D. all of the above
   E. A and B only
4. When dealing with a hostile patient it is very important to:
   A. gain control of the situation with a loud, firm voice
   B. use nonverbal behavior to show disapproval
   C. close the door and calm the patient
   D. limit confusion by dealing with the situation alone
   E. ask for help before the situation escalates

5. Individuals with decreased LOC should be kept under observation because they:
   A. are not responsible for their actions or answers
   B. tend to be violent when regaining consciousness
   C. need to remember and follow instructions
   D. cannot hear while unconscious
   E. need help going to the bathroom
6. When dealing with children, it is important to:
   A. calm them by giving them lots of choices
   B. let them know who is in charge
   C. keep directions simple, direct, and honest
   D. get written permission for immobilization
   E. tell a crying child, "Stop that, or we can't take all the pictures!"
7. Dealing with death or loss may be characterized by expressions of:
   A. anger
   B. bargaining
   C. denial
   D. depression
   E. all of the above
8. Cultural differences may result in differing perceptions of which of the following behaviors?
   A. eye contact
   B. nodding one's head
   C. a casual hug
   D. a loud, firm voice
   E. all of the above

CRITICAL THINKING EXERCISES

1. Adam, age 4, has been brought in for radiography of an injured hand and is very frightened. How can you communicate successfully to Adam that he is in a safe place so that he will cooperate? What kinds of nonverbal signals can you use to support your verbal message? How would you validate the effectiveness of your communication?
2. What urgent situations might require you to rapidly retrieve information from a patient's chart?
3. Allison Jones, age 3 , has swallowed a quarter, and the emergency department physician has ordered chest and abdomen x-rays. Both Allison and her mother are upset and worried. What can you do to calm Mrs. Jones and enlist her help in obtaining Allison's x-rays?
4. Can you review a sample chart and identify the subjective, objective, assessment, and plan components? If these items are not in a SOAP format, make a sample progress note using the SOAP system.
5. What are the possible consequences to the patient and to the radiographer when a radiographer fails to be objective and accountable in record keeping?

CHAPTER 4

Safety, Transfer, and Positioning

OBJECTIVES

At the conclusion of this chapter, the student will be able to:

- List four important electrical safety precautions.
- List in sequence the steps to be taken if you discover a fire in or near the radiology department.
- List three common infractions of fire safety rules in hospitals.
- Discuss hazards caused by obstructions and spills.
- List two steps to be taken to ensure accuracy of patient identification.
- Demonstrate safe techniques for patient moving and transferring, using the principles of good body mechanics:
  - Assist patient with sitting from a recumbent position.
  - Assist patient into and out of wheelchair.
  - Perform two-person transfer of patient from bed to stretcher and stretcher to bed.
- List four complications that may arise from improper patient positioning.
- Demonstrate the use of pillows and positioning blocks to ensure the patient is comfortable on the x-ray table.
- List three situations when the patient's head should be elevated.
- Demonstrate proper use of safety straps, side rails, restraints, and compression bands.

98

VOCABULARY

base of support
body mechanics
center of gravity
debilitated
decubitus ulcers
emesis

kyphotic
line of gravity
lordotic
orthostatic hypotension
sedation
spontaneous combustion

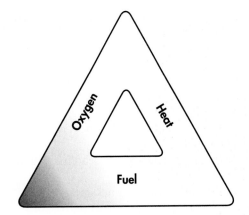
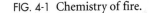

FIG. 4-1 Chemistry of fire.

THIS CHAPTER FOCUSES ON safety in the imaging department and in the hospital setting as a whole. Here you will learn precautions to minimize risks and procedures to follow in situations that may be hazardous. While patient safety is a primary concern for all radiographers, you will note that this chapter also provides information to help ensure your own safety as you care for patients.

Health care facilities are required to have written policies and procedures to ensure patient safety. The Occupational Safety and Health Administration (OSHA), a federal agency governing safety in the workplace, provides guidelines to ensure a high level of safety for hospital workers, and these guidelines are a part of the safety procedures in hospitals. It is your duty to be familiar with the established safety procedures for your employment situation.

FIRE HAZARDS
Fire Prevention

Nothing strikes more terror in a hospital than the word *fire*. Our first discussion of safety practices is centered on fire prevention, which is obviously preferable to coping with a fire. An awareness of potential hazards is the first step toward prevention.

Three components must be present for a fire to burn: a flammable substance (fuel), oxygen, and heat (Fig. 4-1). Fire can be avoided by ensuring that these three elements never occur in the same place at the same time. Once started, a fire can be stopped if one of the elements can be removed from the situation. We use this principle when we fight a fire by adding water (lowering the temperature) or by smothering

(removing oxygen), as when we wrap a blanket around a person whose clothing has ignited. Most hospital fires are traceable to one of four causes:

- Spontaneous combustion
- Open flames
- Cigarette smokers
- Electricity

Spontaneous combustion

Spontaneous combustion occurs when a chemical reaction in or near a flammable material causes sufficient heat to generate a fire. This is a relatively infrequent cause of hospital fires, since hospital safety standards, as well as state and local safety regulations, control the types of chemicals and cleaning products used.

Of particular concern in this regard is the practice of recycling hazardous materials and the regulatory requirements for their safe disposal. Laboratories and maintenance departments now retain chemical, plastic, and glass materials for recycling or disposal in areas that may not have been designed for this purpose. Spontaneous combustion may also occur during renovations when paint products, solvents, and cleaning rags may be stored temporarily in a closed environment or too near a heat source. Oily or paint-soaked waste should be placed in tightly covered containers near the maintenance department.

Open flames

Open flames that burn out of control are a common source of fires in homes, but relatively few hospital fires begin in this way. Those that do usually occur in kitchens or laboratories where open burners are used. Precautions include:

- Keeping flammable substances a safe distance from the flame
- Using strict standards of cleanliness in kitchen areas
- Never leaving open flames untended

Smoking

Smoking has essentially been eliminated in hospitals today and is seldom a potential cause of fires. As health care providers, hospitals promote positive health habits by prohibiting smoking, and most hospitals are designated as nonsmoking facilities. This practice reduces the incidence of this type of fire, but danger still exists from covert smoking. People who smoke tend to cope with the stress of hospitalization by smoking, but hospitals are no longer equipped to accommodate them. They must be directed to the designated smoking area, which may be outside the building.

Electrical failures

Electrical fires are potential sources of fire hazard and are of special concern in radiology departments, where there is much electrical equipment. For this reason, we emphasize avoiding electrical hazards and preventing electrical fires (Box 4-1). The same principles apply in any area where electrical equipment is used, especially in the emergency department and the intensive care unit.

A short circuit in an x-ray control panel, especially in older units, may result in fire. This is usually preceded by smoldering wire insulation, which causes smoke and an unpleasant odor. It is usually readily detectable before an actual fire.

If you suspect a fire hazard from an electrical malfunction:

- Turn off the electricity at the main power source.
- Call for qualified assistance.
- Stand by with the proper fire extinguisher.

BOX 4-1

ELECTRICAL SAFETY RULES

- All electrical equipment and appliances must be approved for hospital use.
- Follow equipment manufacturer's instructions.
- Equipment used on or near patients or near water must have grounded plugs.
- Inspect equipment regularly, paying attention to cords and plugs. Arrange for repairs as needed.
- Do not overload circuits by connecting too many devices to a single outlet or outlet group.
- Unplug or turn off electrical equipment before exposing internal parts.
- Do not attempt to repair equipment unless you are trained to do so.
- Use only extension cords approved for the intended purpose.
- In case of electrical fire, use a Class C or carbon dioxide fire extinguisher.

All radiographers should be aware of the locations of fire extinguishers and instructed in their use. During your education as a radiographer you will learn to use a wide variety of complex electrical equipment. Do not let familiarity with electrical items lull you into a false sense of security.

Oxygen by itself does not burn, but it does support combustion. Since the presence of oxygen greatly increases the fire hazard, it is important to exercise extreme care when it is in use. There should be no smoking, no open flames, and no ungrounded appliances. Be familiar with the location and operation of oxygen shut-off valves in your area (Fig. 4-2).

Be Prepared

Hospitals are required to observe certain fire safety precautions to maintain their accreditation. In most hospitals the head of the maintenance department or the chief engineer is responsible for initiating fire safety programs. These include clearly defined plans for staff action in the event of a fire, fire drills every calendar quarter, and frequent in-service classes on

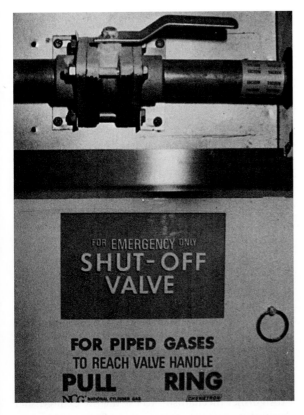

FIG. 4-2 Oxygen shut-off valve, an important location to remember.

fire-fighting procedures and equipment. The radiographer must be familiar with the fire plan for the hospital, especially for the radiology department. Be sure you know the evacuation route from your area and at least one alternate route. In addition, have at least a general knowledge of your facility's floor plan, and take special note of the locations of fire alarms, fire extinguishers, and fire doors.

A coded communication is usually used in the event of a fire to notify the staff without alarming the patients. This may be a code number announced over the paging system: "Attention all staff, there is a code 100 on Three East." Some hospitals use a special message, such as, "Dr. Redfern, report to Third Floor East." This same code is commonly used for fire drills.

Fire drills must be taken seriously. Take full advantage of fire drills and in-service classes to gain confidence in evacuation procedures and the use of fire extinguishers. If you are well prepared for a fire, your self-confidence will allow you to function effectively and will reassure those around you.

According to professional fire marshals, the most frequent infractions of fire safety rules include:
- Blocking fire doors to prevent them from closing
- Storing equipment in corridors, hindering evacuation
- Improperly storing flammable items
- Using extension cords not approved for hospital use

Fire doors in hospitals are marked for easy identification. They are designed and constructed to restrict the spread of a fire to a small area. For this reason, fire doors should never be blocked open. They should remain closed unless they are designed to close automatically when the fire alarm is activated.

Since radiographers often use mobile stretchers, wheelchairs, carts, and x-ray machines, care must be taken to avoid obstructing passages and doorways. Corridors should not be used to store equipment; if some items need to be placed there temporarily, keep them on the same side and make sure room is available to pass easily. Ask yourself the question, "If we had to evacuate the area, would this piece of equipment be a problem in this location?"

In Case of Fire

If you discover a fire, your primary responsibility is to evacuate everyone in the immediate area to a safe location beyond at least two intervening fire doors. Second, report the fire and location using the prescribed code procedure. A small wastebasket blaze may be extinguished with a nearby pitcher of water or smothered with a pillow, but do not waste precious minutes in futile attempts. Report the fire as soon as the immediate area is evacuated so that hospital personnel trained in fire fighting can assess the situation and direct an appropriate course of action.

The following steps apply whether the fire is in your area or in another part of the building:
- Close all doors.
- Shut off all electrical equipment.

- Shut off main oxygen valves.
- Prepare patients for further evacuation while awaiting instruction.

If the fire is in or near the radiology department, a staff member will direct patients to a safe area. During evacuation it is especially important to remain calm, use a low voice, and try to avoid using the word *fire*. Instead, you might say, "Mrs. Jensen, there is a little smoke in one of the rooms and we are going to move you outside until we can see how serious it is." Box 4-2 lists the steps to follow in case of fire.

Again, no substitute exists for knowing the location of the fire extinguishers, fire alarms (Fig. 4-3), and fire doors. Although this is usually included as part of your hospital orientation, familiarity with this information is your personal responsibility. Thorough knowledge of the prescribed procedure for reporting a fire is also essential.

Fire extinguishers

Fires are classified according to the type of fuel involved:

- Class A fires involve solid combustibles such as paper or wood.
- Class B fires involve flammable liquids or gases.
- Class C fires involve electrical equipment or wiring.

Fire extinguishers are marked to indicate the class or classes of fire for which they are appropriately used. A multipurpose, dry chemical extinguisher is suitable for all three classes of fires and is the type most often found in hospitals and other public buildings.

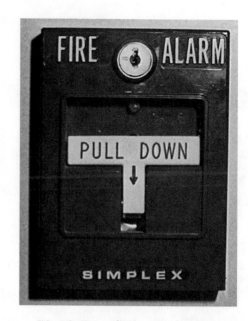

FIG. 4-3 Know this location by heart.

Fig. 4-4 shows a close-up view of a typical fire extinguisher mechanism. To use the fire extinguisher correctly, remember the acronym *PASS:*

- **P**ull the pin.
- **A**im the nozzle.
- **S**queeze the handle.
- **S**weep. Use a sweeping motion from side to side.

Do not aim the fire extinguisher steadily at the flame. A sweeping motion is more effective and covers a wider area, decreasing the likelihood that the fire will spread. Stand back so as not to endanger yourself; fire extinguishers have considerable force and are effective at a safe distance from the fire (Fig. 4-5).

Fire extinguishers must be inspected regularly and recharged periodically. A tag attached to the unit should indicate the dates of the last inspection and the last recharge. The last inspection should be no longer than 1 year ago. When an extinguisher has been used, it must be returned to the maintenance department to be recharged and replaced immediately with a fresh unit.

BOX 4-2

IN CASE OF FIRE

Remain Calm.
1. Evacuate everyone from the immediate area.
2. Report the fire and precise location.
3. Close all doors.
4. Shut off main oxygen valves.
5. Shut off all electrical equipment.
6. Stand by for further instruction from authorized personnel.

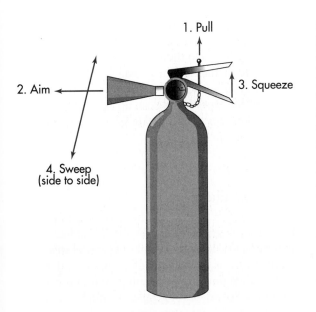

1. Pull

2. Aim

3. Squeeze

4. Sweep
(side to side)

FIG. 4-4 Fire extinguisher mechanism.

OTHER COMMON HAZARDS
Electric Shock

Electric shock may pose a serious hazard to both patients and personnel if safety precautions are not observed. This is especially true with x-ray equipment, which carries an electrical potential in excess of 100,000 volts. The hazard of lesser circuits should not be underestimated, however, since shocks from standard 110-volt outlets may prove fatal under certain circumstances. The rules for electrical safety are listed in Box 4-1. Adherence to these rules greatly reduces the possibility of electric shock. In addition, use extreme caution when using electricity around water. Never stand on a wet floor or use wet hands to perform tasks involving the use of electricity.

Falls and Collisions

Reducing the risk of falls and collisions is a major safety concern in hospitals. Caution is needed for the safety of both patients and personnel. Be especially conscious of hazards when moving stretchers and other mobile equipment, and do not store or "park"

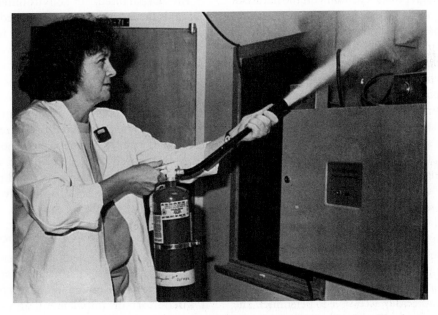

FIG. 4-5 Use fire extinguisher in a sweeping motion from side to side. Stand back at a safe distance.

this equipment where it might cause a problem. Equipment too close to a corner may be an unseen obstruction to someone hurrying from an intersecting hallway or carrying a bulky object.

Storage areas are common sources of accidents when items are not placed properly and secured when necessary. Heavy items stored on high shelves are an invitation to an accident; they should be placed near the floor. Don't stack items precariously. Any item that could cause harm should be situated so that it will not shift unexpectedly.

Do not string electrical cords across doorways or other traffic patterns, and try to position equipment as close as possible to a suitable outlet. If a cord must cross a traffic path temporarily, secure it to the floor with tape to minimize the possibility of someone tripping over it. If hazardous, makeshift electrical connections are a common problem, use the chain of command to suggest a safe, permanent remedy.

Precautions for avoiding patient falls are addressed in detail later in this chapter under Patient Transfer.

Spills

Spills deserve the special attention of the safety-conscious radiographer. Depending on the nature of the substance, spills may pose a chemical hazard in addition to the risk of injury from falls. Chemicals may be as simple as household cleaning agents or as complex as radioactive testing materials. Familiar substances such as household bleach or concentrated darkroom chemicals may cause eye damage or skin burns. Appropriate cleaning measures are needed to avoid potentially serious problems. Your work area should have a spill kit that includes nitrile gloves, a container of kitty litter, heavy plastic bags, a broom, and a dustpan. The litter absorbs spilled liquid so that it can be safely swept up and placed in plastic bags for disposal.

Your hospital has written policies and procedures to follow in determining appropriate action in the event of a chemical spill. OSHA requires that all chemicals be properly labeled and that Material Safety Data Sheets (MSDSs) for all hazardous materials be on file and easily accessible to personnel. The MSDS for any chemical will indicate the required equipment and procedure for safe handling in the

event of a spill. The following steps help to ensure safety when a spill occurs:

- Limit access to the area.
- Evaluate the risks involved.
- Determine whether you have both the equipment and the expertise to clean up the spill safely.
- If you can proceed safely, clean up the spill immediately.
- If you lack the necessary skill or equipment, call your supervisor or the appropriate department.

Darkroom Chemicals

The developer and fixer solutions used to process radiographs are classified by OSHA as hazardous materials. OSHA requires that personnel wear protective aprons, splash-proof goggles, and nitrile gloves when pouring or cleaning up film processing solutions. Splash-proof goggles fit snugly against the face to provide greater eye safety than common industrial safety goggles, which are designed only for protection from airborne debris. Nitrile is a special substance that is impervious to many hazardous chemicals. *Note that common latex gloves are not considered to be adequate protection.*

The Department of Environmental Quality (DEQ) is the federal agency concerned with the safe disposal of hazardous waste. Together with local officials responsible for landfill and sewage treatment facilities, the DEQ sets standards for waste disposal that provide safety for the environment. Used fixer solution contains silver and is not permitted in the sewage system, so environmental standards require that used fixer be processed for silver removal before disposal. If your department does not reclaim the silver from used fixer, it must be drained into suitable heavy plastic containers and picked up for recycling. This service is commonly provided by companies that supply the chemicals.

Eye Splashes and Eyewash Protocol

Prompt treatment is essential for chemical splashes in the eyes. When a chemical eye splash occurs, flood the eye with running water for a full 5 minutes. If discomfort or impairment of vision persists following eyewash, see an ophthalmologist immediately.

An eyewash station is a first aid station for chemical eye splashes that provides a spray of water to the eye from a convenient height. Some are activated by a foot pedal, leaving the hands free to hold the eye open. If a chemical eye splash occurs in the vicinity of an eyewash station, this is obviously the best approach. On the other hand, immediate treatment is essential, so do not waste time and endanger your eyesight by searching for an eyewash station when a splash occurs. Become familiar with the location and operation of eyewash stations in your facility before the need arises. OSHA requires that eyewash stations be within 15 minutes' access of areas where hazardous chemicals are usually handled, but if an eyewash station is not convenient, any running water is satisfactory.

ERGONOMICS AND BODY MECHANICS

Ergonomics is the study of the human body in relation to the working environment. Ergonomic awareness and education in the workplace have reduced job injuries in recent years, but there is still cause for concern. Studies indicate that ongoing education programs and appropriate responses by employers to the ergonomic concerns of their workers is the right approach. Work injury is also minimized when proper equipment is available and is used correctly and when workers help one another.

The U.S. Bureau of Labor Statistics reports that workplace injury rates for hospital workers are similar to those for industrial workers. The most common injuries reported by health care workers are musculoskeletal disorders, especially back strains from lifting and moving patients or equipment. Radiographers also experience strains of the shoulder and neck when reaching overhead to move the x-ray tube. Technologists who perform computerized modalities are more likely to experience spinal stress from sitting at a console for long periods and repetitive stress injuries (RSIs) from intensive keyboard work. Sonographers commonly report RSIs to the hands and wrists as a result of gripping the transducer and repeatedly applying pressure from the same positions. Stress caused by repetitive motion, over-reaching, and maintaining the same positions for long periods can cause microtrauma to muscle tissue. Microtrauma may produce chronic discomfort and lead to more significant injury. Frequent break periods and changes in position help to minimize both positional and repetitive stress.

The principles of proper body alignment, movement, and balance are referred to as **body mechanics.** The application of these principles minimizes the energy required to sit, stand, and walk. When you use these principles to perform tasks that require stooping, lifting, pushing, pulling, and carrying, your effective strength is increased and you are less likely to injure yourself. When you injure yourself on the job, you place a greater burden on the other team members. If you injure yourself while lifting a patient, you may injure the patient as well. Severe strains may require hospitalization and long-term therapy involving considerable pain, inconvenience, and expense. Applied principles of body mechanics prevent the muscle strains that are common among hospital workers, including the types of work injuries most frequently reported by radiographers.

Three concepts are essential to understanding the principles of body mechanics (Fig. 4-6):

1. **Base of support.** This is the portion of the body in contact with the floor or other horizontal surface. It may be represented by a horizontal line linking the points of contact, such as between the feet when the body is erect. A broad base of support provides stability for body position and movement.
2. **Center of gravity,** or center of body weight. This is the point around which body weight is balanced. It is usually located in the midportion of the pelvis or lower abdomen, but the location may vary somewhat depending on body build. Any object you hold adds to the weight on the base of support, so a load's size and position affect the location of your center of gravity. The body is most stable when the center of gravity is nearest the center of the base of support.
3. **Line of gravity.** This is an imaginary vertical line passing through the center of gravity. The body is most stable when the line of gravity bisects the base of support.

With the use of these concepts, the principles of body mechanics can be stated in the five simple rules

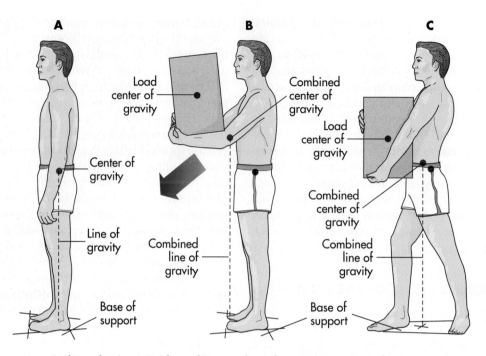

FIG. 4-6 Body mechanics. **A,** With good posture, line of gravity bisects base of support. **B,** When load is held away from the body, line of gravity does not bisect base of support. **C,** A wide stance with load held close to the body allows combined line of gravity to bisect base of support.

printed in Box 4-3. Memorizing them is easy. Smooth performance requires practice.

Bending and twisting the back while lifting is a common cause of back strain (Fig. 4-7). A broad and stable base of support can be easily accomplished by standing with feet apart and one foot slightly advanced. Remember that your thigh muscles are among the strongest in your body. Good body mechanics uses the combined strength of your legs, arms, and abdomen to protect the shorter, more vulnerable back muscles. Think ahead, and use the resources available to you when anticipating a task that may cause muscle strain. These resources include adjusting the height of your work surface, using a cart to move a heavy load, or obtaining help to lift heavy objects. Note the proper use of body mechanics as you study the sections on patient transfer later in this chapter.

POSITIONING FOR SAFETY AND COMFORT

Common body positions have names. It is easier to communicate with other members of the health care team and to follow physicians' orders if you are familiar with these terms (Fig. 4-8).

The term *recumbent* refers to any position in which the patient is lying down. *Supine* (Fig. 4-8, *A*) defines the position in which the patient is lying on his or her back. This is the usual position for

---

BOX 4-3

RULES OF BODY MECHANICS

1. Provide a broad base of support.
2. Work at a comfortable height.
3. When lifting, bend your knees and keep your back straight (see Fig. 4-7, *B*).
4. Keep your load well balanced and close to your body (see Fig. 4-6, *C*).
5. Roll or push a heavy object. Avoid pulling or lifting.

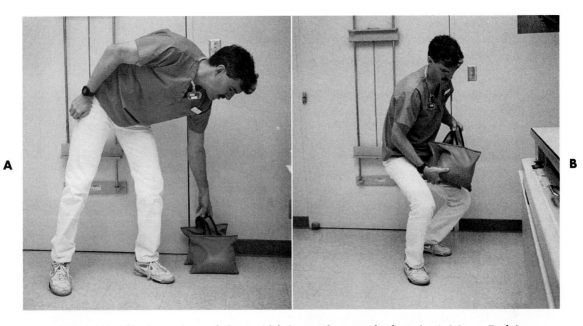

FIG. 4-7 Good body mechanics helps avoid fatigue and prevent back strain. **A,** Wrong. Back is bent and twisted. **B,** Right. Knees are flexed, and back is straight.

stretcher transfers and is also a common radiographic position. When lying face down, the patient is said to be *prone* (Fig. 4-8, *B*). *Lateral recumbent* denotes that the patient is lying on one side. This term may be modified by adding *right* or *left* to indicate which side is in contact with the bed or table. The patient in Fig. 4-8, *C* is in the left lateral recumbent position. The Sims' position (Fig. 4-8, *D*) is a comfortable position that is sometimes used for rectal examination and for taking a rectal temperature; it is the best position for enema administration. Fowler's position (Fig. 4-8, *E*) is a modification of the supine position in which the patient's upper body is elevated. The semi-Fowler's position (Fig. 4-8, *F*) is a modification of the Fowler's position in which the upper body is only partially elevated. In the Trendelenburg position (Fig. 4-8, *G*), the patient's head is lower than the feet. Usually the table is tilted approximately 15°. This position is used during some radiographic and fluoroscopic procedures and is helpful in the treatment of patients suffering from shock. The knee-chest position (Fig. 4-8, *H*) and the lithotomy position (Fig. 4-8, *I*) are not commonly used by radiographers,

but are standard positions used by physicians and nurses in diagnostic examinations and therapeutic procedures.

Support and Padding

When lying on a hard surface such as a radiographic table, patients are more comfortable with radiolucent sponges or cushions strategically placed for support. If a cushion or pillow under the head will not be a hindrance to the examination, it can enable the patient to see what is occurring and thus help relieve apprehension. Elevation of the patient's head also relieves neck strain, allows easier breathing, and helps avoid the uncomfortable sensation that the head is lower than the feet.

A bolster under the knees of a supine patient relieves lumbosacral stress by straightening the **lordotic** (concave) lumbar curve. This is especially comforting to arthritic and **kyphotic** patients (those with a pronounced convex curvature in the upper back) and to most elderly persons. Bolsters are essential for patients with spine injuries and those who have recently undergone spinal or abdominal surgery. Patients with abdominal pain must have the

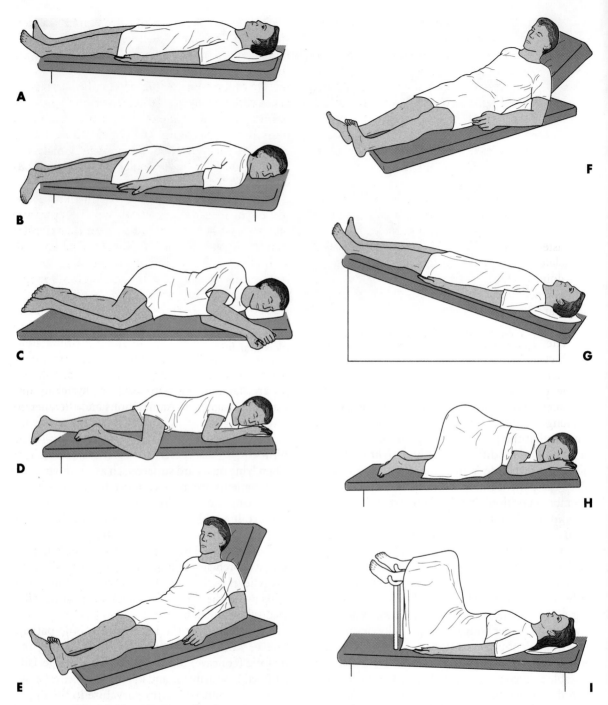

FIG. 4-8 Identification of body positions. **A,** Supine. **B,** Prone. **C,** Lateral recumbent. **D,** Sims'.
E, Fowler's. **F,** Semi-Fowler's. **G,** Trendelenburg. **H,** Knee-chest. **I,** Lithotomy.

head elevated and a bolster under the knees to relieve strain on the abdomen.

The measures used to promote comfort are frequently the same interventions designed to prevent complications. When the body is supine, the weight of the abdominal contents pushes the diaphragm up into the thoracic cavity, making it more difficult to take a deep breath. This is no problem for most of us, but patients who become short of breath when supine must be assisted to sit up immediately.

Patients who are nauseated also need to have their heads elevated, since this position helps control nausea and prevents aspiration of **emesis** if the patient vomits. Patients who become nauseated and cannot be assisted to the Fowler's position should be rolled into a lateral recumbent position.

Padding placed under body prominences, such as the sacrum, heels, or midthoracic curvature, is important for several reasons (Fig. 4-9). One reason is that if patients are reasonably comfortable, they are better able to maintain the positions needed for an effective examination, even on a hard surface. Another reason is that many older or **debilitated** (feeble) patients develop ulcerated areas over prominent bony structures when pressure is exerted for any length of time. These lesions are referred to as **decubitus ulcers** or bedsores.

The cause of decubitus ulcers is simple to understand and important to remember. Pressure on a limited area of tissue inhibits circulation, depriving the cells of oxygen and nutrition. The cells in the middle of the area are affected first. If the pressure is not relieved and circulation restored within a few minutes, the cells in the central portion die and an ulcer forms. Weak or debilitated patients may be in a poor nutritional state and have impaired circulation. Thus the ulcers frequently do not heal well and may even require skin grafting.

A circle or "doughnut" ring is an ineffective type of padding to use. Although it does prevent pressure on a specific bony prominence, it restricts circulation to the central area by placing the pressure all around it. It is preferable to distribute weight over as large an area as possible. Sets of radiolucent sponges in various shapes and sizes are available in the radiology department for this purpose (Fig. 4-10).

If a patient will be in one position on the x-ray table for longer than 10 minutes, a full-size radiolucent pad should be used. This is an important consideration for patients undergoing extended studies such as small bowel series or excretory urograms for obstructive urinary conditions. If a debilitated patient must be left on the table or on a stretcher for an extended time, the radiographer should assist the patient in changing positions periodically to relieve pressure and maintain circulation.

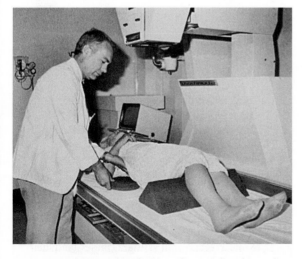

FIG. 4-9 Padding provides comfort and safety when positioning older patients.

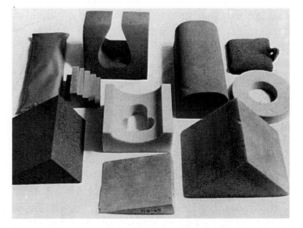

FIG. 4-10 Assortment of positioning aids.

Empathy for patients is enhanced by experiencing what they feel during an x-ray examination. Practice positioning with your classmates until comfort and positioning are part of the same action.

Skin Care

Precautions must be taken to protect the skin while moving and positioning patients. Rough handling or sliding against the table surface may injure the skin of elderly or debilitated patients. A subcutaneous fat layer cushions the skin of young persons, but this underlying padding decreases as we age and may be nonexistent in the elderly. When the subcutaneous fat layer is lost, any shear pressure can cause the skin to tear and bleed. The skin of the feet and legs is especially delicate on patients whose circulation is compromised; you must pay special attention to avoid bumping this skin. Do not wear jewelry on hands or wrists that could injure a patient during the process of moving or positioning. Even very minor contusions or abrasions may increase the likelihood of decubitus ulcer formation.

For the same reason, you must keep the patient clean and dry. Patients who perspire heavily or who are incontinent of urine or feces may develop skin irritation that predisposes to ulcer formation.

PATIENT TRANSFER

When patients are moved from one place to another in the hospital, wheeled transport is required. Patients may believe they can walk to the radiology department, but they must not be allowed to do so. If an ambulatory patient becomes weak or faint in a corridor or elevator during the trip, there is no safe way to cope. Likewise, infants and small children should not be carried to the radiology department. A change in the patient's status may require that you have both hands free to deal with the problem or to obtain help.

The usual method of transport is to use a wheelchair for patients who can stand and sit with safety and comfort, and to use a stretcher for those who cannot. Patients who cannot stand, and those who have not stood or walked since an accident, surgery, stroke, or heart attack, should not be transported by wheelchair. These patients must not be allowed to stand or walk in the radiology department, even if they believe they are capable of doing so. A stretcher is also the best means of transfer for patients who have had recent trauma and/or surgery to the spine.

When a patient's condition makes it extremely difficult or hazardous to move onto a stretcher, the patient may be moved in the bed. Bed transfers require at least two people because the bed is heavy and cumbersome, and patients who must be transferred in bed require careful attention to their physical status during transfer. They may also require considerable auxiliary equipment.

Active infants and toddlers are often transported in their cribs. The high sides of the crib provide greater safety than the side rails of the stretcher, and the crib provides a safe place if the child must be left unattended at any time. Premature infants may be transported in an Isolette.

Preparation for Transfer

The steps of preparing for patient transfer are summarized in Box 4-4. Always check with the nursing station, and obtain the patient's chart before transferring a patient to the radiology department. The nursing service must be advised because they are responsible for knowing the patient's whereabouts

---

BOX 4-4

PREPARING FOR SAFE PATIENT TRANSFER

1. Check with nursing service, and obtain the chart.
2. Check patient identification.
3. Plan what you are going to do, and prepare your work area.
4. Obtain equipment, and check it for safety and function.
5. Enlist the patient's help and cooperation. Remember to tell the patient what you are doing as you proceed.
6. Obtain additional help when necessary. Check to make certain your assistants understand their role in the transfer plan.

at all times. In addition, nurses can often provide you with helpful information about the patient's transfer requirements, and they may also provide assistance in the transfer if needed.

The next step in safely moving a patient is to be certain that you have the right patient. Check the identification bracelet against the requisition, and ask the patient to tell you his or her name as a double check.

A brief visit with the patient will assist in assessing how much the patient can help with the transfer, allowing you to plan for additional hands if needed to ensure a safe move. Decide on the safest, easiest method of moving your patient, obtain the necessary equipment, and check that it is functional and safe. The person transporting the patient is responsible for ensuring that the buckles on safety straps are secure, that side rails lock in the "up" position, and that brakes work properly. Move any furniture or obstacles that may be in the way.

Take note of any special equipment that may need to be transported with the patient, such as monitors or medication pumps. A urine collection bag may need to be detached from the bed. Portable oxygen equipment may be needed if the patient is currently receiving oxygen from a wall outlet. Other equipment may need to be disconnected or rearranged before patient transfer, but consult with the nursing service before disconnecting any equipment.

Next tell the patient what you plan to do, and explain his or her role in the transfer. Since patients can often anticipate painful errors, the radiographer should listen carefully and allow the patient to participate in the plan.

Once the patient is safely moved to the stretcher or wheelchair, check that safety rails or straps are in place and that the patient is comfortable and adequately covered for warmth and modesty. Have you forgotten anything? An emesis basin or a small box of tissues may be handy along the way. Don't forget the chart!

Wheelchair Transfers

Transferring a patient from a bed to a wheelchair may seem elementary, but it is a common cause of falls and accidents. The correct technique makes this procedure safer and easier (Fig. 4-11).

Start by lowering the bed to the level of the wheelchair seat and elevating the head of the bed. Position the wheelchair parallel to the bed with wheels locked and footrests out of the way. Place one arm under the patient's shoulders, one under the knees, and in a single, smooth motion, raise and turn the patient to a sitting position with his or her feet dangling over the side.

Take a moment to assist the patient with slippers and a robe and allow time for the patient to regain a sense of balance. After long periods of rest, many patients have **orthostatic hypotension,** a mild reduction in the oxygen supply to the brain that occurs with changes in body position and may cause them to feel light-headed or faint when rising suddenly.

At this point, most competent patients are able to stand and move to the wheelchair with little assistance, although a steadying hand at the patient's elbow is a good practice. The weak patient needs additional help.

If assistance is required, stand facing the patient, reach around the patient and place your hands firmly over the scapulae; the patient's hands may rest on your shoulders. On your signal, lift upward and help the patient rise to a standing position. Alternatively, a transfer belt around the patient's waist will provide a secure handhold for you to use in helping the patient stand. Remember to use a broad base of support and keep your back straight.

Now instruct and assist the patient to pivot a quarter turn so that the edge of the wheelchair is touching the back of the patient's knees, and ease the patient into a sitting position in the chair. Position the footrests and leg rests, and cover the patient's lap and legs with a sheet or bath blanket to provide warmth and comfort and protect the patient's modesty.

To move the patient from wheelchair to x-ray table, follow the steps illustrated in Fig. 4-12. Place the wheelchair parallel to the table, lock the brakes, and move footrests out of the way. At this point the procedure will vary, depending on whether you are fortunate enough to have an x-ray table that is adjustable in height.

If the height of the x-ray table is adjustable, lower the table to chair height. In this instance the transfer

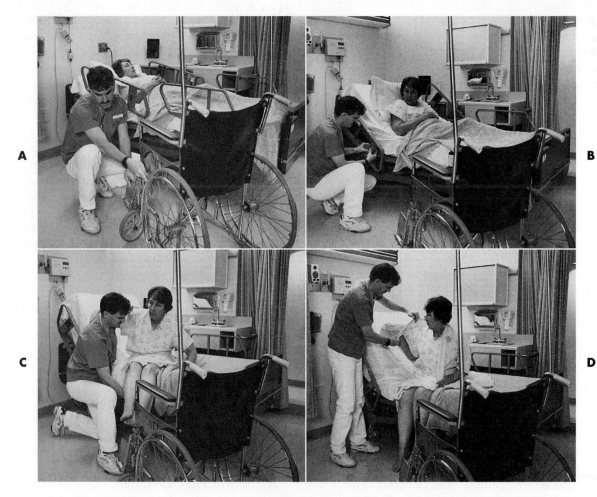

FIG. 4-11 Wheelchair transfer. **A,** Position wheelchair parallel to patient's bed with wheels locked and footrests out of the way. **B,** Lower bed and side rails; lift patient to a sitting position. **C,** Pivot while lifting, allowing patient's legs to clear edge of bed. **D,** Allow patient to rest briefly before standing.

to the x-ray table is the reverse of the transfer from the bed. Using the face-to-face assistance explained previously, help the patient to stand and pivot with the patient's back to the table. Then ease the patient into a sitting position on the edge of the table.

If the table height is stationary, position a step stool with a tall handle nearby. Have the patient place one hand on the stool handle, put one arm on your shoulder, and step up onto the stool, pivoting with the back to the table. Now ease the patient to a sitting position.

Once the patient is seated on the table, place one arm around the patient's shoulders and one under the knees. With a single, smooth motion, place the patient's legs on the table while lowering the head and shoulders into the supine position.

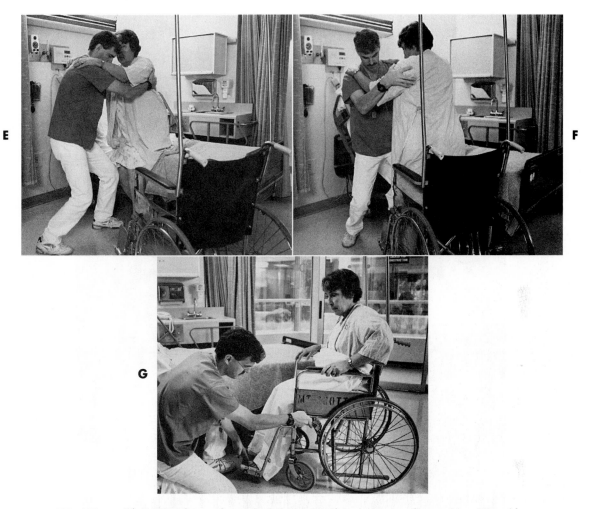

FIG. 4-11—cont'd **E,** Using face-to-face assist, help raise weak patient to standing position. **F,** Provide support as patient eases into wheelchair. **G,** Cover patient's lap and legs; adjust leg and footrests.

The most common type of fall associated with wheelchair transfer occurs when the patient backs into the wheelchair to sit down. The patient may miss the edge of the seat or tip the chair by sitting too near the edge. To avoid such an accident, be sure to lock the wheels of the chair and assist the patient until seated securely.

Special considerations for wheelchair transfers

Stroke. Stroke patients typically have weakness of one side of the body. Determine which side is the patient's weak side, and position yourself on that side. Brace the patient's weak leg with your knee as the patient stands as illustrated in Fig. 4-12, *A.* When moving from the wheelchair to a bed or table, position the patient with the strong side adjacent to the bed or table and instruct the patient to lead with the strong leg. If the patient is totally paralyzed, a two- or three-person lift (see p. 116) from the wheelchair is required; a stretcher is preferred.

Fractures of the lower extremity. Lower-extremity fractures limit the patient's ability to bear weight, but as recovery progresses a patient may be able to bear weight on an extremity that is immobilized in a cast

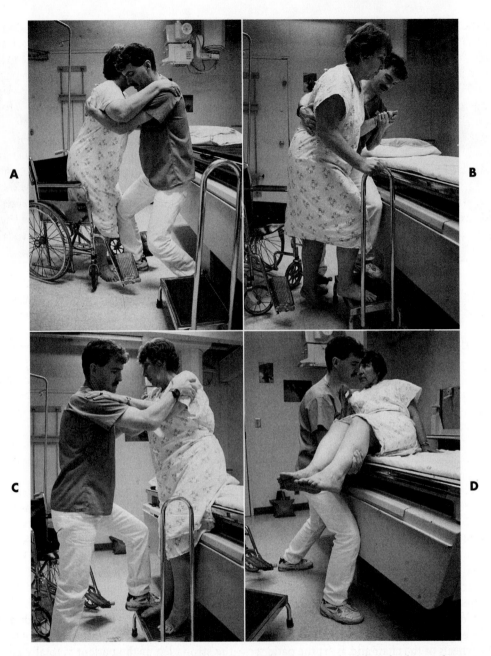

FIG. 4-12 Assisting patient onto radiographic table. **A,** Lock wheelchair brakes and move footrests. Assist patient to stand. **B,** Assist patient with step stool, if necessary. **C,** Assist patient to pivot and sit on table. **D,** Support patient's shoulders while raising legs onto table; ease to supine position.

or splint, thus permitting transport by wheelchair. Skills used to assist the stroke victim are also useful in this case. Support the patient from the affected side and encourage the patient to lead with the strong leg. Elevate the leg rest of the wheelchair to support the injured leg during the transfer, and help the patient lift the leg when changing position. Take care that the fractured limb is not twisted or bumped during transfer. Similar precautions are appropriate for the patient with an undiagnosed leg injury who is sufficiently stable to permit wheelchair transfer.

Joint replacements. Joint replacement surgery demands that the patient receive special care, especially when being transferred during the recovery period. Restrictions vary in accordance with the surgical approach that was used (Box 4-5). Motion must be restricted to avoid stress on muscles that have been surgically disrupted, so always check the chart to determine a patient's limitations.

Hip replacement. Patients who have undergone hip replacement via the anterior surgical approach are able to sit upright in a chair at a 90° angle. Do not permit the patient to adduct, abduct, or rotate the affected leg, and avoid hyperextension, especially when walking.

Patients who have undergone hip replacement via the posterior approach, which is most common, are able to tolerate abduction but must not be allowed to cross the affected leg over the midline; both adduction and internal rotation must be avoided. In addition, *these patients must not flex at the hip beyond 90°.* These restrictions prevent stress on the posterior capsule, which needs time to heal and strengthen

after surgery. During the first month after surgery, patients will be transported by stretcher. If they need to sit up for any reason, take care that they do not bend forward, since most dislocations occur when the patient bends forward past 90°, as when getting up from a low chair. Patients are at some risk of dislocation for up to a year after surgery.

Knee replacement. Knee replacement surgery requires similar considerations when transferring the patient. Weight bearing is usually tolerated, but a walker should be used if the patient will be taking more than one or two steps. Move the patient toward the strong side and place support under the calf and knee of the affected leg to provide comfort and safety.

Spine trauma or spinal surgery. Patients suffering from spinal trauma or recovering from recent spinal surgery should generally be transferred by stretcher. As recovery progresses, wheelchair transfer may be tolerable and safe. Moving from a supine position to a sitting position, or from sitting to supine, places considerable stress on the spine. It is preferable for the patient to sit from the lateral recumbent position. When lying down, the patient should lie first on one side and then turn to the supine position with the knees flexed. Provide support and assistance to the patient while extending the legs, and place a bolster or pillow under the knees for support when supine.

Paralyzed patients. Inpatients who are paralyzed or unable to stand for any reason are always transported within the hospital by stretcher, but outpatients who are paralyzed or unable to stand may arrive at the hospital in a wheelchair. Depending on

BOX 4-5

PRECAUTIONS FOR PATIENTS WITH HIP REPLACEMENTS

SURGERY VIA THE ANTERIOR APPROACH
May sit upright
Weight bearing is usually tolerated (check chart)
Avoid abduction
Avoid adduction
Avoid internal or external rotation
Avoid hyperextension

SURGERY VIA THE POSTERIOR APPROACH
Must not flex hip beyond 90°
Weight bearing is usually tolerated (check chart)
Abduction is permitted
Avoid adduction
Avoid internal rotation

the design of the chair and the requirements of the procedure, extremity examinations and chest radiography may be performed with the patient seated in the wheelchair, but most procedures will require that the patient be placed on the radiographic table. This requires a two- or three-person lift.

Two-person lift. If the patient is not too heavy, two people can perform the lift from the wheelchair to the table (Fig. 4-13). The stronger of the two is the primary lifter and the second person assists. First place the wheelchair parallel to the table and lock the wheels. Then remove the chair arm that is nearest the table if possible. Instruct the patient to cross both arms across the chest. The primary lifter then stands behind the chair and reaches around the patient, extending his or her arms through the patient's axillae and grasping the patient's forearms from the top. The assistant kneels on one knee near the patient's feet and cradles the patient's thighs in one arm and the lower legs in the other. On signal, both lift together and place the patient gently on the table.

Three-person lift. The three-person lift is similar to the two-person lift and is safer if the patient's weight is too much for two people to lift easily (Fig. 4-14). In this case, remove both arms of the wheelchair and position the first two lifters as for the two-person lift.

The third lifter kneels on one knee at the side of the chair farthest from the table, placing one arm around the patient's waist and the other under the buttocks. Then all lift together on signal. The role of the third lifter is primarily to assist in raising the patient from the chair. The wheelchair will block any forward motion of the third lifter, so the first two lifters must complete the transfer.

If your facility has a hydraulic lift, this is the safest method for lifting a paralyzed patient or a very obese patient. Specially trained personnel will usually bring this equipment and operate it when it is needed. Do not attempt to use this equipment until you have been properly instructed in its safe use.

Stretcher Transfers

A stretcher, sometimes called a cart or gurney, should be used to transport any patient who is unable to stand safely. This is also the method of choice for patients who cannot sit comfortably for an extended period. Remember that the patient may have to wait in the imaging department before or after the examination. A weak patient who cannot stand may be under a physician's order to sit in a chair as part of the daily routine. A visit to the radiology department should not be seized as an opportunity to meet this requirement. Such patients can be moved from chair

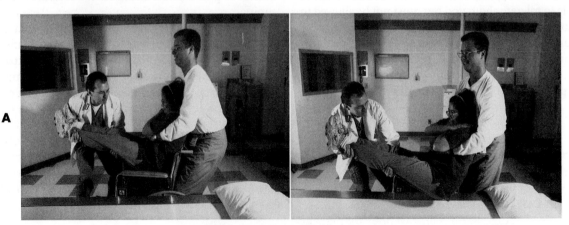

A   **B**

FIG. 4-13 **A,** Primary lifter stands behind the chair and reaches around the patient, extending his arms through the patient's axillae and grasping her arms from the top. The assistant kneels on one knee, cradling the patient's thighs and legs. **B,** On signal, both lift together and place the patient gently on the table.

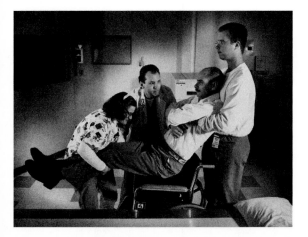

FIG. 4-14 Three-person lift is much like the two-person lift, with the third person helping to raise the patient's hips until they are clear of the chair.

to bed more easily than from chair to x-ray table, especially if the x-ray table height cannot be adjusted. If you have any doubt about the patient's ability to transfer safely from the chair to the table, be safe and start with a stretcher.

If the patient's safety or comfort requires elevation of the head, select a stretcher that provides upper body support. The following stretcher transfer techniques may be used to move patients to the stretcher from either the bed or the radiographic table. If the patient is able to assist and is not too heavy, you may be able to accomplish the stretcher transfer by yourself. Obtain the help of one or more other persons if the patient is obese or very weak.

Provide for the patient's privacy by closing the door to the hallway or drawing the curtain around the bed. Start with the patient near the edge of the bed in the supine position with knees flexed and feet flat. Adjust the bed and the stretcher to the flat horizontal position, and adjust the height of the bed to the height of the stretcher. Position the stretcher parallel to the bed and lock the wheels. Check to be certain that oxygen lines, intravenous tubing, and urinary catheters are free and will not be pulled during the transfer.

If you are working alone, lean across the stretcher, placing one arm under the patient's shoulders and

the other arm under the pelvis. On your instructions, have the patient push with feet and elbows as you lift and pull the patient toward the stretcher. Do not attempt to make the transfer in a single motion. The maneuver may be repeated several times until the transfer is complete.

If you are working with an assistant, one person supports the head, neck, and shoulders while the second person lifts at the pelvis and knees (Fig. 4-15). Both use the lift-pull motion with the patient's assistance until the patient is safely positioned on the stretcher.

As soon as the patient is safely situated on the stretcher, cover the patient and secure the safety straps or side rails. Elevate the head of the stretcher, if needed. Before you leave the room, check to be certain you have everything else you will need. The patient's chart may be slipped under the pillow and other equipment may be placed at the foot of the stretcher beside the patient's feet.

To reverse this transfer, position the stretcher parallel to the bed, lock the wheels, and lower the side rails. Return the stretcher to the flat horizontal position if the head has been elevated; move any equipment out of the way. Since beds are wider than stretchers, it may be easier to work from the stretcher side. Position and support the patient as before. This time, on signal, the patient pushes toward the bed while you assist with a lift-push motion. Repeat as required until the transfer is complete. This same method may be applied to transfers from the stretcher to the x-ray table, but it may be easier to reach across the table and pull the patient toward you.

Various techniques are used for stretcher transfers, depending on the patient's weight and ability to assist. With problem transfers, it is best to obtain experienced help. Two methods of transfer involve the use of draw sheets and slide boards. These are often useful when the patient is unable to assist with the transfer. Practice these transfers in class before attempting to use them with patients.

Draw sheet transfers

Patients who need frequent help with moving are often placed on a "draw" or "pull" sheet. This is a single sheet folded in half that is placed under the

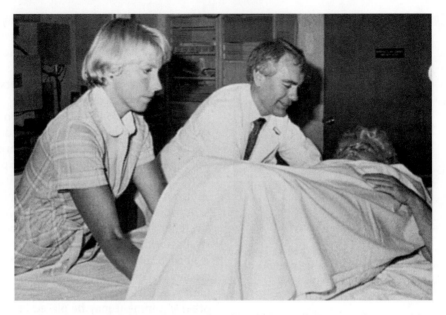

FIG. 4-15 Conventional stretcher transfer. Allow patient to help as much as possible.

patient and over the middle third of the bed. When moving the patient, the edges of the draw sheet are loosened from the bed and rolled up close to the patient's body (Fig. 4-16). The rolled edge provides a handhold for lifting and pulling the patient. Care must be taken that the patient's head and feet move safely with the trunk of the body, which requires two or more persons.

Slide board transfers

The slide board transfer is a variation of the draw sheet method that employs a strong sheet of smooth plastic large enough to support the patient's body with handholds cut into the edges. The patient is rolled to one side and the board is slipped below the draw sheet and about halfway under the patient's body (Fig. 4-17). The remaining width of the board covers the space between the stretcher and the bed. With the patient's arms folded safely across the chest, two persons grip the draw sheet and slide the patient safely and smoothly across the board.

Note: Flexible slide boards must not be used in place of rigid backboards for spinal immobilization.

Safety straps and rails

Stretchers are equipped with safety straps or side rails to ensure that patients will not fall or attempt to climb off without assistance. This is especially important when the patient's state of consciousness is impaired because of **sedation** (calming medication), intoxication, shock, or senility. Application of straps or side rails during transport is such an important safety practice that it must be followed without exception (Fig. 4-18).

RESTRAINTS AND IMMOBILIZATION

Restraints and immobilization methods are used to ensure patient safety and to prevent undesired motion during imaging procedures.

Patients who are active and disoriented may require physical restraints. These may consist of wrist and ankle bands and/or a vest with straps tied to the bed or stretcher. Student radiographers sometimes feel uncomfortable about using such measures, especially when patients find them objectionable. It is helpful to remember that their purpose is to aid and protect the patient. Although restraints

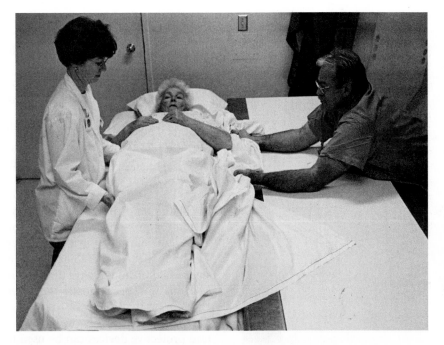

FIG. 4-16 Draw sheet transfer.

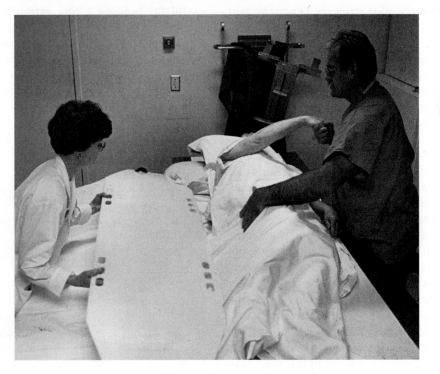

FIG. 4-17 Slide board eases stretcher transfer.

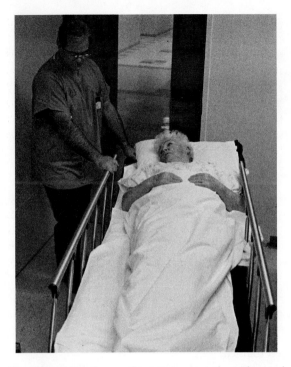

FIG. 4-18 Side rails or safety straps must always be used on stretchers.

may be annoying to patients, they are neither painful nor harmful when properly used. Restraints are almost always fitted before the patient comes to the radiology department. The same restraints used by the nursing service may be employed by the radiographer. *Remember that the application of these physical restraints on an adult patient requires a physician's order.* Liability for a charge of false imprisonment may result from the unauthorized use of restraints.

Safety straps or side rails are used on beds and stretchers to prevent falls when patients are asleep, weak, disoriented, or sedated. Safety straps or compression bands may be used on the x-ray table during waiting periods as a precaution against falling. Patients whose motion is restricted by safety devices must be monitored carefully. Never leave a patient who is unable to change position unattended. Difficulty breathing or the need to cough or vomit may require an immediate position change. The patient's inability to respond to this need may pose a serious hazard; so if you must leave the room,

another qualified person must be assigned to attend the patient. When patients are coherent and cooperative and are neither sedated nor in distress, the decision to leave them alone for a brief period must be based on existing hospital or departmental policy. Some departments have rules that do not allow any patient ever to be left unattended.

Several methods may be used to aid in the immobilization of adults who have difficulty remaining still. When tremors complicate the procedure, it is useful to support the patient as comfortably as possible. Placing either a compression band across the abdomen or the knees or a sandbag across an extremity proximal to the area of interest can provide stabilization during radiography.

Although it is preferable to win the confidence of small children and to have them submit willingly to examination, occasionally you must immobilize children for their safety or to meet technical procedure requirements. The weight of a sandbag or of lead protective devices can be used to aid in maintaining position. Sheets of translucent plastic are useful for holding a tiny extremity in position against a cassette. Tape can also be used to maintain a position if it is not in direct contact with the patient's skin. Tape will hold a tiny finger in position on a cassette, or strap a small patient's hips to maintain a supine position on the x-ray table. Be certain that cloth or a tissue protects the skin from the

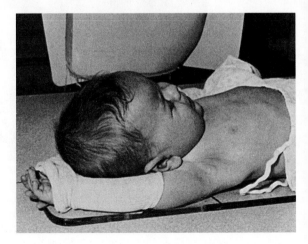

FIG. 4-19 Stockinet may be used to immobilize arms or legs.

adhesive surface of the tape, or twist the tape so that the nonadhesive side is against the patient. Stockinet can be used to immobilize the legs or applied to keep the patient's arms above the head (Fig. 4-19).

Fig. 4-20 demonstrates the mummy wrap method to immobilize an infant or a small child. Fold down the top edge of a small sheet or lightweight blanket to form an inverted triangle. Place the child supine with shoulders just below the fold. Pull one point of the sheet across one arm, tuck it behind the back, and pull it through to the opposite side. Wrap this same point around the second arm, and tuck it securely under the patient. Then grasp the second point and wrap it across the chest, and tuck it behind the back.

Immobilization equipment, such as circumcision boards and other specialty devices, is commercially available to help immobilize children simply and effectively. Fig. 4-21 demonstrates the Tame-Em Immobilizer, an adjustable device with Velcro straps that is helpful in positioning and holding infants. Fig. 4-22 shows the Papoose Board for children 2 to 6 years old. The Pigg-O-Stat infant chair (Fig. 4-23) holds infants and toddlers firmly in the correct upright position for chest radiography. This device incorporates a film holder and gonad shielding.

ACCIDENTS AND INCIDENT REPORTS

Any fall, accident, or occurrence that results in injury or potential harm must be immediately reported to the departmental supervisor and/or the radiologist. As soon as the victim has been attended

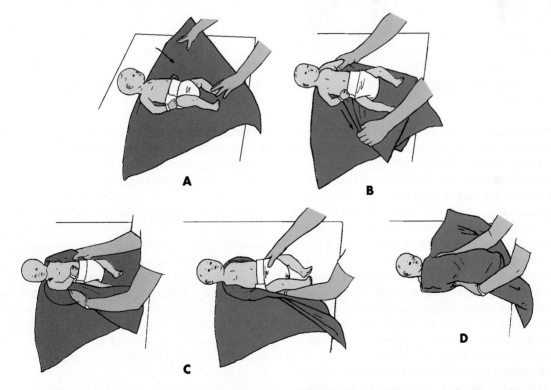

FIG. 4-20 Mummy wrap technique for infant immobilization. **A,** Fold the sheet on the diagonal to make a triangle. **B,** Wrap one corner up over an arm, tuck it under the body, and pull it through to the other side. **C,** Wrap the first corner under the second arm, and tuck it under the body. **D,** Wrap the second corner over the chest, and secure it under the body.

Continued

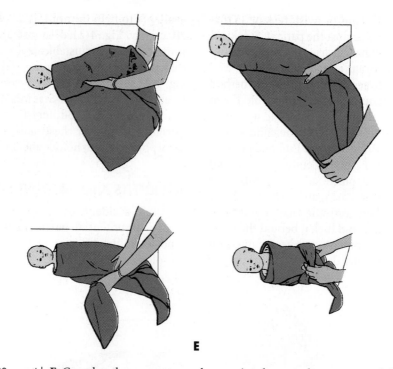

E

FIG. 4-20—cont'd **E,** Complete the mummy wrap by securing the second corner around the child.

to properly, an incident report (sometimes called an unusual occurrence form) must be completed. Reporting incidents is essential whether the victim is a patient, a visitor, or a member of the hospital staff. Do not hesitate to report incidents in which you are injured, even if the injury may seem minor at the time. If the injured person is a patient, the details of the incident must also be recorded in the patient's chart.

Incident reports are crucial to the institution's risk management program. They aid in establishing or limiting the institutional liability for any injury and in documenting the need for changes that may improve safety practices in the future. Appendix E provides an example of a hospital incident report form.

Occasionally a very minor incident may not seem to require the formal procedures of an incident report. It is always a good idea to keep a record of any unusual occurrence in case it should later turn out to be of greater consequence than was originally apparent. Making a note of such events in the patient's chart or on the requisition form provides an important record if questions or consequences develop regarding the event.

The decision as to whether a particular occurrence merits an incident report is a judgment call. For example, a simple sneeze should not prompt an incident report; a severe asthmatic attack is a reportable occurrence. A very mild asthmatic episode that is successfully self-treated by an outpatient with the patient's own medication is an example of a situation where judgment will vary with individuals. The ability to make these kinds of judgments develops with experience. The student radiographer should consult a supervisor when such questions arise. When in doubt, err on the side of caution by filing a report.

CONCLUSION

Safety is the principle underlying everything discussed in this chapter. With safety in mind, think

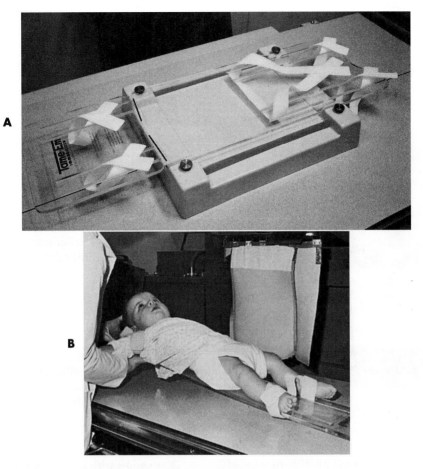

FIG. 4-21 **A,** Tame-Em adjustable infant immobilizer made of Lucite with Velcro straps.
B, Device in use.

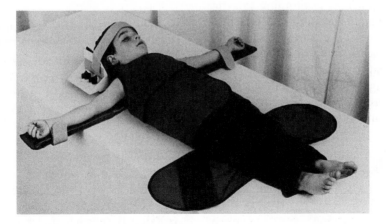

FIG. 4-22 Papoose Board provides selective restraints for children 2 to 6 years of age.

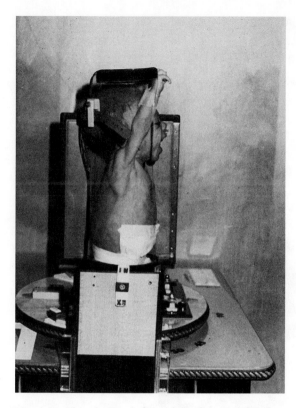

FIG. 4-23 Pigg-O-Stat infant chair for upright chest radiography.

before you act, be conscious of hazards, and plan to avoid accidents.

Knowledge of safety rules is indispensable to the radiographer. Whether responding to a fire, transporting a patient, or positioning a patient on the x-ray table, the objective is to protect patients when they are unable to protect themselves.

When an accident or something unusual occurs, protect your patient, yourself, and your institution by responding appropriately and by documenting the event with the prescribed forms and procedures of your institution.

REVIEW QUESTIONS

1. The most likely cause of a fire in an imaging department is:
   A. spontaneous combustion
   B. open flames
   C. cigarette smoking
   D. electrical problem
   E. heating system
2. Which of the following positions is considered safe for a patient who is nauseated and may vomit?
   A. supine
   B. prone
   C. Fowler's
   D. lateral recumbent
   E. both C and D
3. A slide board can be used to:
   A. evacuate the area
   B. immobilize a child
   C. facilitate a stretcher transfer
   D. provide comfort on the x-ray table
4. A spill kit should contain:
   A. nitrile gloves
   B. dustpan
   C. kitty litter
   D. plastic bags
   E. all of the above
5. Which of the following is NOT a responsibility of the radiographer in case of fire:
   A. assess the situation and direct the activities of others
   B. evacuate the immediate area
   C. report the fire using the proper procedure
   D. stand by with the appropriate fire extinguisher
   E. reassure patients so that they do not become alarmed

CRITICAL THINKING EXERCISES

1. List ways that you can use principles of good body mechanics recommended at work to increase your safety at home.
2. Your supervisor has sent you to bring Elizabeth Nelson to the radiography department for a lower gastrointestinal series. List considerations that would help you determine whether to transfer Ms. Nelson by wheelchair or by stretcher. How would you get the information to make this decision?
3. Ralph Barnes has undergone hip replacement surgery within the past week and has been

brought to the radiography department by stretcher for follow-up x-rays of his hip. How would the surgical approach (anterior or posterior) affect requirements for assisting Mr. Barnes from the wheelchair to the radiographic table? How would you know which type of surgery Mr. Barnes had undergone? Describe the precautions needed following both types of surgery.

4. While you are helping Ella Christopherson into a wheelchair, she puts her weight on the footrest causing the chair to tip and bump her leg. Mrs. Christopherson says, "Ouch!" and rubs her leg; but when you ask whether she is all right, she smiles and insists that she is fine. Should you file an incident report? Why or why not?

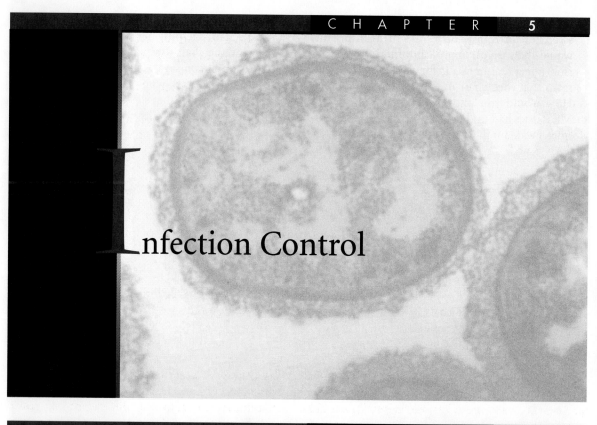

CHAPTER 5

Infection Control

At the conclusion of this chapter, the student will be able to:

- Define medical asepsis, disinfection, and sterilization.
- List six factors involved in the cycle of infection.
- State five examples of personal hygiene that help to prevent the spread of infection.
- Demonstrate techniques for effective hand hygiene.
- Describe the correct method of linen disposal using medical asepsis principles.
- Name the agent and state the dilution used for disinfecting radiographic equipment, as recommended by the Centers for Disease Control and Prevention (CDC).
- Demonstrate proper disposal of contaminated equipment in the clinical area.
- Contrast isolation techniques for infectious and immunodeficient patients.
- Demonstrate removal and disposal of gowns, gloves, and masks without breaking isolation principles.
- List and describe six main routes of infection transmission.

V O C A B U L A R Y

airborne contamination	nosocomial infection
asepsis	opportunistic infection
autoclave	pathogen
direct contact	phagocytosis
disinfection	spore
droplet contamination	sterile conscience
endospore	sterile field
epidemic	sterilization
fomite	vector
immunosuppressant	vehicle
microbial dilution	virulence factors

BECAUSE HOSPITALS ARE GATHERING PLACES for the sick, they are also focal points for the transmission of disease. Anyone with a health problem is more susceptible to infection, and therefore infection control is of critical importance in patient care.

As a member of the health care team, it is your professional duty to follow established infection control policies. This will promote the safety of patients, yourself, and other members of the health care team. The emergence of new diseases, the return of old ones, and the development of hospital-acquired, multidrug-resistant infections make it even more important for these policies to be followed and for everyone to play a role in preventing the spread of infection.

MICROORGANISMS

Microorganisms are living organisms that are too small to be seen with the naked eye. They include bacteria, viruses, protozoa, prions, and fungi. Most microorganisms do not cause disease and are essential for our well-being. Microorganisms that live on or inside the body without causing disease are referred to as normal microbial flora. They aid in skin preservation and digestion and protect us from infection. Microorganisms that cause disease are called **pathogens,** and their harmful effects will be discussed later in this chapter (see Infectious Organisms).

Bacteria

Bacteria are very small, single-cell organisms with a cell wall and an atypical nucleus that lacks a membrane (Fig. 5-1). The cell wall is essential for survival of the bacterium, making it the target for destruction by some antibiotics.

Bacteria grow independently and do not need a host cell to replicate. They are classified according to shape, and most have one of three distinct shapes: spherical, called cocci; rod-shaped, called bacilli; and spiral, classified as either spirilla or spirochetes (Fig. 5-2). Cocci may be further classified based on how the cells are grouped. They may exist singly, in groups of two, in long chains, or in clusters. Bacilli occur as single cells, in pairs, or in chains.

By using staining processes, bacteria can be subclassified as gram-positive or gram-negative, and as acid-fast or nonacid-fast. Following the gram-stain process, bacteria are identified as gram-positive if they retain the dye when treated with alcohol. If the alcohol washes out the dye, they are called gram-negative. To determine if bacteria are acid-fast, a different staining process is used. The bacteria are stained, heated, and treated with an acid alcohol to remove the color. If the bacterium resists decolorization, it is classified as acid-fast positive, indicating that acid-fast bacteria are present. If decolorization occurs, the bacterium is acid-fast negative. Streptococci and staphylococci are gram-positive. *Escherichia coli,* a bacillus, is gram-negative, and *Mycobacterium tuberculosis,* a bacillus, is acid-fast positive, often simply called "acid fast."

Bacteria are also grouped based on their oxygen requirements. Some require oxygen to grow and are called obligate aerobes, while others will not grow in the presence of oxygen and are called anaerobes. Bacteria that can adapt and grow under either aerobic or anaerobic conditions are called facultative organisms.

Some types of bacteria have the ability to generate **endospores,** a resistant form of the bacterium that is formed within the cell when environmental conditions are unfavorable. Most endospore-forming bacteria live in the soil, but they can reside almost anywhere. Endospores are resistant to destruction and can remain viable for many years, often being

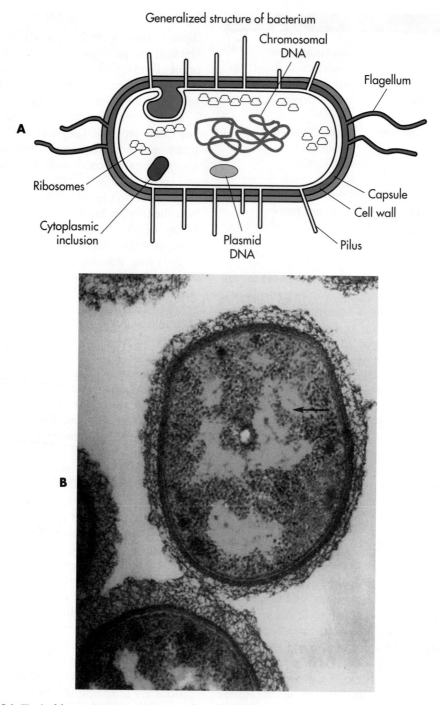

FIG. 5-1 Typical bacterium. **A,** Diagram of structure. **B,** Photomicrograph. Note absence of nuclear membrane *(arrow).*

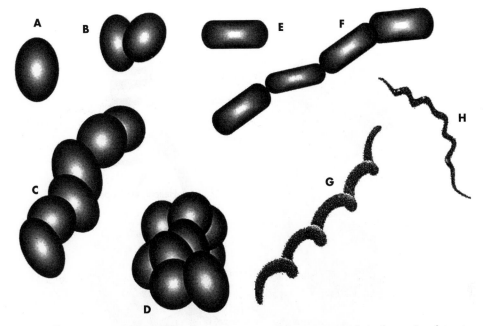

FIG. 5-2 Bacterial forms. Cocci: **A,** single coccus; **B,** diplococcus; **C,** chain formation (strepto-coccus); and **D,** cluster (staphylococcus). Bacilli: **E,** single bacillus; and **F,** chain. Spiral bacteria: **G,** spirillum; and **H,** spirochete.

carried through the atmosphere on invisible dust particles. When conditions improve, endospores can germinate, revitalizing the bacteria.

Bacteria are able to adapt to new conditions and are also able to mutate, allowing them to resist and survive in the presence of antimicrobial drugs.

Significant diseases caused by bacteria include tuberculosis, streptococcal pharyngitis (strep throat), streptococcal Group A necrotizing fasciitis (flesh-eating bacteria), and Lyme disease, as well as infectious diarrhea and hemolytic uremic syndrome, both of which are caused by *E. coli* O157:H7.

Rickettsiae

Although rickettsiae are considered bacteria, they are discussed separately because they are atypical. They are smaller than most bacteria and are just barely visible in an ordinary light microscope. Their most significant identifying feature is that they only grow inside animal cells (e.g., rabbits and rats). Rickettsiae do not survive in the environment and are transmitted among animals by infected arthropod vector

bites (ticks, lice, fleas, and mites). Humans are only accidental hosts. Rickettsiae are causative agents for Rocky Mountain spotted fever and typhus fever.

Viruses

Viruses are subcellular organisms and are among the smallest known disease-causing organisms. Because of their small size, they must be viewed with an electron microscope. A fully developed viral particle, called a virion, is made up of genetic material, DNA or RNA, which is protected by an outer protein coating called the capsid. The capsid may be covered by a lipoprotein envelope that has projecting spikes (Fig. 5-3). Enveloped viruses such as influenza, human immunodeficiency virus (HIV), and hepatitis B use these spikes to attach to host cells. Some viruses, such as the rhinovirus that causes the common cold, lack both the envelope and spikes, so the capsid assists this virus in attaching to the host cell.

Viruses cannot survive independently. A virus invades a host cell for which it has specificity, stimulating it to participate in the formation of additional

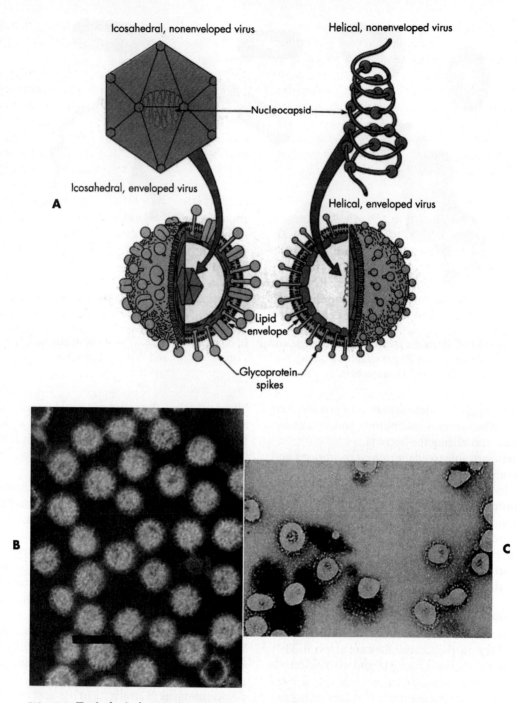

FIG. 5-3 Typical viral structure. **A,** Diagrams of nonenveloped and enveloped viruses. **B,** Photomicrograph, nonenveloped virus. **C,** Photomicrograph, enveloped virus.

virus particles. For example, the hepatitis virus attaches to receptor sites on a liver cell. Because viruses reside in and use the host cell to replicate, it has been difficult to create antiviral drugs that are not also harmful to the host cell. Only a few antiviral agents exist, and these are useful for only a limited number of viruses.

Other common viruses are the Epstein-Barr, which causes infectious mononucleosis, and varicella, which causes chicken pox and herpes zoster (shingles).

Fungi

Fungi (singular, fungus) occur as single-celled yeasts or as long, branched, filament-like structures called molds that are composed of many cells (Fig. 5-4). Some fungi can exist in either form, depending on the environment. Yeasts reproduce by forming buds, while molds reproduce by **spore** formation. There are more than 100,000 diverse species of fungi, many which serve useful purposes. They are a key ingredient in the production of alcoholic beverages, are responsible for the flavor of cheese, give bread its lightness, and produce the antibiotic penicillin. Fungi are also important in nature

because they help decompose dead plants and animals, making these complexes available for plant growth.

Some species of fungi are destructive to products made of natural materials like wood and leather, while others cause diseases in plants, animals, or humans. Fungi cause skin infections in humans, such as athlete's foot and ringworm, respiratory infections such as histoplasmosis and coccidioidomycosis, and **opportunistic infections** (infections due to usually nonpathogenic organisms) such as *Pneumocystis carinii* pneumonia (PCP) and pharyngeal and esophageal candidiasis in individuals with compromised immune systems.

Prions

The smallest and least understood of all microbes is the prion, which was discovered in 1983. Scientists believe that prions may be "infectious proteins." Their method of replication is not understood since prions do not have DNA or RNA, but they are capable of automatically transforming healthy proteins in nerve cells into more prions. Prions are resistant to the body's natural defenses and can

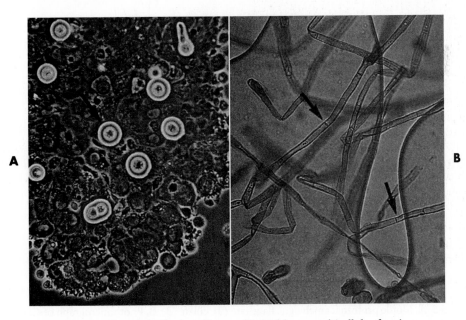

FIG. 5-4 Fungi. **A,** Single-cell yeasts. **B,** Molds are multicellular fungi.

continue to multiply unchecked, causing irreversible neurological damage. They were first identified as the cause of scrapie, a degenerative disease affecting the nervous systems of sheep. It is thought that prions are the cause of Creutzfeldt-Jakob disease in humans and perhaps other conditions characterized by slow deterioration of the nervous system. Further study of prions may help researchers understand the cause of Alzheimer's disease.

Protozoa

Protozoa are complex single-celled animals that generally exist as free-living organisms; a few are parasitic and live within the human body. They may be classified as motile (moving) or nonmotile.

If motile, they are further classified by their method of motility. Some move by changing their shape to form pseudopods (false "feet"); others move using flagella, whiplike formations that move the cell, or cilia, fine, hairlike projections that propel the organism (Fig. 5-5). Most parasitic protozoa produce some type of resistant form, such as a cyst, to survive in the environment outside the host. Other protozoa have complicated life cycles involving alternate existence in the human body and an insect vector. This is true of the protozoan that causes malaria. Protozoa can infect the gastrointestinal, genitourinary, respiratory, and circulatory systems. Common protozoal diseases include amebiasis, giardiasis, toxoplasmosis, and trichomoniasis.

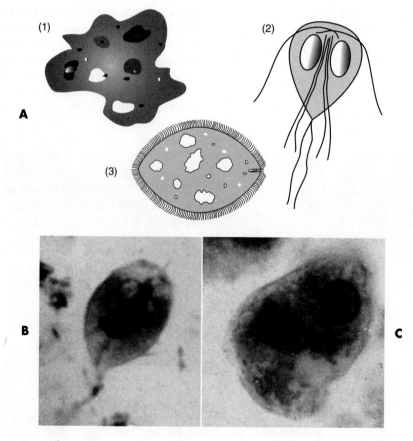

FIG. 5-5 **A,** Motile protozoa: ameba *(1),* flagellate *(2),* ciliate *(3).* **B,** Photomicrograph of *Giardia lamblia,* a flagellate. **C,** Photomicrograph of *Entamoeba histolytica,* an ameba.

CYCLE OF INFECTION

The factors involved in the spread of disease are sometimes called the cycle of infection (Fig. 5-6). For infections to be transmitted, there must be an infectious organism, a reservoir of infection, a portal of exit, a susceptible host, a portal of entry, and a means of transporting the organism from the reservoir to the susceptible individual.

Infectious Organisms

Microorganisms capable of causing disease are called pathogenic organisms or pathogens. They possess certain properties called **virulence factors** that distinguish them from nonpathogenic organisms or normal flora. These factors enable bacteria to destroy or damage host cells and resist destruction by the host's cellular defenses. Bacterial pathogens have an affinity for a certain type of cell in the body and attach to these cells, excreting protein substances called toxins that kill or injure the host cells. They can destroy red and white blood cells and activate enzymes in the host cell that enable them to spread through tissues. They usually inhibit recognition by the host cell and resist destruction by white blood cells. Their destructiveness and resistance

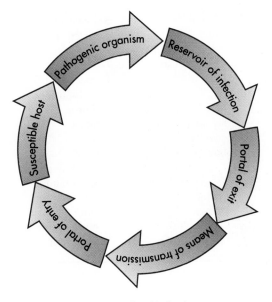

FIG. 5-6 Cycle of infection.

allow them to grow and cause the signs and symptoms of disease. The pathogens that cause diphtheria, pertussis, typhoid fever, and dysentery have these virulence factors. Table 5-1 provides other examples of pathogens.

Normal flora are capable of causing disease when they are not confined to their usual environment, when an individual's resistance is weakened, or when broad-spectrum antibiotics disrupt the ecological balance of the resident flora. *E. coli*, normal flora of the gastrointestinal tract, can become pathogenic if it enters the bladder. This occurs more often in the female due to the shorter urethra. *Candida albicans* may be found in the throat or gastrointestinal tract of many healthy persons, yet this same organism can assume a pathogenic role, causing vaginal infections in females when competing bacteria are destroyed by antibiotic treatment. *Candida* is an opportunistic organism that proliferates when immunity is compromised, causing both esophagitis and respiratory infections in patients with acquired immunodeficiency syndrome (AIDS).

Reservoir of Infection

The reservoir or source of infection may be any place where pathogens can thrive in sufficient numbers to pose a threat. Such an environment must provide moisture, nutrients, and a suitable temperature, all of which are found in the human body. A source of infection might be a patient with hepatitis, a radiographer with an upper respiratory infection (URI), or a visitor with staphylococcal boils.

Since some pathogens live in the bodies of healthy individuals without causing apparent disease, a person may be the reservoir for an infectious organism without realizing it. These persons are called carriers. Many of us have throat cultures that are positive for *Staphylococcus aureus*, but we do not have a sore throat. A susceptible patient with an open wound could contract a life-threatening infection if sufficiently contaminated with this organism. The classic example of a carrier of infection is Typhoid Mary, a "healthy" food handler. Hundreds of cases of typhoid fever were attributed to contamination of the meals she helped to prepare. Better sanitation and food-handling education have

TABLE 5-1

SOME EXAMPLES OF PATHOGENS

SYSTEM	NAME	CLASSIFICATION	DISEASE(S)	MODE OF TRANSMISSION
Respiratory tract	*Bordetella pertussis*	Bacterium	Whooping cough	Droplet
	Candida albicans	Fungus	Pneumonia, thrush in infants	Droplet
	Corynebacterium diphtheriae	Bacterium	Diphtheria	Droplet
	Mycobacterium tuberculosis	Bacterium	Tuberculosis	Airborne
	Mumps virus	Virus	Mumps	Droplet
	Streptococcus pneumoniae	Bacterium	Pneumonia, sinus infections	Droplet
	Streptococcus pyogenes	Bacterium	Strep throat	Droplet
Gastrointestinal tract	*Entamoeba histolytica*	Protozoan	Amebic dysentery	Vehicle, contact
	Escherichia coli O157:H7	Bacterium	Infectious diarrhea	Vehicle, contact
	Giardia lamblia	Protozoan	Giardiasis	Vehicle, contact
	Poliomyelitis virus	Virus	Poliomyelitis	Vehicle, contact
	Salmonella species	Bacterium	Salmonellosis	Vehicle, contact
	Shigella species	Bacterium	Shigellosis (bacillary dysentery)	Vehicle, contact
Genitourinary tract	*Escherichia coli*	Bacterium	Cystitis, nephritis	Contact
	Herpes simplex, type 2	Virus	Genital herpes	Sexual contact
	Neisseria gonorrhoeae	Bacterium	Gonorrhea	Sexual contact
	Nonhemolytic *Streptococcus (Enterococcus)*	Bacterium	Cystitis, nephritis	Contact
	Treponema pallidum	Bacterium	Syphilis	Sexual contact
Skin	Varicella	Virus	Chicken pox, disseminated herpes zoster	Contact, airborne
	Herpes simplex, type 1	Virus	Fever blisters	Contact (and predisposition)
	Measles virus (rubeola)	Virus	Measles	Airborne
	Nonhemolytic *Streptococcus (Enterococcus)*	Bacterium	Surgical wound infection	Contact
	Staphylococcus aureus	Bacterium	Boils, wound infection	Contact
	Tinea capitis, Tinea pedis	Fungus	Ringworm, athlete's foot	Contact (and predisposition)
Blood	*Plasmodium* species	Protozoan	Malaria	Vectors (mosquitoes)
	Salmonella typhi	Bacterium	Typhoid fever	Vehicle, contact

reduced the incidence of foodborne diseases. Today an example of a carrier of infection is the asymptomatic individual infected with HIV who spreads the disease through sexual intercourse or by sharing contaminated needles with intravenous drug users (IDUs).

Although the human body is the most common reservoir of infection, any environment that will support the growth of microorganisms has the potential to be a secondary source. Such sources include contaminated food or water or any damp, warm place that is not cleaned regularly.

Portal of Exit

The portal of exit from the human body may be any route through which blood, body fluids, excretions, or secretions leave the body. Examples include the respiratory, urinary, and gastrointestinal tracts; an infected wound; and the bloodstream.

Susceptible Host

Susceptible hosts are frequently patients who have a reduced natural resistance to infection. In addition to the primary problem that caused their hospitalization, they may develop a **nosocomial infection** (hospital-acquired infection). Approximately 2 million patients admitted to hospitals each year acquire nosocomial infections. Although many of these infections are not life-threatening, the CDC estimates that 90,000 patients die each year of hospital-acquired infections and that most of these are preventable. Typical sources of nosocomial infections include the contaminated hands of health care providers, contaminated instruments, and urinary catheters, which can allow microbes to gain easy entrance into the body.

There are several nosocomial infections that greatly concern health care providers and their hospitalized patients because they are multidrug–resistant. Methicillin-resistant *Staphylococcus aureus* (MRSA) and vancomycin-resistant enterococci (VRE) contribute to surgical wound infections. Penicillin-resistant *Streptococcus* and *Pseudomonas aeruginosa* cause respiratory infections. The overuse of antimicrobial agents and poor infection control practices have been implicated in the emergence and

spread of these multidrug-resistant infections. These pathogens are very difficult to treat, and intensive infection control is required to limit their spread. Even as we write, other organisms are adapting to the drugs used to treat them and will soon emerge to present new infection control threats in health care facilities, so this problem will be with us for some time.

Hospital infections also pose a threat to health care workers. When contracted by health care workers, these infections are called occupationally acquired rather than nosocomial infections. The hepatitis B and C viruses are the biggest concerns, since both are spread by blood and blood products. Hepatitis B is more infectious than hepatitis C, and the risk of developing clinical hepatitis from a needlestick with infected blood is as high as 30%. Although a needlestick injury is the most efficient method of transmitting the hepatitis B virus (HBV), another mode of transmission is through nonintact skin contact with infected blood on environmental surfaces. HBV has been demonstrated to survive in dried blood on environmental surfaces for at least a week. This means you can contract HBV if you have an open wound and touch a contaminated surface. There is no evidence to support that hepatitis C can be transmitted through contact with infected dried blood. For a discussion of these and other important infections, see the section on Infectious Diseases that follows.

In December 1991 the Occupational Safety and Health Administration (OSHA) published regulations that require health care employers to provide HBV immunizations to employees as well as procedures and equipment to prevent the transmission of HIV and other bloodborne diseases to which employees are exposed. Because of vaccinations the number of cases of hepatitis B in the general population has decreased sharply since 1985. Currently there is no vaccine for hepatitis C, so the best protection from contracting this disease is to follow the infection control procedures established for other bloodborne infections.

Hospital workers are exposed to many pathogens. In a single day a radiographer may care for ambulatory outpatients, hospital patients in isolation, and emergency trauma patients with "dirty" wounds. The radiographer who must work when resistance is low because of fatigue, stress, or a low-grade infection has increased susceptibility to contagious diseases. A healthy, well-rested body is your best protection.

Portal of Entry

The portal of entry is the route by which microorganisms gain access into the susceptible host. Examples include the respiratory, urinary, and gastrointestinal tracts; an open wound or break in the skin; the mucous membranes of the eyes, nose, or mouth, and the bloodstream.

Transmission of Disease

The most direct way to intervene in the cycle of infection is to prevent transmission of the infectious organism from the reservoir to the susceptible host. To accomplish this you must understand the six main routes of transmission.

The first route is **direct contact.** This transmission mode requires that the host is touched by an infected person and that the organisms are placed in direct contact with susceptible tissue. For example, syphilis and HIV infections may be contracted when infectious organisms from the mucous membrane of one individual are placed in direct contact with the mucous membrane of a susceptible host. Also, skin infections often occur among hospital workers because of the frequent contact with patients who have staphylococcal and streptococcal diseases. The five other principal routes of transmission are indirect and involve transport of organisms by way of fomites, vectors, vehicles, airborne means, and droplet contamination.

An object that has been in contact with pathogenic organisms is called a **fomite.** A contaminated urinary catheter is a typical example. Other fomites in the radiology department might include the x-ray table, vertical bucky, cassettes, and positioning sponges contaminated with infectious body fluids.

A **vector** is an arthropod in whose body an infectious organism develops or multiplies before becoming infective to a new host. The bite of such infected insects can transmit diseases to humans. Some examples of vectors are mosquitoes that transmit malaria or dengue fever, fleas that carry bubonic plague, and ticks that spread Lyme disease or Rocky Mountain spotted fever.

A **vehicle** is any medium that transports microorganisms. Examples include contaminated food, water, drugs, or blood.

Airborne contamination occurs either by dust containing spores or by droplet nuclei, which are particles of evaporated droplets measuring 5 microns (micrometers, μm, .001 millimeter) or smaller containing microorganisms that remain suspended in the air for long periods. These particles may be dispersed by air currents and may be inhaled by a susceptible host. Special air handling and ventilation are required to prevent airborne transmission of these infected particles. *Mycobacterium tuberculosis,* rubeola, and the varicella viruses are examples of airborne infections.

Droplet contamination often occurs when an infectious individual coughs, sneezes, speaks, or sings in the vicinity of a susceptible host. Droplet transmission involves contact of the mucous membranes of the eyes, nose, or mouth of a susceptible person with large droplets (greater than 5 microns) containing microorganisms. These particles do not remain suspended in the air and travel only short distances, usually 3 feet or less. Influenza, meningitis, diphtheria, pertussis, and streptococcal pneumonia are examples of illnesses that spread by means of droplet contamination.

Although many organisms are fragile, requiring continuous warmth, moisture, and nutriment to exist, the endospores formed by some bacteria are resistant to heat, cold, and drying and can live without nourishment. Endospores can float through the air and lurk in dusty corners waiting for the opportunity to invade a susceptible host. Spore-forming bacterial organisms are responsible for serious but relatively uncommon diseases such as tetanus, anthrax, and botulism. The spores are transmitted to a host through inhalation, ingestion, or contact. The host provides the moisture, warmth, and nutrients that enable the endospore to germinate into a bacterial cell again.

Epidemiological studies have shown that some viruses can resist drying for weeks. The virus that causes herpes (both oral and genital) is an example. It is apparent that the need for cleanliness as a defense against infection from both spores and viruses cannot be overstated.

THE BODY'S DEFENSE AGAINST INFECTION

The human body is protected from the invasion of microorganisms in three ways: natural resistance and defenses, acquired resistance (also known as active immunity), and short-term passive immunity.

Natural Resistance

Mechanical barriers such as intact skin and mucous membranes provide natural resistance. The importance of intact skin in preventing infection is easily understood when severe burns, cuts, and abrasions disrupt this protective barrier and allow microorganisms to pass into tissues and proliferate.

The mucous membranes of the respiratory, urinary, gastrointestinal, and reproductive systems secrete mucus, which traps foreign particles. Additionally the respiratory tract is lined with cilia that transport mucus containing dust and microorganisms out of the body. The urinary tract is protected from ascending infections by the composition and outward flow of urine.

Chemicals, such as lysozyme in human tears and acids of the stomach, vagina, and skin, also help destroy invading microorganisms. The pH, salt content, and dryness of the skin limit the number of bacteria that will reside there, and beneficial normal flora prevent the overgrowth of undesirable organisms.

In spite of these barriers, microorganisms do gain access into the body. This occurs as a result of common daily activities such as brushing one's teeth and shaving. This invasion initiates our second line of defense, the inflammatory response. Inflammation increases blood flow to the site and permits the passage of fluids and white blood cells into the tissues to engulf and destroy the invading pathogens. This process is called **phagocytosis.**

When viruses infect the body, virus-infected cells produce interferons, small protein molecules that protect the uninfected cells from invasion by the original virus as well as others. Interferons are species-specific and are currently being produced in laboratories for the treatment of herpes and chronic hepatitis B and C.

Acquired Immunity

Humans are born with a certain amount of immunity, but most humans become resistant to a disease by becoming infected with a specific organism. This infection may or may not manifest itself as an obvious illness. Immunity can also be conferred from vaccines made from dead or weakened strains of microorganisms for a specific infection or from an inactivated toxin. This state of being resistant to a specific infection is called acquired immunity. Acquired immunity occurs because the body is able to distinguish itself from foreign protein substances that enter the body. These substances are called antigens. Antibodies are protein substances formed in response to specific antigens. They are produced by a specific white blood cell, the B-cell, that works with other white blood cells to destroy invading foreign substances and prevent reinfection by a particular antigen. Because the body forms its own antibodies to the specific antigen, acquired immunity is long term.

Passive Immunity

Passive immunity occurs following an injection of *preformed* antibodies to a particular infection. This is the case when individuals are given pooled immune globulin (human blood and antibodies pooled from the general population) before and after exposure to hepatitis A. The antibodies act immediately and prevent disease but will weaken over time. The newborn is temporarily immune to infections because of the antibodies that are passed from mother to fetus in utero. The infant will continue to receive this passive immunity if breast-fed after birth. Because the body does not produce these antibodies, passive immunity is short term.

INFECTIOUS DISEASES
Emerging Diseases

There are many new diseases in the world and some old diseases once thought to be under control are returning in **epidemic** (widespread) proportions after years of low-level incidence. As a worker in the health care field, you will be on the front line of exposure to both old and new diseases. The infection control department within the hospital is responsible for keeping track of these infections and developing infection control policies to protect you, other staff, and patients, based on recommendations from the CDC. The CDC monitors and studies the types of infections occurring in the nation, compiles statistical data about these infections, and publishes this information in both a weekly report and an annual surveillance summary report. The World Health Organization (WHO) studies, collects, and compiles infection data from every country in the world and makes this information available worldwide.

Emerging diseases include new diseases appearing in the population, preexisting ones that are rapidly increasing in incidence or geographic range, and resurgent or recurrent old diseases caused by an old or mutated pathogen. Disease emergence is precipitated by many factors: increased human exposure to vectors in nature, population growth and migration to crowded cities, rapid international travel and transportation of goods, contact with new strains of dangerous pathogens, pathogen mutation caused by overutilization of antimicrobial agents, a breakdown in public health measures, and bioterrorism.

The outbreak of *Hantavirus* respiratory syndrome (a potentially fatal respiratory disease) in the southwestern United States in 1993 was blamed on a 6-year drought followed by a mild, wet winter and spring. These conditions were favorable for a dramatic rise in the population of deer mice that increased their contact with humans. *Hantavirus* infection is contracted by inhaling dust containing the particles of droppings from these mice.

The unusually warm temperatures in Mexico and southern Texas in 1995 provided ideal conditions for mosquitoes carrying dengue fever to reproduce and transmit this flavivirus. Dengue fever, also called "break-bone fever," is characterized by a high fever, headache, muscle and joint aches, malaise, and often, a rash. The disease may range from a mild illness to a severe, sometimes fatal, condition with hemorrhage and shock.

Reforestation increases populations of deer and deer ticks, the vector for Lyme disease. When humans move closer to these forests, it is easier for the pathogen that causes Lyme disease to spread from its normal host into humans.

Human migration from isolated areas of the world to crowded cities is responsible for the spread of once localized infections such as HIV, cholera, and dengue fever. International travel has the potential to spread many pathogens around the world. Travelers from Asia brought the virus for severe acute respiratory syndrome (SARS) to North America in the spring of 2003; new strains of influenza spread rapidly across the globe as travelers met and exchanged infections. Air transport of used tires from Asia introduced the mosquitoes carrying dengue fever to the United States.

Ingestion of food contaminated with *E. coli* O157:H7 causes diarrhea and hemorrhagic uremic syndrome. This strain of *E. coli* has caused severe illness and death linked to the consumption of undercooked hamburger meat, unpasteurized apple juice, and dried venison.

Medical settings provide an ideal environment for the development and transmission of nosocomial infections. Invasive procedures permit pathogens to enter the bloodstream and overcome the defense mechanisms of immunocompromised patients. The wide and inappropriate use of broad-spectrum antibiotics has led to the development of drug-resistant infections in hospitals as well as in the community. Some of these infections are untreatable because they are resistant to the available drugs. Development of a new drug takes time, is costly, and does not seem to be a lasting solution to this complex problem.

Inadequate public health measures in South America and Africa have resulted in cholera outbreaks due to poor sanitation and insufficient chlorine levels in water supplies. Drastic political change in the former Soviet Union and the resulting deterioration of public health programs accounted for the resurgence of diphtheria there. Russian immigrants reintroduced the disease to the United States. The outbreak of anthrax in the United States in 2001 demonstrated the ease with which terrorists can spread diseases once thought to be under control. This has raised public concern about other diseases that could affect a large portion of our population.

Bloodborne Pathogens

HIV and AIDS

The rapid spread of HIV and AIDS concerns everyone. Public health concern is focused particularly on the number of new HIV infections occurring nationwide. New infections are arising most rapidly among people of color (black non-Hispanics and Hispanics), and women. Women are becoming infected primarily as a result of intravenous drug use and heterosexual contact. Approximately 1 million people in the United States are living with HIV infection, and approximately half of these infections are untreated, according to the CDC. The worldwide estimate is 42 million, which could increase to 67 million by 2010. The annual mortality rate is 3 million, and the worldwide cumulative death toll could reach 100 million by 2020. As of December 2001, a cumulative total of approximately 800,000 cases of AIDS has been reported in the United States and the number of AIDS-related deaths has exceeded 450,000.

While the incidence of AIDS has dropped significantly, the total number of HIV patients continues to rise. This is due not only to new cases, but also to the increasing number of HIV-infected individuals who have avoided converting to AIDS by the use of new, more effective antiretroviral drugs.

In the early 1980s HIV was identified as the cause of AIDS. Two major types of HIV have been found to infect humans: HIV Type 1 (HIV-1), the predominant type throughout the world, and HIV Type 2 (HIV-2), found primarily in heterosexual populations in West Africa.

HIV is an RNA retrovirus. RNA viruses are called retroviruses because they replicate in a "backward" manner, converting from RNA to DNA once they invade a host cell. HIV can infect a number of different cells in the body, including cells of the central nervous system, but it is the adverse effect on immune system cells that produces the immunosuppression

and manifestations of AIDS. The virus has specificity for the receptors on CD4 lymphocytes, attaching to and invading these cells and becoming a permanent part of their genetic material. Cell replication produces infected CD4 cells and additional HIV.

An HIV-infected individual can transmit the virus to others a few days after infection, even though antibodies to the virus may not be detected in the blood for 3 to 6 months. Without therapy, this individual will pass through several phases of infection over a span of months to years before exhibiting the immunosuppression of full-blown AIDS.

In the early stages of the infection there is usually a brief period of flulike symptoms, often followed by years without symptoms. During the asymptomatic phase the virus is silently replicating in the body and decreasing the number of CD4 lymphocytes. At the end of the asymptomatic period, before the full development of AIDS, the individual will experience night sweats, oral infections, weight loss, persistently enlarged lymph nodes, and low-grade fever. The appearance of AIDS is characterized by a low CD4 count and the occurrence of multiple opportunistic infections and malignant diseases. Some of the opportunistic infections observed are PCP, mucocutaneous *Candida,* disseminated herpes, and cytomegalovirus. There is also increased risk of contracting tuberculosis and developing active disease. Kaposi's sarcoma, a malignancy of pigmented skin cells, is the most common form of cancer affecting AIDS patients.

Although drugs have been developed that prolong the time required for HIV infection to progress to AIDS, at this time no known cure exists. The primary problem in producing a successful vaccine has been the high mutation rate of this virus, but there is continued hope that a vaccine will be developed.

Fortunately the AIDS virus is not acquired by casual contact. Touching or shaking hands, eating food prepared by an infected person, and contact with drinking fountains, telephones, toilets, or other surfaces does not result in transmission of HIV. The routes of transmission are through sexual contact, contaminated blood or needles, fluids containing blood, or from mother to fetus via the placenta. Infection can also be transmitted to infants through breast milk.

As we began the new millennium, men who have sex with other men (MSM) still accounted for the largest number of cases of AIDS in this country, followed by IDUs. AIDS is increasing at a faster rate in the same groups as HIV: non-Hispanic blacks, Hispanics, and women. The higher rate of AIDS in these groups is attributed to poor access to health care and/or failure to follow prescribed drug regimens. This means that in order to continue the decline in AIDS diagnosis and deaths in the future, there will need to be better access to health care, simpler drug regimens, and continued development of effective antiretroviral drugs.

As a health care worker in today's world, you must expect to encounter unidentified or undiagnosed cases of AIDS and other bloodborne diseases. Current controversy surrounds the patient's right to confidentiality regarding the AIDS diagnosis within the hospital setting, preventing you from being informed about diagnosed cases. Diagnosed patients are only the "tip of the iceberg," since many undiagnosed cases exist for every known case. Anxiety about HIV infections is typical and understandable among health care workers, but the occupational risk is not great. The vast majority of health care workers infected with HIV were exposed as a result of activities unrelated to their work. The most common occupational exposure is the needlestick, but according to the CDC the probability of infection following a needlestick injury with blood containing HIV is only 3 out of 1000 exposures or 0.3%. Thousands of needlesticks have been reported over the years, but as of December 2001 only 57 health care workers with no other identified risk factors have been diagnosed as HIV positive. Of these 57 cases, 26 have developed AIDS. The implications here are obvious. Although prevention at work is essential, self-care in terms of safe sexual practice is equally crucial.

Hepatitis

In the 1990s there was some evidence that new forms of hepatitis existed, but researchers are now finding that some of these other viruses do not cause hepatitis or any human illness. For this reason, only the common forms of hepatitis are addressed here. The five common types of hepatitis are classified A through E. Hepatitis A and E are transmitted through food and water contaminated with feces. Hepatitis B, C, and D are bloodborne. Hepatitis E is uncommon in the United States, and hepatitis D appears only as a co-infection to hepatitis B. Hepatitis B can be spread through contact with blood or blood products; with body fluids such as saliva, semen, and vaginal secretions; and through maternal-fetal contact. Hepatitis C is primarily spread by contact with blood or blood products. The risk for contracting this virus is greatest for persons with large or repeated percutaneous exposures to blood, such as IDUs, whose risk is 60%. The risk is lowest in sporadic percutaneous exposures such as health care workers, whose risk following a needlestick is 1% to 2%. The risk is 15% to 20% for sexual transmission and 5% to 6% for maternal-fetal transmission.

The manifestations of all forms of hepatitis are similar: jaundice, fatigue, abdominal pain, loss of appetite, nausea, vomiting, and diarrhea. Because hepatitis C is a more silent infection, there may be no symptoms or awareness of the infection until there is liver damage. Both hepatitis B and hepatitis C have the potential to develop into chronic infections and cirrhosis, although the risk is greater with hepatitis C. Following infection with hepatitis C, about 85% develop chronic infection, approximately 70% develop liver disease, 10% to 20% develop cirrhosis, and 1% to 5% develop liver cancer. These sequelae take place over a 10- to 20-year period.

The number of new cases of both hepatitis B and C has decreased due to immunizations for hepatitis B, decreased needle sharing among IDUs, and blood donor screening for both B and C viruses. However, the incidence of hepatitis A has shown periodic increases. Large nationwide outbreaks of type A usually occur once each decade, with the last outbreak occurring in 1989.

Health care workers can protect themselves against hepatitis B by taking a vaccine, which usually provides immunity for 7 to 10 years. There is also a vaccine for hepatitis A, but it is indicated only in certain situations: for individuals with medical, behavioral, occupational, or other indications, such as for travelers to Third World countries. Protection from hepatitis A and C can be achieved by following the established infection control practices in your institution. Hepatitis A remains the most common form of the disease and is best controlled by practicing good personal hygiene, especially hand hygiene.

Management of occupational exposures to bloodborne pathogens

If an accidental needlestick occurs or the skin is broken by a contaminated object, allow the wound to bleed under cold water and wash with soap. If your eyes, nose, or mouth are splashed with a patient's bodily fluids, rinse these mucous membranes with water. An incident report must be filed, even though the injury or incident might seem insignificant. In addition to the incident report, most hospitals now ask that a baseline blood sample be drawn to help rule out infection acquired before the occupational exposure. You will also be advised by the medical provider about post exposure prophylaxis (PEP) therapy following a puncture with a contaminated needle. If treatment is recommended, it should be administered within 2 hours of the blood exposure. Currently, for most HIV exposures that warrant PEP, a 4-week, two-drug regimen is recommended and several drug options are available. At the same time you are tested for HIV, you will also be tested for hepatitis B and C. If you have not had the hepatitis B vaccine series, it will be initiated along with hepatitis B immune globulin for immediate immunity. There is no effective prophylactic therapy for hepatitis C at this time, so if testing reveals you were exposed to an HCV-positive source, follow-up HCV testing will be necessary to see if infection develops. Since HIV infection may not be apparent in the blood for approximately 3 months, another sample is tested for HIV at 6 months.

Tuberculosis

Tuberculosis (TB) is a lung disease caused by the acid-fast bacillus *Mycobacterium tuberculosis,* also referred to as tubercle bacillus. Historically this disease was called consumption because of the victim's tendency to lose weight steadily and "waste away." In the past, the incidence of TB in the United States was spread across all economic groups. Today the highest rate of active cases is seen among the homeless, recent immigrants, and immunosuppressed individuals. While the incidence of cases in this country is much lower now than it was before 1950, the appearance of resistant strains of the bacteria has raised grave concern.

Pulmonary TB is spread through airborne droplet nuclei that are generated when an infected person coughs or speaks. These particles are 1 to 5 microns in size and are easily transmitted through the air. The probability that a susceptible person will be infected depends upon the concentration of the infectious droplet nuclei in the air.

The vast majority of those infected with the tubercle bacillus do not develop a clinical disease and become infectious. Within 2 to 10 weeks following infection, the body aided by its immune system begins walling off the infection, preventing its multiplication and spread. When walled off, the disease is inactive or dormant but can be reactivated at any time. Reactivation may occur when an individual's immune response is weakened as it is in old age, illness, or malnutrition, or with **immunosuppressant** therapy involving drugs that decrease the body's normal immune response.

Patients in a weakened or immunosuppressed state, such as with HIV, progress rapidly to active disease. Symptoms of active disease include productive or prolonged cough, fever, chills, loss of appetite, weight loss, fatigue, and night sweats. As the bacilli multiply, they cause tissue necrosis that results in lung cavities as illustrated in Fig. 5-7. These spaces are major reservoirs for the infection that can then be spread by coughing. Severe cases can be fatal.

Extrapulmonary TB, which infects bone or organs other than the lung, accounts for a small percentage of TB infections. Patients with extrapulmonary infection and no active pulmonary disease do not require airborne precautions.

The simplest and most common method of testing for TB infection is the tuberculin skin test. This test involves an intradermal injection on the anterior forearm. The wheal that is produced is inspected 48 to 72 hours later to determine whether the individual has been exposed to tuberculosis. A negative test indicates that the person has never been

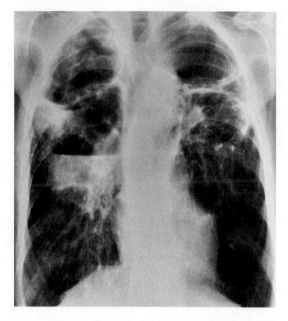

FIG. 5-7 Chest radiograph demonstrates advanced tuberculosis with many large cavities exhibiting air-fluid levels. Note also chronic fibrous changes and upward retraction of the hila.

infected with tuberculosis. A positive result indicates that a person has at one time been infected and has developed antibodies to the organism. Since few people develop clinical symptoms or become infectious, many people have a positive skin test without having active disease. This test is frequently administered if a person is known to have been exposed to TB and has not already tested positive.

If the skin test is newly recognized as positive or if symptoms are present, a chest radiograph is ordered to rule out active disease. When there are symptoms, sputum smears and cultures are tested for acid-fast bacilli (AFB). Positive results are definitive proof of active disease and are an indication to begin treatment.

Screening is often mandatory for those who work in contact with vulnerable or high-risk populations. For example, schoolteachers, corrections officers, and health care workers are often required to have pre-employment tuberculin skin tests.

In 2002 the CDC reported that there were approximately 15,000 new cases of tuberculosis diagnosed in the United States. This number represents a 5.7% decrease from 2001 and is the lowest number of reported cases since national reporting began in 1953. Although TB rates have declined in both American born and immigrant populations, this decline has been substantially less among immigrant or foreign born populations. The continued decline in the number of reported cases since 1992 reflects improvements in TB prevention and control programs by state and local health departments, but this falls short of the national goal the CDC has set to eventually eliminate this disease from our population.

Although we have seen a decline in the number of new cases in the United States, tuberculosis is still a worldwide problem. One third of the world's population is infected with TB. There are 9 million new cases and over 2 million deaths attributed to TB each year. In 2002, for the first time, the number of foreign born persons with TB in the United States slightly exceeded the number of American born persons, according to the CDC. If global TB control is not achieved, this disparity in TB incidence in the United States will continue to rise.

Early identification, isolation, and treatment are required to minimize transmission of tuberculosis. Health care workers are at risk of contracting this disease if the patient is exhibiting symptoms of active TB. The diagnosed patient will be isolated in a room with negative pressure (air flows from the hallway into the room) and more than six air exchanges per hour. Personnel and visitors must wear special masks and follow all precautions and procedures designated by the institution for the care of patients with airborne infections.

According to OSHA's standard on TB, infection control experts within the health care facility are to assess the actual risk for transmission of TB in inpatient and outpatient settings. If the findings reveal risk, they are to develop TB infection control interventions. These include free TB skin tests, the provision of personal respirator equipment, the operation of one or more isolation rooms with negative air pressure and special ventilation or circulation, annual employee training about the disease, and implementation of effective work practices. OSHA estimates that the average lifetime occupational risk of TB infection may be as high as 386 infections per 1000 workers exposed to TB on the job. The average lifetime occupational risk of developing active TB disease ranges from 3 to 39 cases per 1000 workers exposed to TB.

Severe Acute Respiratory Syndrome

As of this writing, severe acute respiratory syndrome (SARS) epidemics that occurred in the spring of 2003 are thought to be under control and the World Health Organization travel advisories warning of SARS dangers in Toronto, Canada and several Asian cities have been rescinded. SARS certainly continues to be a cause of concern, however, because it is highly contagious and potentially fatal. The disease has resulted in the contamination of some health care facilities that treated patients infected with the SARS virus, making it necessary to close them temporarily.

SARS is caused by a novel form of coronavirus. The incubation period is approximately 2 to 7 days. Individuals are suspected of having SARS if they have the symptoms listed here and have recently traveled to an affected region of the world or have had close contact with someone who is known to have SARS. The usual symptoms include a fever (temperature greater than 100.5° F [38° C]), muscle aches, a dry cough, and difficulty breathing. Victims may need mechanical ventilation to receive adequate oxygen. SARS is fatal to about 3% of victims, and those who are aged or infirm are at greatest risk. Caring for those who either have been exposed to the disease or are suspected of having SARS requires strict precautions to avoid transmission of this virus. The CDC recommends a combination of Standard Precautions, airborne precautions, and contact precautions as described in the following section. This disease is so new that relatively little is known as this book is published. If one or more patients in your facility are suspected of having SARS infection, it will be very important for you to obtain and follow the latest information from your infection control department.

PREVENTING DISEASE TRANSMISSION
Historical Perspective

When infectious disease was rampant, those infected were often "quarantined," meaning all members of the household were prevented from leaving the home or allowing others to enter. This practice helped to confine the infection to one family. Although quarantine is no longer commonly used, the United States Public Health Service still has the legal authority to detain and quarantine individuals when necessary to prevent the spread of certain serious infections. Diseases for which quarantine is currently authorized include cholera, diphtheria, infectious tuberculosis, plague, smallpox, yellow fever, viral hemorrhagic fevers, and SARS.

Decades ago, hospitals developed policies that involved separating patients admitted with infectious diseases from other patients. Contacts with other persons were rigidly controlled. This "isolation" was a logical outgrowth of the practice of quarantine. These techniques provided for specialized methods of asepsis when the danger of disease transmission was exceptionally great. Although isolation techniques were effective when used correctly, no mechanism existed for the prevention of serious diseases carried by asymptomatic individuals such as HBV and HIV carriers.

Universal precautions

In acknowledgment that many patients with bloodborne infections are not recognized, the CDC introduced a system in 1985 known as Universal Precautions (UP). Under this system all patients are treated as potential reservoirs of infection. The system is based on the use of barriers for all contacts with blood and certain body fluids known to carry bloodborne pathogens, rather than focusing on the isolation of a patient with a diagnosed bloodborne disease. The need to use barriers such as gloves and masks depends on the nature of the interaction with the patient rather than on the specific diagnosis. Emphasis is placed on blood and certain body fluids being potential sources of infection, regardless of diagnosis.

Body substance precautions

Because Universal Precautions placed emphasis on bloodborne infections and did not include precautions for contamination by feces, nasal secretions, sputum, sweat, tears, urine, and vomitus (unless contaminated with visible blood), a new system was introduced in 1987 called Body Substance Precautions (BSP). This system focused on the use of barriers for all moist and potentially infectious body substances from all patients. The system was developed to protect health care workers from acquiring and transmitting infections from all pathogens. In 1996 the CDC recommended a new system that synthesized the features of UP and BSP. This is the current system, and it is called Standard Precautions.

Standard Precautions

Standard Precautions are designed to reduce the risk of transmission of unrecognized sources of bloodborne and other pathogens in health care institutions. Standard Precautions apply to:

- Blood
- All body fluids
- Secretions and excretions (except sweat), regardless of whether they contain visible blood
- Nonintact skin
- Mucous membranes

Standard Precautions also reduce the risk of transmission from recognized sources of infection by including precautions for three modes of transmission: airborne, droplet, and contact. These transmission-based precautions are discussed later in Isolation Techniques.

You must decide when to take the extra time to protect both yourself and your patients. How you assess these risks and respond to them will vary with the setting and your level of experience. As a beginning student, your level of precautions should be very high. Although you may observe more experienced workers taking fewer precautions, do not think you must follow their example. At this stage in your education, it is far better to take too much precaution than to use too little.

Remember that the key to effective protection is using a consistent approach to all contact with all body substances of all patients at all times.

OSHA bloodborne pathogens standard

Previously it was stated that OSHA published the Occupational Exposure to Bloodborne Pathogens standard in 1991 to protect workers exposed to blood and other potentially infectious materials. As a result of this standard, employers are required to develop an exposure control plan for the work site describing employee protection measures. The plan must include how an employer will use a combination of engineering and work practice controls, ensure the use of personal protective clothing and equipment, provide signs and labels to identify biohazard materials, and take other measures to protect workers. Employers must also provide annual bloodborne pathogen training, hepatitis B vaccinations, and medical care in the event of an occupational exposure.

In response to the concern for the high number of needlesticks that occur annually involving contaminated sharps, Congress passed the Needlestick Safety and Prevention Act in November 2000 directing OSHA to revise this bloodborne pathogen standard and expand their definition of engineering controls. The revision defines engineering controls as use of effective and safer medical devices, such as sharps with engineered sharps injury protections and needleless systems. This revision became effective in 2001. Some of these devices are illustrated and discussed in Chapter 7. As part of this new policy, employers must document the process used for consideration and selection of these safer devices and involve employees in this process.

Medical Asepsis

Medical **asepsis** deals with reducing the probability of infectious organisms being transmitted to a susceptible individual. The healthy human body has the ability to overcome a limited number of infectious organisms, but this resistance can be overwhelmed by a massive exposure. On the other hand, a reduced resistance caused by disease, cancer chemotherapy, immunosuppressants, or extremes in age may result in infection after only minimal exposure. The fewer organisms to which a patient is exposed, the more likely it is that he or she will resist infection. The process of reducing the total number of organisms is called **microbial dilution** and can be accomplished at several levels.

Simple cleanliness measures avoid transmitting organisms when proper cleaning, dusting, linen handling, and hand hygiene techniques are used. The second level is **disinfection** and involves the destruction of pathogens by using chemical materials. The third stage is surgical asepsis, or **sterilization.** This involves treating items with heat, gas, or chemicals to make them germ-free. They are then stored in a manner that prevents contamination.

You can easily find examples of poor aseptic technique in most clinical settings, but the results of carelessness are seldom traced to the culprit. It is the patient acquiring a nosocomial infection who suffers. Armed with the knowledge of disease transmission, how can you fight the spread of infection?

- Stay home when you are ill if possible. If you *must* work, definitely avoid contact with immunocompromised patients.
- Use a tissue to cover your mouth when you sneeze or cough.
- Wear a clean uniform daily, and remove it immediately when you go home.
- Perform hand hygiene frequently.
- Use established precautions when handling patients, linens, or items contaminated with body substances.
- Practice good housekeeping techniques in your work area.
- When in doubt about the cleanliness of any object, do not use it.
- Dispose immediately of linens, instruments, or other items that touch the floor. The floor is always considered contaminated.
- Ask patients who are coughing or sneezing to cover mouth and nose with tissues.

Hand hygiene

The first three principles just listed are simple and self-explanatory. Handwashing also may seem obvious but is frequently overlooked in many hospital settings. Medically aseptic handwashing is an easy and effective method to control the transmission of infections (Fig 5-8). Unfortunately, evidence shows that most physicians, nurses, and other health care workers do not wash their hands often enough or well enough. There are several reasons attributed to the poor adherence to regular handwashing in health care facilities: inaccessibility to sinks, lack of time in between patients, lack of role models, and the concern that handwashing is irritating to the skin and causes dryness.

As previously addressed, the CDC estimates that each year nearly 2 million patients in the United States get an infection in the hospital, and about 90,000 patients die as a result. In an effort to address this adverse outcome, the CDC issued a revised hand hygiene guideline in 2002. An important part of the guideline is the recommended use of an alcohol-based hand rub (an alcohol containing preparation in the form of a gel, rinse, or foam containing 60% to 95% isopropanol or ethanol alcohol). The alcohol-based hand rubs have some benefits that the CDC believes will improve compliance with hand hygiene. Use of an alcohol-based hand rub requires about 15 seconds of time versus about a minute to walk to a sink and another 30 to 60 seconds to complete the handwashing procedure. An alcohol-based hand rub is more accessible than a sink because it can be carried in the health care worker's pocket or is located at the patient's bedside. Additionally, it has been found to be more efficacious than soap and water in reducing nosocomial infections. It is very effective against many microorganisms (gram-negative, gram-positive, *Mycobacterium tuberculosis*, fungi, and some viruses) including multidrug-resistant organisms. However, it will not destroy bacterial spores such as *Clostridium difficile* and *Bacillus anthracis*. Handwashing with soap and water is still recommended to physically remove spores from the surface of contaminated hands. Alcohol-based hand rubs are also less irritating to the skin, especially when skin-conditioning agents are added to the formulation.

Alcohol-based hand rubs should not replace handwashing with soap and water when hands are

FIG. 5-8 ASEPTIC HANDWASHING TECHNIQUE

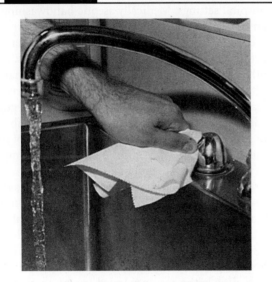

A Sink is contaminated. Use paper towel to handle controls unless there are foot or knee levers.

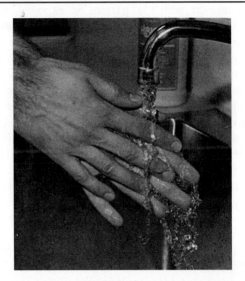

B Wet hands thoroughly. Keep hands lower than elbows so water will drain from clean area (forearms) to most contaminated area (fingers).

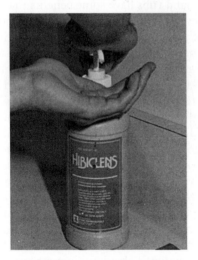

C Apply antimicrobial soap.

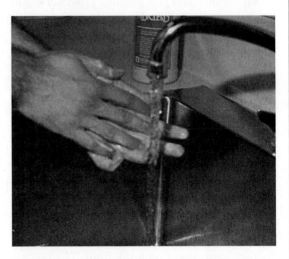

D Lather well. Rub hands and fingers together with firm rotary motion for 20 seconds. Friction is more effective than soap in removing microorganisms from skin. Rub palms, backs of hands, and areas between fingers.

FIG. 5-8   ASEPTIC HANDWASHING TECHNIQUE—cont'd

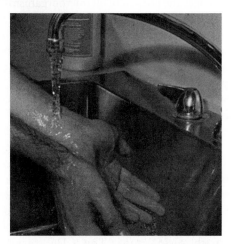

E Rinse, allowing water to run down over hands. Repeat steps to cleanse wrists and forearms.

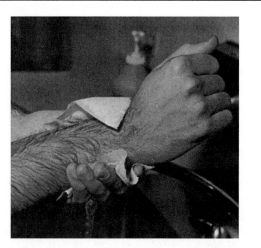

F Use paper towel to dry thoroughly from fingertips to elbows.

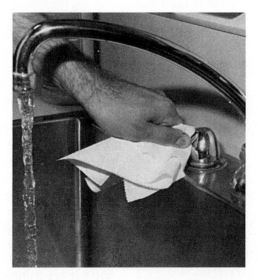

G Turn off water with paper towel to avoid contaminating hands.

visibly soiled or contaminated with blood or body secretions or excretions. Gloves should always be worn to prevent contact with the patient's blood or other body fluids. Following removal of the gloves, the hands should be decontaminated through use of an antiseptic hand rub or antiseptic hand wash to reduce bacterial counts.

Studies reveal that health care workers who wear artificial nails are more likely to harbor bacteria at the fingertips below the nails than those who have natural nails, both before and after hand hygiene. Therefore many health care institutions do not permit health care workers to wear artificial nails. According to the CDC, artificial fingernails or extenders should not be worn by health care workers who have direct contact with patients at high risk, such as those in the intensive care unit and in the operating room. Additionally, the tips of natural nails should be kept less than ¼-inch long.

Throughout this text you will find reminders to perform hand hygiene. Hand hygiene refers to decontamination of the hands using soap and water, an antiseptic hand wash, or an alcohol-based hand rub. The CDC recommendations for the use of alcohol-based hand rubs in the clinical setting are listed in Box 5-1.

Housekeeping

Good housekeeping in the workplace reduces the incidence of airborne infections and the transfer of pathogens by fomites. A clean, dry environment discourages the growth of all microorganisms. Much of the cleaning in the radiology department may be done at night by the housekeeping staff, but the radiographer is responsible for inspecting the work area regularly and maintaining high standards of medical asepsis.

Several general principles apply whenever cleaning is required:

- Always clean from the least contaminated area toward the more contaminated area and from the top down.
- Avoid raising dust.
- Do not contaminate yourself or clean areas.
- Clean all equipment that comes in contact with patients after each use. Use a cloth moistened with disinfectant. The CDC recommends sodium hypochlorite bleach (Clorox) as an inexpensive, effective disinfectant for preventing the spread of HIV.
- Mix bleach in a 1:10 solution daily, because its effectiveness declines rapidly when diluted.

Most hospitals have detailed written procedures concerning preferred cleansing agents and the extent of responsibility for disinfecting rooms (see Appendix F). Consult the infection control procedure for your clinical area.

Handling linens

Objects or linens soiled with body secretions or excretions are considered contaminated and may serve as fomites even when no stains are apparent. Any linens used by patients should be handled as little as possible. To prevent airborne contamination, fold the edges of linens to the middle without shaking or flapping, and immediately place loosely balled linens in the hamper. Never use any linen for more than one patient.

Most institutions today handle all linen the same way, regardless of the degree of contamination. The linen is placed in plastic bags, and laundry handlers follow established precautions to prevent infection transmission. Many hospitals provide laundry bags that dissolve in hot water, reducing the number of times linen must be handled by laundry personnel.

> **BOX 5-1**
>
> ### CDC GUIDELINES FOR THE USE OF ALCOHOL-BASED HAND RUBS IN THE CLINICAL SETTING
>
> When to use:
> 1. Use before and after patient contact as long as the hands are not visibly soiled or contaminated.
> 2. Before donning gloves.
> 3. After removal of gloves.
> 4. After contact with inanimate objects (including medical equipment) in the immediate vicinity of the patient.
>
> How to use:
> Apply product to palm of hand, and rub hands together, covering all surfaces of hands and fingers, until they are dry. Follow the manufacturer's recommendations regarding the volume of product to use.

From the Centers for Disease Control and Prevention, *Morbidity and Mortality Weekly Report* (MMWR, October 25, 2002 51/RR-16:1-44), www.cdc.gov/handhygiene.

Handling and disposal of contaminated items and waste

A modern hospital uses many disposable items, from simple objects such as paper cups and tissues to more complex items such as catheterization sets. Disposable items are designed to be used only once and then discarded. The only exception to this rule involves the immediate reuse of an unsterile item (e.g., emesis basin) by the same patient.

Each hospital has a protocol for discarding disposable items. Some separate glass, plastic, and paper into covered containers, while others place everything together. Follow the procedure for your institution. Regulations demand that objects contaminated with blood or body fluids be discarded in a suitable container and marked with the biohazard symbol (Fig. 5-9).

Used needles and syringes are placed in special containers designed to receive the syringe without recapping it (Fig. 5-10). OSHA's new requirement for safer medical devices may reduce the high number of needlesticks that previously occurred when workers had greater contact with unprotected

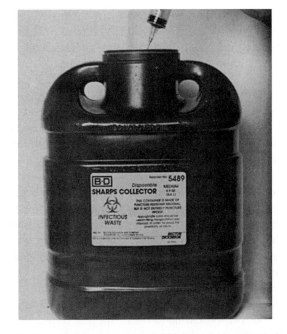

FIG. 5-10 Sharps container is bright red in color. Safe disposal practices prevent rehandling of needles and syringes.

sharps. A broad array of these safer medical devices is available. Some provide a sheath that slides forward to shield the contaminated needle, and others have a retractable needle. The health care worker can retract the needle into the syringe after removing the needle from the vein. It is important to use these safety features to prevent accidental needlesticks. A needleless system provides the greatest protection from needlesticks and should be used to introduce medications and contrast media after initial venous access is established (see Chapter 7).

Contaminated bandages and dressings are handled with gloves and placed directly into red plastic biohazard bags, which are sealed and discarded.

Before sending specimens to the laboratory, place them in clean containers with secure caps and slip them inside a plastic bag labeled with a biohazard symbol.

Always wear gloves when assisting patients with bedpans or urinals. Be sure to empty these at once

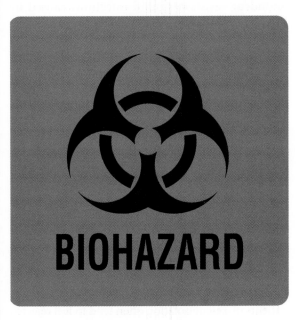

FIG. 5-9 Biohazard symbol.

unless a specimen is needed. Rinse them well over the hopper or toilet and discard them, or put them in the proper place to be sterilized unless they are to be reused immediately by the same patient.

Isolation Technique

Diagnosis or suspicion of communicable disease was the reason for isolation prior to the development of Universal Precautions. When it was recognized that *all* patients were potentially infectious, Universal Precautions and then Body Substance Precautions were established (see pp. 143-144). Hospitals began using these new precautions in combination with their isolation policies. Therefore this text identifies the various types of isolation systems that have been previously used and describes the current CDC recommendations.

Formerly the guidelines for isolation precautions in hospitals recommended that each hospital adopt one of two systems: a category-specific system with seven different types of isolation or a disease-specific system. The current guidelines replace both of these systems. The CDC document *Recommendations for Isolation Precautions in Hospitals* is reprinted in Appendix G, together with the *Synopsis of Types of Precautions and Patients Requiring the Precautions.*

Transmission-based precautions

The current CDC recommendation for isolating patients is called Transmission-Based Precautions. This system collapses the old category-specific and disease-specific precautions into three sets of precautions based on routes of transmission. These sets are designed to reduce the risk of airborne, droplet, and contact transmission, respectively. They may be used singularly or in combination for diseases that have multiple routes of transmission, and they must be used with Standard Precautions. Refer to Fig. 5-11 for examples of precaution cards used with this system.

Airborne precautions. Airborne precautions are designed to reduce the risk of transmitting dust particles containing the infectious organism or airborne droplet nuclei (5 microns or smaller) to a susceptible person. Airborne precautions are used to prevent diseases such as tuberculosis and measles (rubeola). Health care workers and visitors entering the room of an infectious person must wear particulate respirators approved by the National Institute for Occupational Safety and Health (NIOSH). These masks must be capable of filtering particles 1 micron in size and have a 95% efficiency (Fig. 5-12). Patients under airborne precautions are placed in rooms with negative airflow and special air circulation with more than six air exchanges per hour to the outdoors or through high-efficiency particulate air (HEPA) filters. The doors to these rooms must always remain closed.

Droplet precautions. Droplet precautions are designed to reduce the contact of large-particle droplets (greater than 5 microns) with the conjunctivae or with mucous membranes of the nose and mouth of a susceptible person. Droplet precautions are used to prevent the transmission of diseases such as diphtheria and influenza. Health care workers and visitors coming in close contact with these patients must wear surgical masks, but no special air circulation is required in these rooms.

Contact precautions. Contact precautions are designed to reduce the risk of transmitting pathogens by direct skin-to-skin contact or indirect contact with a contaminated object. Contact precautions are used to prevent transmission of diseases such as multidrug-resistant wound infections caused by MRSA and VRE, the new strain of *E. coli* (O157:H7) that causes gastrointestinal and renal problems, and various skin infections such as impetigo. Health care workers who come in close contact with infected patients must wear gloves and a gown.

Combination airborne and contact precautions. Combination airborne and contact precautions are designed to reduce the risk of transmitting pathogens by both airborne droplet nuclei and direct skin-to-skin contact. These precautions are used to prevent transmission of the virus that causes SARS and the varicella virus that causes chicken pox and disseminated herpes zoster. Health care workers who have not had chicken pox should avoid contact with infected patients. Previously infected personnel need not wear masks.

Radiography of isolation patients

Patients placed in isolation often tend to feel rejected and "untouchable." You can help alleviate these

STANDARD PRECAUTIONS
FOR THE CARE OF ALL PATIENTS

Includes Blood, Body Fluids, Secretions, Excretions, and Contaminated Items

A

1. Wash hands BEFORE and AFTER patient care, regardless of whether gloves are worn. Wash hands immediately after gloves are removed and between patient contacts.

2. Wear gloves when touching blood, body fluids, secretions, excretions, and contaminated items. Put on clean gloves just before touching mucous membranes & nonintact skin.

3. Wear mask and eye protection or a face shield to protect mucous membranes of the eyes, nose and mouth during procedures and patient care activities that are likely to generate splashes or sprays of blood & body fluids.

4. Wear gown to protect skin and prevent soiling of clothing during procedures and patient care activities that are likely to generate splashes or sprays of blood & body fluids. Remove soiled gown as promptly as possible & wash hands.

5. Take care to prevent injuries when using needles, scalpels and other sharp instruments or devices; when handling sharp instruments after procedures; when cleaning used instruments; and when disposing of used needles.

Use mouthpieces, resuscitation bags, or other ventilation devices as an alternative to mouth-to-mouth resuscitation.

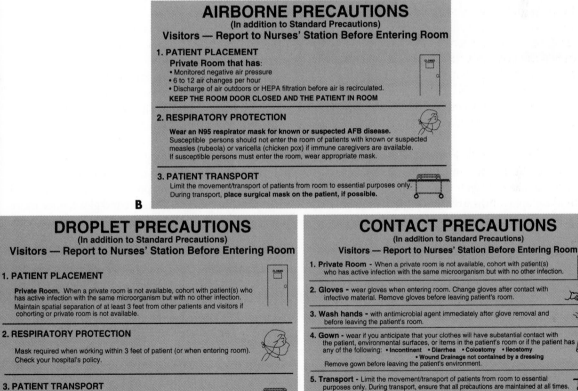

AIRBORNE PRECAUTIONS
(In addition to Standard Precautions)
Visitors — Report to Nurses' Station Before Entering Room

B

1. PATIENT PLACEMENT

Private Room that has:
- Monitored negative air pressure
- 6 to 12 air changes per hour
- Discharge of air outdoors or HEPA filtration before air is recirculated.

KEEP THE ROOM DOOR CLOSED AND THE PATIENT IN ROOM

2. RESPIRATORY PROTECTION

Wear an N95 respirator mask for known or suspected AFB disease.
Susceptible persons should not enter the room of patients with known or suspected measles (rubeola) or varicella (chicken pox) if immune caregivers are available. If susceptible persons must enter the room, wear appropriate mask.

3. PATIENT TRANSPORT

Limit the movement/transport of patients from room to essential purposes only. During transport, **place surgical mask on the patient, if possible.**

DROPLET PRECAUTIONS
(In addition to Standard Precautions)
Visitors — Report to Nurses' Station Before Entering Room

1. PATIENT PLACEMENT

Private Room. When a private room is not available, cohort with patient(s) who has active infection with the same microorganism but with no other infection. Maintain spatial separation of at least 3 feet from other patients and visitors if cohorting or private room is not available.

2. RESPIRATORY PROTECTION

Mask required when working within 3 feet of patient (or when entering room). Check your hospital's policy.

3. PATIENT TRANSPORT

Limit the movement/transport of patients from room to essential purposes only. During transport, **place surgical mask on the patient, if possible.**

CONTACT PRECAUTIONS
(In addition to Standard Precautions)
Visitors — Report to Nurses' Station Before Entering Room

1. **Private Room** - When a private room is not available, cohort with patient(s) who has active infection with the same microorganism but with no other infection.

2. **Gloves** - wear gloves when entering room. Change gloves after contact with infective material. Remove gloves before leaving patient's room.

3. **Wash hands** - with antimicrobial agent immediately after glove removal and before leaving the patient's room.

4. **Gown** - wear if you anticipate that your clothes will have substantial contact with the patient, environmental surfaces, or items in the patient's room or if the patient has any of the following: • Incontinent • Diarrhea • Colostomy • Ileostomy • **Wound Drainage not contained by a dressing** Remove gown before leaving the patient's environment.

5. **Transport** - Limit the movement/transport of patients from room to essential purposes only. During transport, ensure that all precautions are maintained at all times.

6. When possible, dedicate the use of noncritical patient-care equipment to a single patient. If common equipment is used, clean and disinfect between patients.

FIG. 5-11 **A,** Standard precautions. **B,** Visible reminders for staff and visitors.

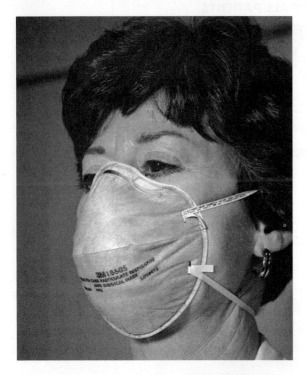

FIG. 5-12 Particulate respirator provides defense against airborne infections.

feelings by expressing a friendly interest in the patient and by avoiding any display of fear or revulsion as you perform your duties.

Radiography of the isolation patient requires two people, preferably, two radiographers. The "dirty" member of the team positions the patient, and the "clean" member handles the equipment. Although both radiographers must follow all designated isolation precautions, the "clean" member has no direct contact with the patient, the bed, or any items the patient may have touched. This radiographer is the only one who handles the x-ray machine and the uncovered cassettes. This team method minimizes contamination of x-ray equipment, which is difficult to disinfect completely.

Before you and your teammate enter the isolation room, prepare the necessary cassettes by placing each one in a smooth-fitting plastic bag or pillowcase and don your lead apron. Remove your jewelry and watch and place them in your pocket or pin them to your uniform. At the door you will find the necessary supplies for the required precautionary measures (e.g., disposable gloves, gowns, masks). Use the posted isolation guidelines for the designated type of isolation, and don protective clothing (Fig. 5-13). If the room was well designed for isolation, this procedure may take place in a vestibule adjoining the patient area.

Now you are ready to approach the bedside. Greet the patient, make introductions, and explain the procedure. The dirty member of the team places the cassette appropriately, making certain that the exposure side is toward the x-ray tube (Fig. 5-14). The clean teammate positions the machine, sets the controls, and makes the exposure. As each exposure is completed, the cassette is retrieved and the protective cover partially removed. It is then offered to the clean teammate with the edge exposed (Fig. 5-15). The contaminated cover is placed in the proper container, and the cassette is stored in the machine compartment.

When the examination is completed, make certain that the patient is comfortable and secure before removing isolation attire. The procedure for removing contaminated isolation attire is illustrated in Fig. 5-16. First untie your waist belt and remove your gloves. Pull off the first glove by gripping its contaminated side and inverting it as you remove it. Discard it directly into the container provided. Insert your clean fingers inside the cuff of the second glove, once more inverting it as it is removed. Perform hand hygiene. Then untie the neck strings of your gown and your mask strings. Remove the mask without touching the contaminated face portion, hold it by the strings or rubber band, and place it in the container provided. Next remove your gown, taking care to hold it away from you. Fold the contaminated sides together and place it in the hamper. Repeat hand hygiene.

Clean the mobile x-ray unit thoroughly before taking it back to the radiology department. If additional films might be needed, you may leave the mobile unit in a safe location just inside the isolation area and postpone cleaning until the films are processed. When no further exposures are needed, push the unit into the corridor for cleaning.

FIG. 5-13   PREPARATION FOR EXAMINATION IN ISOLATION

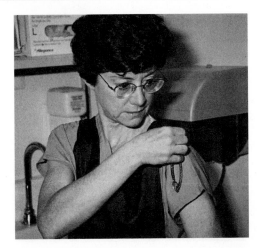

A Wearing lead apron, remove jewelry and attach to uniform.

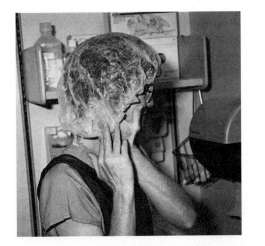

B Don cap or hood, making sure that all hair is covered.

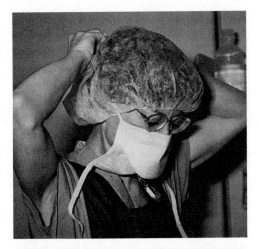

C Don mask, making certain that nose and mouth are completely covered and nose piece fits snugly.

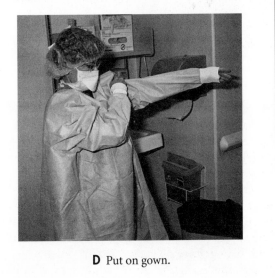

D Put on gown.

Continued

Isolation patients in the radiology department

If it is necessary to transport an infectious patient to the radiology department, the first step is to identify the isolation category involved and prepare for the examination accordingly. Cover the stretcher or wheelchair with a sheet, then with another sheet or cotton blanket. Depending on the isolation category involved, you may need to protect yourself and your uniform by wearing a gown, mask, and gloves. The patient with respiratory disease should wear a mask while being transported (Fig. 5-17).

FIG. 5-13   PREPARATION FOR EXAMINATION IN ISOLATION—cont'd

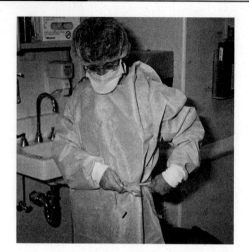

E Fasten gown securely, making sure that uniform is completely covered.

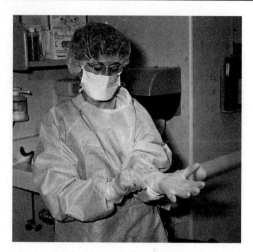

F Don protective gloves.

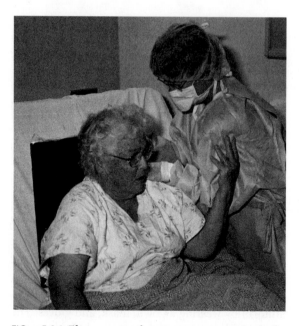

FIG. 5-14 Place covered cassette as required for radiographic examination.

Transfer the patient to the wheelchair or stretcher, folding the inner cover around the patient, then the outer cover, and tucking them both in securely.

When you arrive at the radiology department, take the patient directly into the x-ray room. Protect the table with a sheet. Work with a partner so that one radiographer handles the patient and the other handles the equipment and controls as previously described. Position the patient, and make your exposures as efficiently as possible. Return the patient to the wheelchair or stretcher, rewrapping the sheet and blanket. Place the sheet from the table and any other contaminated linens in the linen bag. Place tissues, caps, and other disposable contaminated materials in the proper container. Tissues, masks, and other disposable contaminated materials that are not soaked with blood or body fluids can be placed in the regular trash. Anything wet and contaminated with blood or body fluids must be placed in a red bag or a special container marked with a biohazard symbol.

After returning the patient to the bed, remove your gloves, perform hand hygiene, and remove your gown as previously described. Clean the wheelchair

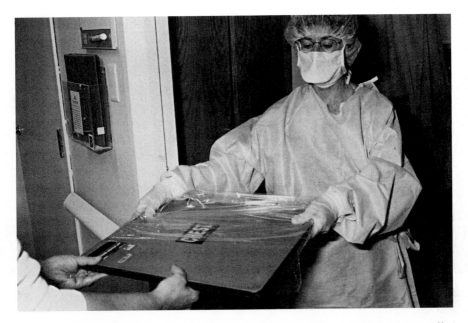

FIG. 5-15 Following exposure, pull back contaminated cover without touching cassette, offering "clean" cassette to teammate.

FIG. 5-16	REMOVING ISOLATION ATTIRE

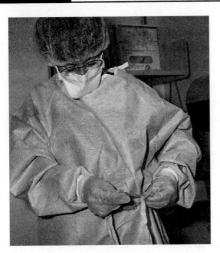

A First, unfasten waist tie.

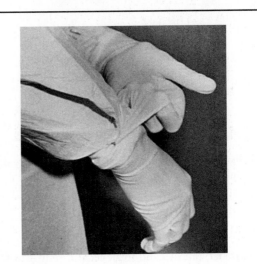

B Grasp the first glove from the outside, and pull it off.

Continued

FIG. 5-16   REMOVING ISOLATION ATTIRE—cont'd

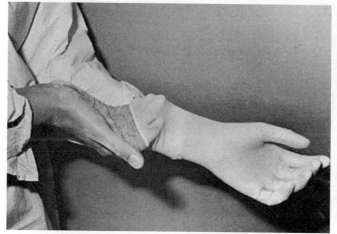

C Insert your clean fingers inside the cuff of the second glove, and remove it.

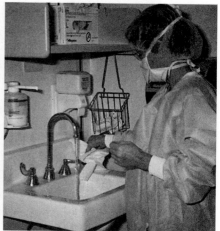

D Perform hand hygiene.

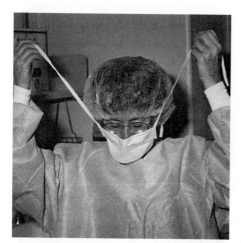

E Mask is contaminated. Remove by handling ties only.

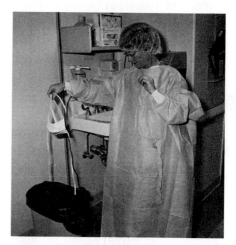

F Discard mask.

or stretcher, repeat hand hygiene, and return to the radiology department. During this period your partner should finish cleaning any other equipment used, including the table, and should then complete the task with hand hygiene.

Precautions for compromised patients

The compromised patient has very limited immunity and requires special precautions to avoid exposure to potential infection. These patients may have undergone organ transplants and may be taking

FIG. 5-16   REMOVING ISOLATION ATTIRE—cont'd

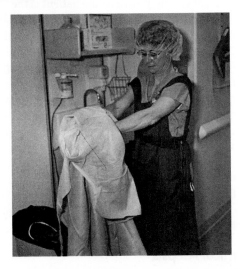

G Remove gown, folding contaminated surface inward. Discard.

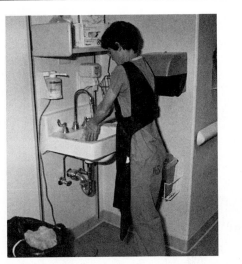

H Repeat hand hygiene.

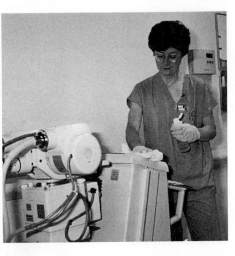

I Disinfect mobile x-ray unit when procedure is complete.

immunosuppressant medications. Burn patients and neonates at risk may also require these precautions. These precautions are sometimes used for patients receiving chemotherapy that reduces their resistance.

These precautions were once referred to as reverse isolation or protective isolation. Federal isolation guidelines published in 1983 eliminated the category of protective isolation, largely because the purpose and procedure are the opposite of those for other

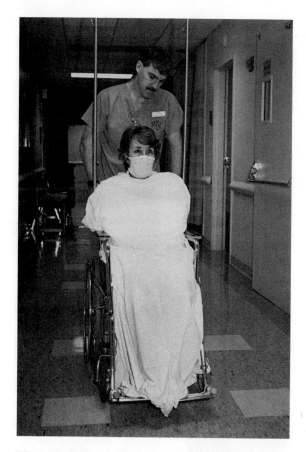

FIG. 5-17 Patient under respiratory isolation is transported to imaging department.

Under the system of protective precautions, the radiographer who positions the patient is the "clean" member of the team. Wearing the proper protective clothing, this radiographer avoids contact with uncovered cassettes, the x-ray machine, and other potentially contaminated articles. To cover the cassette properly, this radiographer folds back the edges of the sterile cassette cover and holds it open while the second radiographer places the cassette inside. Care must be taken not to contaminate the outside of the cover (Fig. 5-18). The "clean" radiographer touches only the patient, the bed, the covered cassette, and "clean" or sterile items, whereas the dirty radiographer touches only the equipment. This is the exact opposite of the procedure for isolation technique.

Surgical Asepsis

Earlier in this chapter we defined medical asepsis as a method of reducing the number of pathogenic microorganisms in the environment and intervening in the process by which they are spread. Surgical

isolation categories. The basic principles are unchanged, and you may find that these terms are still used in the clinical setting.

Precautions for the compromised patient require that the equipment be cleaned *before* entering the patient's room. Hand hygiene is required before touching the patient, the bed, or articles handled by the patient. Masks, caps, sterile gowns, and gloves may be worn in the same manner used in the operating room, or a modification of surgical technique may be indicated. The modified technique results in a very high degree of medical asepsis without requiring the rigorous protocol of sterile technique. Specific precautions are posted outside the patient's room.

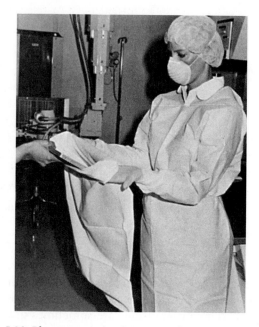

FIG. 5-18 Place cassette in clean cover for protection of patient with compromised resistance.

asepsis, on the other hand, is the complete destruction of all organisms and spores from equipment used to perform patient care or procedures. The sterile linens, gloves, and instruments used in surgery may be the first examples brought to mind, but many other procedures require sterile equipment. Examples include lumbar punctures, catheterizations, and injections, as well as the care of some immunocompromised patients.

It should be clarified that although the surgical suite is a sterile environment, radiographers who are called to this area to obtain radiographs or operate the C-arm fluoroscope do not wear sterile attire. Before entering, they dress in clean scrub clothes and wear a cap and surgical mask. Sterile dress is not required because the radiographer avoids contact with the sterile field. Radiography in surgery is discussed in greater detail in Chapter 11.

Sterile items used in the radiology department are usually obtained from central sterile supply. Most disposable items, such as small syringes, intravenous sets, and catheterization sets, are sterile when purchased and are protected by a paper or plastic wrap. Reusable items such as instruments and glass syringes are wrapped, sterilized, and reissued by central sterile supply.

Sterilization

Although the radiographer is seldom directly involved in the process of sterilization, it is helpful to understand the methods that may be involved. Five methods of sterilization are used, some of which are more reliable than others: chemical, dry heat, gas, gas plasma technology, and autoclaving (steam).

Chemical sterilization. Chemical sterilization involves the immersion and soaking of clean objects in a bath of germicidal solution followed by a sterile water rinse. The effectiveness of this process depends on solution strength and temperature and the immersion time, all of which are difficult to control accurately. Contamination of the solution or the object being sterilized may occur and is not easily detectable. For these reasons, chemical sterilization is one of the less satisfactory methods for providing surgical asepsis and is not recommended. If chemical sterilization must be used, follow the chemical manufacturer's instructions completely. Chemical sterilants are often used to achieve high-level disinfection of devices that come in contact with the mucous membranes, such as flexible, fiberoptic endoscopes. High-level disinfection can be accomplished in less than an hour and is effective at destroying microorganisms but will not kill spores.

Dry heat. Dry heat such as that in an oven is required to sterilize some sharp instruments, certain powders and greasy substances. The amount of time needed for this type of sterilization varies from 1 to 6 hours at a temperature range of 329° to 338° F (165° to 170° C).

Conventional gas sterilization. Items that would be damaged by high temperatures are usually sterilized with a mixture of gases (freon and ethylene oxide) heated to 135° F (57° C). Gas sterilization is used primarily for electrical, plastic, and rubber items, and for optical ware. Telephones, stethoscopes, blood pressure cuffs, and other equipment used in isolation rooms may be sterilized in this manner. This treatment is very effective but has one drawback. The gases used are poisonous, so they must be dissipated by means of aeration in a controlled environment. Because aeration is a slow process, it is important to send items for gas sterilization to central sterile supply well in advance of the time they will be used. A note indicating the date and hour the item is needed will help the staff plan their workload effectively.

Gas plasma technology. Due to the toxic fumes and residues of ethylene oxide sterilization, a new and safer method of sterilizing heat- and moisture-sensitive items is being used in hospitals. Items are cleaned, wrapped and placed in a compact mobile unit where low-temperature hydrogen peroxide gas plasma diffuses through the wrapped instruments and effectively kills both microorganisms and spores. Gas plasma is formed within this sterilizing unit when vaporized hydrogen peroxide is subjected to radio-frequency energy, changing the vapor into a low-temperature plasma. The plasma then breaks down into free radicals (atoms with unpaired electrons in outer shells). These free radicals destroy the microorganisms by stripping their atoms of electrons. Upon completion of the sterilization cycle the remaining free radicals are converted into nontoxic byproducts, primarily water and oxygen.

Because the gas plasma system uses very low heat and moisture, it can effectively sterilize endoscopes, fiberoptic devices, microsurgical instruments, and powered instruments. Another advantage is greater safety for central sterile supply department workers because there are no toxic fumes, byproducts, or residues, and no handling of chemicals. For these reasons, gas plasma technology has significantly reduced the use of ethylene oxide, but it cannot completely replace this method. Gas plasma cannot sterilize instruments that have long, narrow lumina, and it cannot be used for powders, liquids, or any cellulose materials, such as paper, cotton, linen, or muslin.

Autoclaving. An **autoclave** is a device that provides steam sterilization under pressure, the most commonly used sterilization method. It is also the quickest and most convenient means of sterilization for items that can withstand heat and moisture. High temperatures (250° to 275° F [121° to 135° C]) can be achieved under pressure, making this an extremely effective method.

Sterility indicators. Most forms of hospital sterilization use chemical indicators to identify that a pack has been sterilized. Indicators are placed inside the pack as well as outside to show that the gas, heat, steam, or gas plasma has penetrated to all surfaces. Indicators change color when the required conditions have been met. Radiographers are responsible for correctly recognizing the sterilization indicators used in their clinical facility.

In addition to chemical indicators, hospitals use biological indicators (BIs) to ensure all forms of microbial life are destroyed during the sterilization process. BIs are closed containers that contain different species of nonpathogenic spore-forming bacilli, each resistant to a specific sterilization process. The appropriate container is placed inside the unit with the instruments during sterilization. Inability to culture the spores following sterilization confirms that the instruments are free of all microbial life. BIs are used in each load that includes implantable devices, and on a routine daily or weekly basis, depending on hospital policy.

Suppliers of commercial packs use ionizing radiation from cobalt-60 or an electron beam to destroy microorganisms and spores. Commercial packs also contain indicators and expiration dates to confirm their sterility.

Sterile fields

A **sterile field** is a microorganism-free area prepared for the use of sterile supplies and equipment. The first step in preparing a sterile field is to confirm the sterility of packaged supplies and equipment (Fig. 5-19). Packages are considered sterile if they meet the following criteria:

- They are clean, dry, and unopened.
- Their expiration date has not been exceeded.
- Their sterility indicators have changed to a predetermined color, confirming sterilization.

Preparations must be made before starting a procedure that requires sterile technique, and the radiographer may be responsible for assembling the needed equipment. Most procedures today use disposable equipment wrapped in paper or plastic. Directions on the packages are usually clear and precise, and the time taken to read them in advance increases self-confidence when assisting the physician. Nondisposable equipment that has been processed by central sterile supply is double-wrapped in cloth or heavy paper and sealed with indicator tape. All packs are wrapped in a standardized manner and are always opened using the following method (Fig. 5-20):

- Place the pack on a clean surface within reach of the physician.
- Just before the procedure begins, break the seal and open the pack.
- Unfold the first corner away from you; then unfold the two sides.
- Pull the front fold down toward you and drop it. Do not touch the inner surface.
- The inner wrap, if there is one, is opened in the same manner.
- You have now established a sterile field.

Nondisposable sterile items wrapped separately may now be added to the sterile field. Standing back from the table, grasp the object through the wrapping with one hand. With the other hand, unseal the wrappings, allowing them to fall down over your wrist. Hold the edges of the wrapper with your

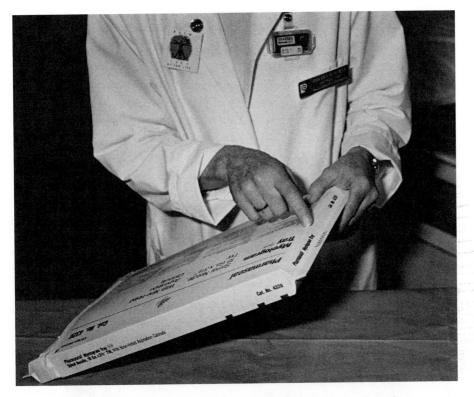

FIG. 5-19 Always check expiration dates before opening sterile packs.

free hand, and drop the object onto the sterile field without releasing the wrapper (Fig. 5-21).

Disposable sponges, gloves, and other small items are supplied in "peel-down" paper wraps and may be added to the sterile field. Following the instructions, separate the paper layers, invert the package, and allow the object to fall onto the sterile field without contaminating the object or the sterile field (Fig. 5-22).

It may be necessary to add a liquid medium such as Betadine to a sterile tray. After reading the label three times, position the label toward your hand, open the spout, squirt the first few drops into the wastebasket or sink, pour the required amount into the sterile receptacle on the tray, show the physician the label, and close the spout. By discarding the first small amount poured, you "wash" the container's lip and avoid the possibility of contaminating the tray (Fig. 5-23).

When a radiographer must manipulate items in a sterile field, a sterile transfer forceps is used. Unwrap the forceps, grasping the handles firmly without touching the remainder of the instrument. Keep the forceps above your waist and in your sight at all times. After use, place the tips in a sterile field with the handles protruding so you can use them again. Do not reach across the sterile field.

If a procedure must be postponed, do not open the tray. If it is already open, cover it immediately with a sterile drape or discard it, since airborne contamination is just as serious as a break in sterile technique.

Upon completion of the procedure, don gloves and thoroughly clean all reusable items before returning them to central sterile supply. Items must be free of all residue so that the sterilizing agent can penetrate to all surfaces. Thorough cleaning is very important and is

FIG. 5-20 ESTABLISHING A STERILE FIELD

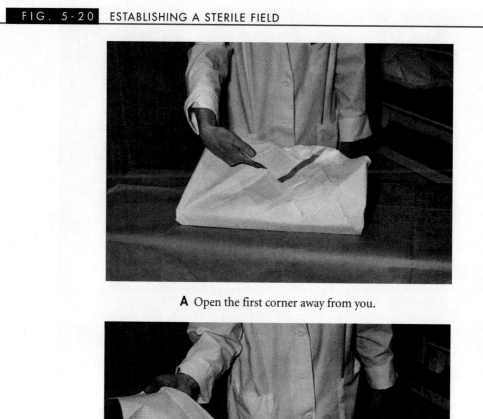

A Open the first corner away from you.

B Open one side by grasping corner tip.

most easily accomplished when done promptly. Discard disposable items, placing needles in the sharps container and the remainder in a biohazard bag. Box 5-2 summarizes the principles of surgical asepsis.

We cannot overemphasize the importance of developing a **"sterile conscience."** This refers to an awareness of sterile technique and the responsibility for telling the person in charge whenever you contaminate a field or observe its contamination by someone else. The inconvenience of reestablishing a sterile field may make a beginning student reluctant to speak out about apparent breaks in

FIG. 5-20   ESTABLISHING A STERILE FIELD—cont'd

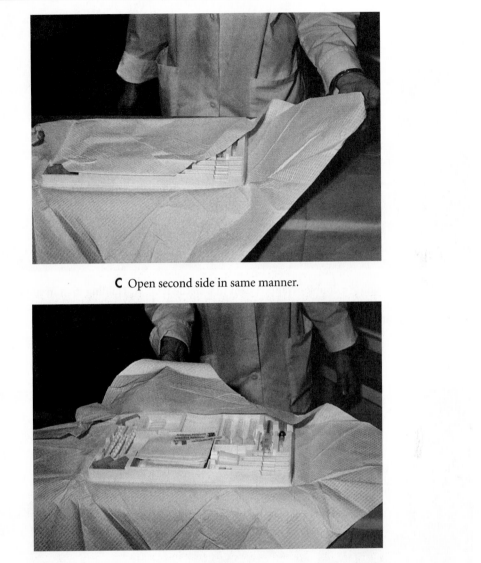

C Open second side in same manner.

D Pull remaining corner toward you. If there is an inner wrap, open it in the same manner. A sterile field is now established.

technique. Physicians and coworkers may not seem to appreciate your challenge at the moment, but your professionalism and concern for the patient's welfare will be reflected in the confidence that team members place in your aseptic technique.

Skin preparation

Procedures that involve puncture or incision of the skin require special skin preparation to prevent pathogens from entering the body. Skin preparation must sometimes be performed in medical imaging

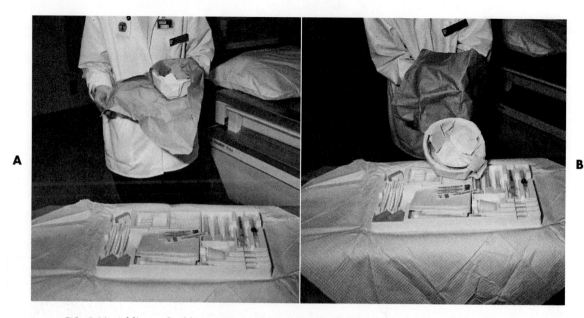

FIG. 5-21 Adding a double-wrapped item to a sterile field. **A,** Holding item in nondominant hand, open outer wrap; open first fold away from your body. **B,** Avoid contamination of field by holding corners of outer wrap while dropping item onto tray.

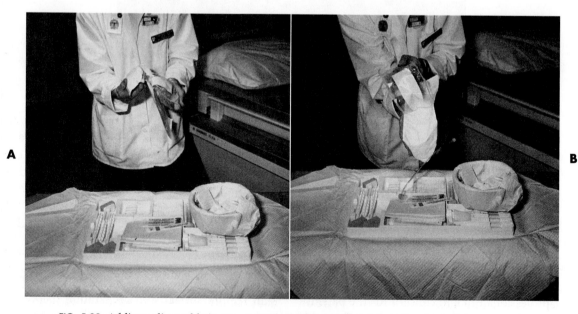

FIG. 5-22 Adding a disposable item to a sterile field from a "peel down" wrap. **A,** Separate wrap according to package instructions. **B,** Invert package, allowing item to drop onto field.

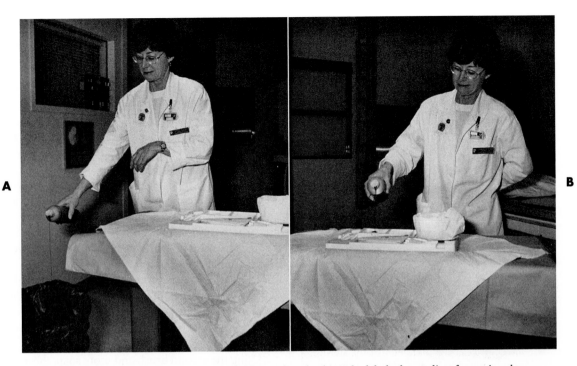

A

B

FIG. 5-23 Adding liquid to a sterile field. **A,** After checking the label, cleanse lip of container by squirting small amount into waste container. **B,** Pour required amount into receptacle on tray, taking care not to contaminate sterile field.

departments and is required for invasive radiologic procedures such as lumbar puncture for myelography and arterial catheterization for angiography. These procedures are described in more detail in Chapters 10 and 12.

The purpose of the skin preparation is to minimize the introduction of pathogens to the body via the puncture or incision, thus reducing the likelihood of infection. Although it is not possible to sterilize the skin, a high degree of microbial dilution is accomplished by means of proper skin preparation. Preparation includes thorough cleansing, and hair removal if necessary, followed by application of an antiseptic solution such as Betadine or Zephiran, and the surrounding of the prepared area with sterile drapes. The prepared area is usually a circle approximately 12 inches in diameter with the puncture or incision site at its center. The physician will specify the exact site. The procedure is outlined in Box 5-3.

Hair removal is not always required for skin preparation, and shaving is done only on the specific order of the physician in charge.

Surgical scrub

The ability to perform a surgical scrub is necessary if the radiographer is asked to assist with a sterile procedure. Prior to donning sterile gown and gloves, the radiographer performs this scrub to remove as many microorganisms as possible from the skin of the hands and forearms through both chemical and mechanical means. You should not scrub (or assist with any sterile procedure) if you do not feel well or if you have an upper respiratory infection. Do not scrub if there are skin problems involving your hands or arms. Wounds and hangnails tend to ooze serum, which encourages rapid bacterial growth and increases the danger of infection to the patient.

STANDARD PRINCIPLES OF SURGICAL ASEPSIS

1. Any sterile object or field touched by an unsterile object or person becomes contaminated.
2. Never reach across a sterile field. Organisms may fall from your arm into the field. Reaching also increases the chance of brushing the area with your uniform.
3. If you suspect an item is contaminated, discard it. This includes items that are damp (moisture permits the transfer of bacteria from the outside to the inside of a wrapped set) and items that have the seal broken or on which the indicator tape has not assumed the correct color.
4. Do not pass between the physician and the sterile field.
5. Never leave a sterile area unattended. If the field is accidentally contaminated (e.g., by a fly or a patient reaching for her glasses), no one would know.
6. A 1-inch border at the perimeter of the sterile field is considered to be a "buffer zone" and is treated as if it were contaminated.

Your institutional policies will govern the selection of materials for the surgical scrub as well as the method to be used. Disposable or reusable brushes may be used, and the brush packages frequently contain a fingernail cleaner. Brushes are sometimes impregnated with soap, or the soap may be in a wall-mounted container controlled by a foot or knee lever. An antimicrobial soap or detergent is used that is effective against both gram-positive and gram-negative microorganisms. These agents act rapidly and continue to inhibit microbial growth in the hours following the scrub. The extent of the scrub may be determined by the timing of the steps or by counting brush strokes.

A properly executed surgical hand scrub using the anatomical counted brush stroke method is illustrated in Fig. 5-24. Before you begin, examine your hands to be certain that the nails are short and free of polish, the cuticles are in good condition, and there are no cuts or skin problems. Remove all jewelry from your hands and forearms. Don a cap or hood to cover all hair, and put on a fresh mask. If goggles or protective eyewear are to be worn, put them on at this point and adjust them comfortably. Open your sterile gown pack and a pack of sterile towels, and obtain two brushes and a disposable fingernail cleaner. Check to be sure your scrub clothes are properly tied and tucked in to avoid contamination from loose garments.

After adjusting the water temperature, wet your hands. Add a few drops of antimicrobial soap and more water as needed to make a lather. Before beginning the actual scrub, wash your hands and forearms thoroughly, use one brush and soap to clean your nails, and clean under your nails with the nail cleaner. Rinse your hands and arms thoroughly, keeping your hands higher than your elbows. Take care to avoid splashing your scrub clothes, since the dampness may later moisten your sterile gown, causing contamination.

Using the second brush and more soap, the actual scrub begins. The prescribed number of brush strokes is usually 30 strokes to the nails and 20 to each area of the skin, which usually takes about 5 minutes. Light friction is effective; too harsh a scrub may cause skin damage with predisposition to infection. The fingers, hands, and arms should be visualized as having four sides, and each side must be effectively scrubbed. Starting with the fingernails, scrub them vigorously, holding the brush perpendicular to them. Then scrub all sides of each finger and the palms and backs of the hands. Use a circular motion to scrub each side of the forearms and elbows, up to 2 inches above the elbows. Keep your hands above your elbows while scrubbing and add small amounts of water as needed to maintain a good lather. When scrubbing is completed, discard the brush and rinse your hands and arms thoroughly. To dry, grasp the corner of a sterile towel and step back from the field, allowing the towel to fall open. Bend forward at the waist and hold your arms away from your body and above your waist. Dry your hands, then your arms, thoroughly, rotating the towel as required. Take care not to contaminate the sterile field, the towel, or your

BOX 5-3

PREPARING THE SKIN FOR STERILE PROCEDURES

1. Obtain a "skin prep set" and a bottle of antiseptic for painting the skin. The preparation set includes a basin, liquid soap such as pHisoderm, gauze sponges, razor, towel, forceps, and medicine cup.
2. Perform hand hygiene.
3. Place the patient in a comfortable position and ensure privacy.
4. Explain what is to be done.
5. Expose an area slightly larger than the preparation site, keeping the patient as completely covered as possible to provide comfort and modesty.
6. Fill the basin with warm water.
7. **Note:** If hair removal is not ordered, omit steps 7 to 11.
8. Using a gauze sponge, thoroughly wet the area to be shaved and apply soap, forming a lather.
9. Shave a small area at a time. Hold the skin taut with one hand and shave with short, firm strokes in the direction of hair growth. Rinse the razor frequently.
10. Rinse the area, removing all the hair.
11. Rinse and refill the basin with warm water.
12. Using soap and a fresh gauze sponge, cleanse the area completely. Starting at the puncture site, use a circular motion and scrub in ever-widening circles. Do not scrub harshly, but remember that friction is more effective than soap in cleansing the skin.
13. Use a sterile gauze sponge to remove the soap and water, again using a circular pattern and starting at the center. This pattern avoids recontamination of the area that has been cleansed.
14. Pour a little of the antiseptic into a waste container to cleanse the lip of the bottle.
15. Fill the medicine cup with antiseptic.
16. Grasp several gauze sponges with the forceps and dip them into the antiseptic.
17. Paint the skin with the antiseptic, starting in the center of the area and working outward in a circular pattern. Discard the sponge.
18. Allow the skin to dry.
19. Repeat steps 16 and 17.
20. Open the pack containing the sterile drape or sterile towels. The physician, wearing sterile gloves, will drape the area surrounding the prepared site.

hands. You are now ready to don your sterile gown and gloves.

In the 2002 CDC guidelines regarding hand hygiene, the CDC recommends that in place of performing a surgical scrub using an antimicrobial soap, the following two-stage surgical scrub may be performed. Begin by washing the hands and forearms using a nonantimicrobial soap, then thoroughly dry the hands and forearms, and apply an alcohol-based surgical hand-scrub product with persistent activity, following the manufacturer's instructions. Wait for thorough drying before donning sterile gloves. This newer method has been very effective in reducing bacterial counts on hands.

Sterile gowning, masking, and gloving

Prior to performing your surgical scrub, put on a mask and a cap and open the package containing the sterile gown or have someone who is not scrubbed assist you. To don the sterile gown the radiographer follows the procedure shown in Fig. 5-25.

There are two methods of gloving for sterile procedures, the open method and the closed method. The closed method is illustrated as a part of the sterile gowning procedure in Fig. 5-25. The open method is used by radiographers when sterile gowning is not required and is depicted in Fig. 5-26.

When removing the gloves, invert them as you pull them off. Perform hand hygiene.

Removing and applying dressings

In many health care institutions today, radiographers are called upon to perform skills that were once performed solely by nurses. You may be directed by a physician to remove a patient's dressing, and it may also be your duty to apply a fresh dressing when the examination has been completed.

When a dressing is to be removed, perform hand hygiene, don gloves, and inform the patient of what you are about to do. Use care in removing the dressing to prevent cross contaminating the wound and yourself. Remove the dressing gently to avoid hurting the patient. Place the soiled dressing in a plastic bag and seal it before adding it to the biohazard container. Remove your gloves following the same procedure used with isolation techniques, and perform hand hygiene.

The application of a new dressing requires sterile technique. Begin by preparing your supplies: sterile gloves, sterile drape, sterile gauze, and tape. You may also need some normal saline to clean the area around the wound. When everything you will need has been assembled, proceed as follows:

- Tell the patient what you plan to do.
- Perform hand hygiene.

FIG. 5-24 STERILE SCRUB PROCEDURE

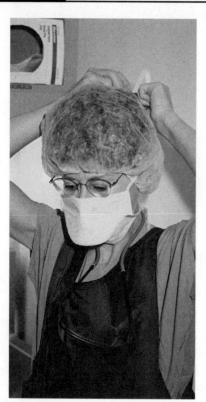

A Don cap or hood, mask, and protective goggles.

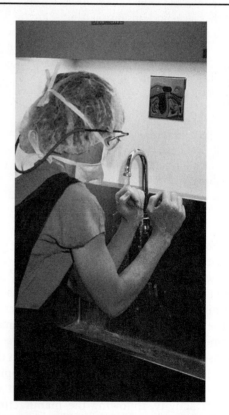

B Using foot or knee lever, adjust water flow and temperature. With hands above elbows, wet hands and forearms. Avoid splashing your clothing.

FIG. 5-24 STERILE SCRUB PROCEDURE—cont'd

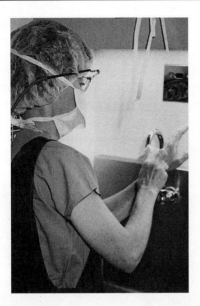

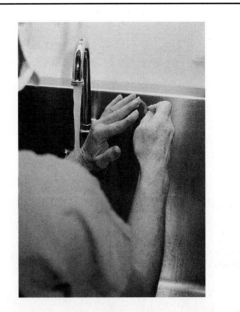

C Add antimicrobial soap and more water as needed to make a lather. Thoroughly wash hands and arms. Use brush to scrub nails and hands (about 1 minute for each hand). Discard brush.

D Under running water, clean under fingernails with fingernail cleaner.

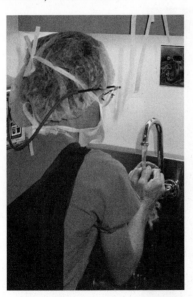

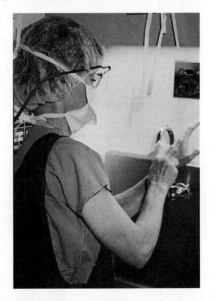

E Rinse hands and forearms.

F With the second brush and antimicrobial soap, scrub fingernails 30 strokes. Using 20 strokes for each skin area, scrub all sides of each finger, the webs between the fingers, and the palms and backs of both hands. Add water as needed to maintain a lather.

Continued

FIG. 5-24   STERILE SCRUB PROCEDURE—cont'd

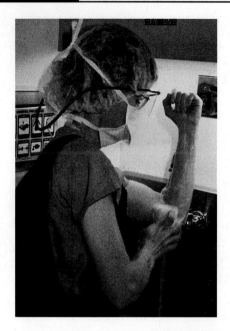

G Use a circular motion with brush to scrub all sides of forearms and elbows, 20 strokes for each area.

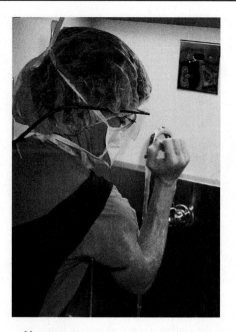

H Rinse, keeping hands above elbows.

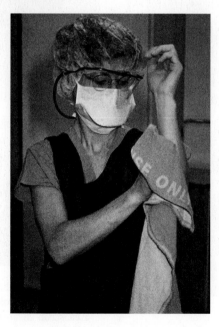

I Dry thoroughly with a sterile towel, starting with the fingers. Avoid contaminating the towel.

FIG. 5-25   STERILE GOWNING WITH CLOSED GLOVING TECHNIQUE

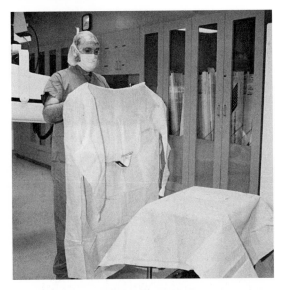

A Lift folded sterile gown, and step back from table. Allow gown to unfold with inside of gown toward you.

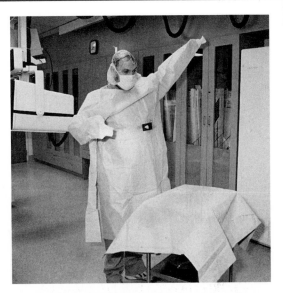

B Insert arms into sleeves. Do not allow hands to protrude through cuffs.

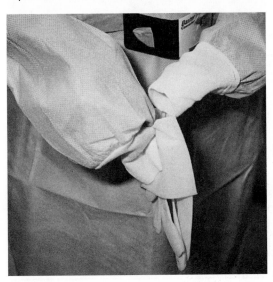

C With dominant hand remaining inside sleeve, pick up glove for nondominant hand.

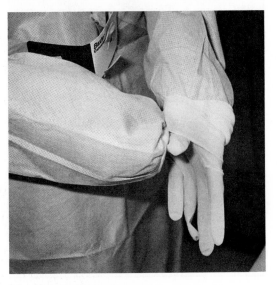

D Insert nondominant hand into glove.

Continued

FIG. 5-25 STERILE GOWNING WITH CLOSED GLOVING TECHNIQUE—cont'd

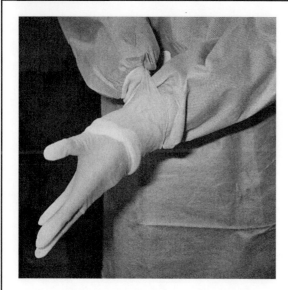

E Stretch cuff of glove over cuff of gown.

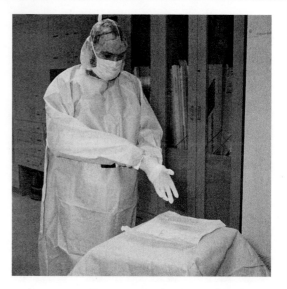

F Adjust fit of glove.

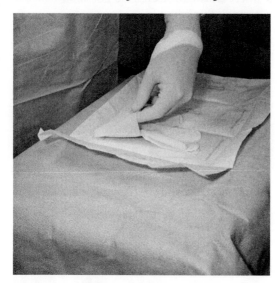

G With nondominant hand, pick up second glove.

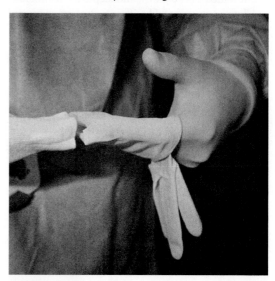

H Insert fingers of dominant hand into open glove.

FIG. 5-25   STERILE GOWNING WITH CLOSED GLOVING TECHNIQUE—cont'd

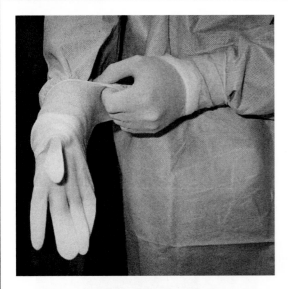

I Stretch cuff of glove over cuff of gown.

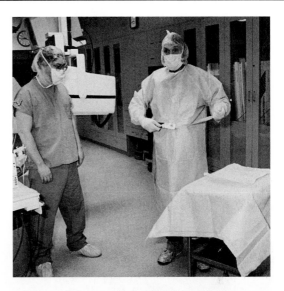

J Separate waist tie from gown.

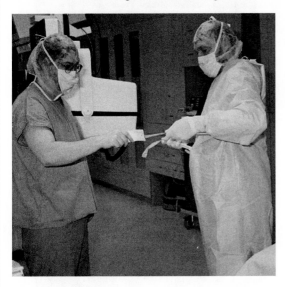

K Pass protective tab to assistant, then turn in a circle to wrap tie around your waist.

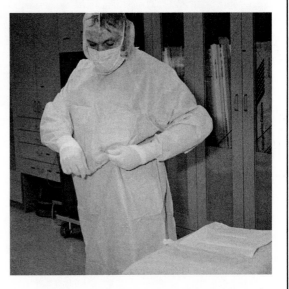

L A sharp tug on the tie will separate it from the contaminated tab, allowing you to fasten the tie without contaminating the gown.

FIG. 5-26 OPEN GLOVING TECHNIQUE

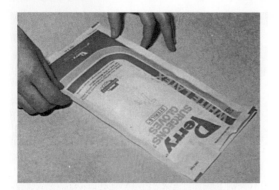

A Perform hand hygiene. Obtain gloves, and check for correct size.

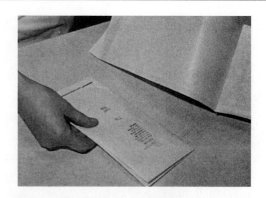

B Open outer wrap to expose folded inner wrap.

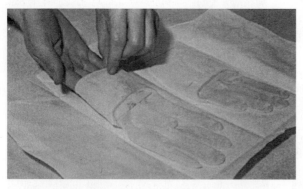

C Expose gloves with open ends facing you.

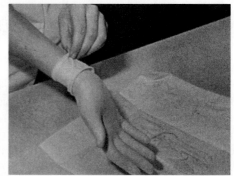

D Put on first glove, touching only inner surface of folded cuff.

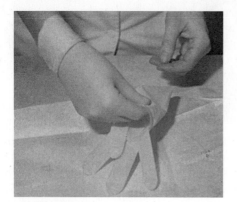

E Using gloved hand, grasp second glove under cuff.

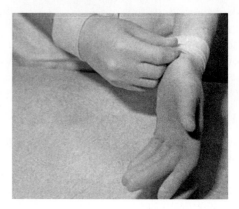

F Put on second glove, and unfold cuff.

FIG. 5-26   OPEN GLOVING TECHNIQUE—cont'd

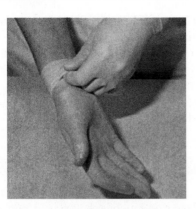

G Insert fingers under cuff of first glove, and unfold cuff.

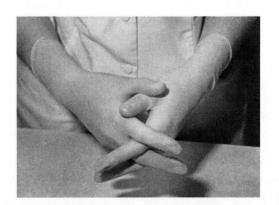

H Gloving complete. Keep hands in front of body and at safe distance from uniform to avoid contamination.

- Tear several strips of tape to a convenient length.
- Open the sterile drape pack, placing the drape near the patient.
- Partially open the drape by pulling from the corners. This creates a small sterile field for your other sterile items.
- Open the dressing package and add the sterile dressing to your sterile field.
- If you will need to cleanse around the wound, drop sterile gauze sponges into your field for this purpose.
- To moisten the gauze sponges, open a small vial of sterile normal saline solution. Recheck the label and pour a small amount of the saline over the sponges. Do not allow liquid to soak through to the sterile towel. Check the label for the third time before discarding the vial.
- Don sterile gloves using the open method described for sterile gloving.
- Use the moist sponges to clean gently around the wound.
- Allow the area to dry completely.
- Apply the dressing over the wound and secure it in place with tape.
- Cover the patient.

- Dispose of any waste.
- Remove your gloves and perform hand hygiene.

CONCLUSION

In the early part of the twentieth century, cleanliness and isolation were our only defenses against infection. Sulfa drugs were developed in the 1930s and penicillin in the 1940s. These "miracle drugs" were followed by powerful, broad-spectrum antibiotic agents plus new antiviral, antifungal, and antiprotozoan treatments. As these medications significantly reduced the suffering and death once caused by infections, the medical profession began to rely on pharmaceutical research for solutions to the lingering problems of infectious disease.

As you have learned in this chapter, many of these problems still exist and some are growing at an alarming rate. There are still no medications to treat many viral infections. Other organisms are mutating rapidly, acquiring immunity against medications that were once highly effective. Asymptomatic carriers of HIV and HBV pose a significant threat to members of the community, including health care workers, who may be exposed to infectious blood or body fluids without being aware that the infection is present. It has become apparent that an emphasis on the prevention of disease transmission, along with the development of both new technology and new policies, must receive at least as much emphasis as the development of new treatments. Disease prevention is clearly preferable to the most efficacious cure.

Infection control covers many situations that include minimizing the spread of the common cold, preventing postoperative infections, and avoiding exposure to HIV from contaminated blood that could lead to death from AIDS.

Radiographers must be aware of both the subtle and the potentially devastating possibilities of infection to themselves and to their patients. A commitment to aseptic technique is demonstrated by the conscientious application of knowledge and skill.

REVIEW QUESTIONS

1. Microorganisms that live on or inside the body without causing disease are referred to as:
   A. pathogens
   B. endospores
   C. microbial flora
   D. parasites
2. Bacteria can be classified or grouped based on:
   A. staining
   B. oxygen requirements
   C. shape
   D. all of the above
3. Under the system of protective precautions, the "dirty" technologist touches the:
   A. x-ray equipment
   B. patient
   C. covered cassette
   D. A and C
4. Tuberculosis is transmitted by:
   A. direct contact or touching the patient
   B. airborne route
   C. droplet route
   D. contact with a fomite
5. The standard principles of surgical asepsis include:
   A. not passing between the surgeon and sterile field
   B. never reaching across a sterile field
   C. discarding items that become contaminated
   D. all of the above

CRITICAL THINKING EXERCISES

1. Billie Cross was recently diagnosed with leukemia and requires a mobile chest x-ray. Upon arrival you find a sign on his door with a warning: "Do not enter—Protective Precautions." Outline the procedure you would follow to complete his exam, and identify the attire you may need to don before entering his room. Apply this to your clinical setting, following the policy in place at your institution.
2. You have been asked to transport Mr. Newton, who is in isolation with bacterial pneumonia, to the x-ray department. What will you need to do before you enter his room, and how will you prepare Mr. Newton to be transported? What procedure will be followed once you arrive in the x-ray department?
3. Mr. Mowrey was admitted through the emergency department with a staphylococcal infection resulting from leg trauma. List some persons who might become contaminated with his microorganisms if proper precautions are not used.
4. Name the type of isolation necessary for Mr. Mowrey, and list the protective attire that should be worn by the health care workers who care for him.

Patient Care and Assessment

At the conclusion of this chapter, the student will be able to:

- State four reasons for learning good evaluation skills.
- Demonstrate how to drain and measure the output from a urinary collection bag.
- List three personal comfort needs common to most patients.
- Demonstrate how to take a history appropriate to a specific procedure.
- Find the admitting diagnosis on the patient's chart.

- Take and record temperature, pulse, and respiration.
- State the normal values for temperature, pulse, respiration, and blood pressure.
- Obtain and record blood pressure readings.
- Describe the difference between a carotid pulse and an apical pulse.
- Use terms such as dyspneic, diaphoretic, and tachycardiac in describing patients' physical status.

V O C A B U L A R Y

apex, apical	hypertension
asystole	hypotension
bradycardia	ileostomy
bradypnea	incontinence
cardioversion	LOC
catheter	metabolism
colostomy	NPO
cyanotic	shock
diaphoretic	sinus rhythm
diastolic	sphygmomanometer
electrocardiogram	stoma
(ECG, EKG)	systolic
emphysema	tachycardia
fibrillation	tachypnea

OBSERVATION, ASSESSMENT, AND EVALUATION are activities so woven into our lives that we take them for granted. Every day we note changes in our environment without making a conscious effort. The house next door has a fresh coat of paint, new shrubs have been planted in the hospital parking area, and so on. We observe a new product at the store that promises increased effectiveness at slightly higher cost. We buy it, assess whether it meets our expectations, and then evaluate whether the difference in performance is worth the price. These same skills, when consciously practiced in the clinical area, will increase your value as a radiographer and help you become more sensitive to the condition of your patients.

PATIENT ASSESSMENT, AN ESSENTIAL SKILL

Many patients are intimidated in a medical environment, and this may prevent them from making complaints about physical needs or discomfort. The patient who is confident that personal needs will be met is more cooperative and receptive to directions.

Patient assessment is important when setting priorities. Radiographers are frequently responsible for scheduling the operation of a specific room and may need to determine how to sequence patients most effectively. Good evaluation skills will allow you to be both comfortable and flexible while arranging schedules to meet the needs of patients who are acutely ill, obviously in pain, or presenting with valid emergencies.

Another aspect of your role as a radiographer is the responsibility for relaying information to the radiologist. Through your ability to take a relevant history and report pertinent observations, you assist the radiologist in making decisions concerning diagnosis and treatment. Most important, by being alert to changes in patient condition, you may help avoid a life-threatening emergency.

ASSESSING PERSONAL CONCERNS OF PATIENTS

Uncertainty about an upcoming procedure, fear of a possible diagnosis, or concern about the effect of illness on family members can cause varying reactions in patients. Sometimes these concerns are expressed as anger and demonstrated by inappropriate speech or rude behavior toward personnel. Other expressions of anxiety may include a need to talk constantly, or conversely, becoming quiet and withdrawn. You may observe fidgeting or other nervous mannerisms. Anxiety can also be caused by a concern over modesty, especially when enemas, catheterizations, or urinary procedures are expected. Reassure patients by providing ample covers, an explanation of the procedure, and a matter-of-fact attitude.

Your presence is comforting to the anxious patient. Touch patients reassuringly, and tell them what to expect. Let them know when you leave the area and when you expect to return. Escort ambulatory patients to the bathroom or back to their waiting area. It can be very distressing to patients if they must wander about in a hospital gown, wondering where to go. Once you start a procedure, try to remain near the patient. If possible, postpone your lunch or break until the procedure is complete. If you must leave and another radiographer takes your place, introduce your substitute and excuse yourself rather than simply vanishing. If patients must wait in an x-ray room or dressing room, let them know that you are within hearing distance and that they may call on you for help. A call button is available in most patient bathrooms. Show patients how to use it, and assure them that someone will assist them promptly if they call.

Physical discomfort adds to tension as well. Remember that most patients will find it hard to remain still during a long procedure on a hard surface. This is especially difficult for a thin patient or an elderly person with kyphosis. An obese patient may have difficulty breathing when lying flat on the table. Note skin temperature when you touch the patient, and inquire whether the patient is warm enough. Use sufficient blankets, and tuck them in to provide both additional warmth and a sense of security. As you move briskly around the room the temperature may seem warm enough to you, but elderly or frail patients may not be active enough to keep warm.

If the patient is coughing or sniffling, offer paper handkerchiefs and position a waste container within reach for the soiled tissues (Fig. 6-1).

If dentures must be removed, place them in a safe and visible location in a suitable disposable

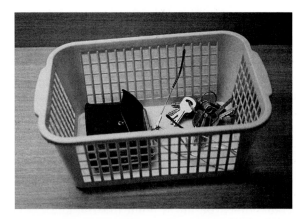

FIG. 6-2 A safe place for valuables within sight of the patient.

container. When you return dentures, rinse them for the patient or direct the patient to a sink. Dentures slide in much more easily when wet. Glasses and hearing aids also require responsible care. These items are essential to activities of daily living and are difficult and expensive to replace or repair. A bright colored plastic box is a useful container for these items. Choose a safe location in view of the patient, use the same place consistently, and point out the location to the patient. This is especially important for outpatients who have not been provided with a locker to secure valuables such as a purse or wallet (Fig. 6-2).

ASSESSING PHYSIOLOGICAL NEEDS
Water

A dry mouth can be caused by medication or may result from anxiety. If an inpatient requests water, first check the chart and note whether oral fluids are permitted. Many patients receiving intravenous (IV) therapy are allowed nothing at all by mouth. The abbreviation for this order is **NPO** (for the Latin, *nil per os,* meaning "nothing by mouth"). This means no food or liquid, not even ice chips or small sips of water, until the physician orders otherwise. If water is permitted, offer it with a straw if the patient cannot sit up. Record the amount taken in the chart.

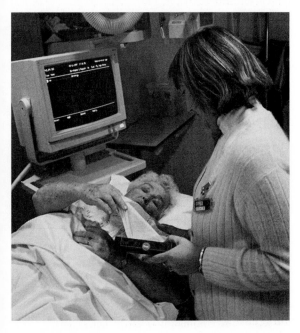

FIG. 6-1 Small comfort measures are greatly appreciated.

Elimination

An urgent need to void can be very bothersome to a patient. A full bladder may cause discomfort, irritability, and difficulty remaining still during the procedure. When this need is ignored in an older or debilitated patient, **incontinence** (loss of bladder or bowel control) may cause acute embarrassment for the patient and cleanup problems for the radiographer. Be especially sensitive to the need for a urinal, bedpan, or bathroom facilities when procedures are prolonged. If the procedure is likely to take considerable time, you might point this out and ask if the patient would like to visit the bathroom before getting onto the table.

When a urine specimen is needed, provide the proper container and cleansing supplies and instructions for obtaining a clean catch midstream (CSMS) specimen. These instructions are printed in Appendix H and are often printed on signs posted in patient restrooms.

When a patient needs to defecate or urinate and is unable to walk or be taken to the bathroom in a wheelchair, a bedpan or urinal is used. Placing a patient on the bedpan or offering the urinal is not a complex task. If you are unfamiliar with this procedure, the chief obstacle to overcome is embarrassment. Learn the location of equipment needed, and practice these procedures before you need to use them in a clinical situation.

There are two types of bedpans. A fracture pan has a flat lip in the front that makes it easy to slide under a patient who is in a cast or any patient who has problems lifting the pelvis for bedpan placement. The regular bedpan is somewhat larger and deeper with a rounded lip designed to support the buttocks (Fig. 6-3). Single-use containers, including bedpans and urinals made of a disposable material, are now available in many emergency departments and other short-stay hospital departments. Special disposal units accept both container and contents, which minimizes handling. To assist a patient with a bedpan, assemble the supplies you will need, don protective gloves, and follow the procedure outlined in Box 6-1.

Be sure that the patient is adequately covered for privacy. Remember when a female patient is placed

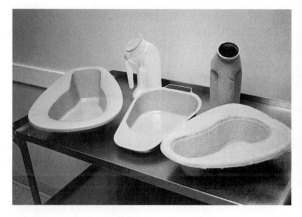

FIG. 6-3 *Left to right:* plastic bedpan, plastic urinal, plastic fracture pan, single-use disposable urinal, single-use disposable bedpan.

BOX 6-1

ASSISTING PATIENTS WITH THE BEDPAN

1. Assemble your equipment: bedpan with cover, toilet tissue, washcloth and towel, and a sheet or blanket.
2. Perform hand hygiene, and don disposable gloves.
3. Close the drapes and/or door to provide privacy.
4. If the patient is on the x-ray table, elevate the torso with pillows or angle sponges. Cover the patient.
5. Ask the patient to bend the knees and raise the hips.
6. Assist the patient by lifting with one hand under the small of the back while you slide the bedpan under the buttocks with the other.
7. Ask the patient to call when finished. Elevate the side rails of bed or stretcher.
8. When the patient is finished, provide toilet tissue, then a wet washcloth and towel for the patient's hands.
9. Ask the patient to raise the hips, and remove the bedpan.
10. Cover the bedpan, and place it aside until the patient is settled and secure.
11. Dispose of the contents in the toilet or hopper; remove gloves, and repeat hand hygiene.
12. Record elimination in the patient's chart.

on the bedpan that the upper torso needs to be slightly elevated to prevent urine from running up her back.

When a patient has restricted mobility, two people may be needed to assist the patient onto the bedpan. If the patient is already on the x-ray table, one person should stand on each side of the table to prevent the patient from falling. Patients may find it difficult to use the bedpan if they feel they are being watched, so remain out of their line of sight if possible while staying close enough to meet safety requirements.

When the patient has finished, you may have to assist with wiping. Wear gloves and have toilet tissue, a wet washcloth, and a dry towel conveniently placed. Assist the patient to lift the hips or roll away from you onto one side while you steady and remove the pan. Place it safely aside and help the patient by wiping from front to back with paper first, and then with a wet cloth before drying. Offer the patient a disposable moist towelette or a clean wet cloth and towel to cleanse the hands.

Male patients may need to use a urinal. If he is unable to use it himself, don protective gloves and spread the patient's legs; lift the sheet with one hand and slide the penis into the urinal with the other. It may be advisable to hold the urinal in position until the patient is finished.

Check the chart *before* emptying bedpans or urinals to see if the patient needs to have a specimen of urine or feces collected, or if intake and output (I&O) need to be measured. The nursing staff should call this to your attention. Make sure the correct container is available, and ask the nursing staff for instructions if you are unfamiliar with the procedure. The exact procedure for specimen collection will vary somewhat with the institution. Patients sometimes require a quantitative test that demands that all specimens be saved, and failure to comply may invalidate an entire 24-hour urine collection. If such a test is needed, a special container should be provided.

If no special tests are ordered, measure and discard the urine and record the amount. Most urinals are marked in milliliters for easy measurement, but urine in a bedpan will need to be emptied into a graduated container for measurement. If stool is present, observe it for obvious blood or diarrhea, and record any such observations. Empty the bedpan or urinal carefully into the hopper or toilet to avoid splashing. Rinse all containers and place them in the correct location for disposal or sterilization. Remember to perform hand hygiene after removing your gloves.

Some patients will have a urinary **catheter** (tube). These tubes are inserted through the urethra into the bladder, allowing urine to be continuously emptied into an attached collection bag. The most common type is called a Foley catheter. It has a small balloon at the tip that can be inflated with water to hold the tip securely within the bladder. When these patients are transferred from the wheelchair or stretcher to the radiographic table, urine collection bags must be held below the level of the patient's bladder to prevent urine in the tube or bag from being siphoned back into the bladder, causing discomfort and allowing bacteria potential access into the bladder.

If the bag is full, it must be emptied and the urine may need to be measured. Some collection bags consist of a rigid measuring container within a flexible plastic reservoir. Urine flows first into the graduated section, and tipping the unit empties the measured urine into the reservoir. Most collection bags have a drainage outlet at the bottom. Wearing protective gloves, open the stopcock and allow the bag to empty into a suitable waste container or a graduated pitcher (Fig. 6-4). Reclose the stopcock! Since most patients with urinary catheters require I&O measurement, be sure to record the amount.

Colostomy care

Occasionally you will encounter a patient who has a **colostomy** or **ileostomy.** These are surgically formed fistulas from the large or small bowel through the abdominal wall that terminate in an external opening called a **stoma.** A temporary colostomy may be performed to rest the bowel and allow it to heal after surgery, massive trauma, infection, or chronic disease. After the bowel is healed, the healthy portions are reconnected (anastomosis) and the temporary opening is closed. A permanent colostomy is one

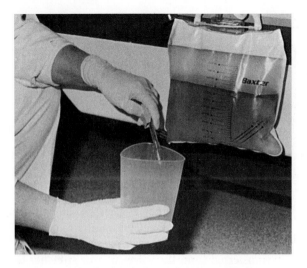

FIG. 6-4 Measuring urinary output.

in which the diseased portion of the bowel is removed.

Patients with colostomies or ileostomies wear an external bag to collect fecal material and may be extremely sensitive about wearing this appliance. Patients with a recent colostomy may find the alteration in body image difficult to accept, and any expression of revulsion on your part may be perceived as disgust and rejection. If you have never seen a colostomy, your first encounter should be as an assistant to an experienced radiographer. More detailed information about colostomies and their care can be found in Chapter 9.

These patients almost invariably carry supplies with them. When patients are scheduled for procedures that require removing a colostomy bag, they should be reminded to bring their own supplies, since brands of colostomy bags vary in size and shape of the opening. If it is necessary to empty a colostomy bag, the patient may prefer to complete this procedure in private. You may need to provide a sealable bag for the used supplies and facilities for hand hygiene. If you must empty the bag, don gloves and empty the bag into the toilet. If the empty bag is disposable, it can be sealed inside a plastic bag and placed in the container for disposal of contaminated waste. Since some patients rely on reusable

colostomy bags, check before you dispose of the used bag. If the patient does not have a clean bag, rinse the used one with cold water and allow the patient to reattach it. Otherwise, empty the reusable bag, rinse, seal it in a plastic bag and return it to the patient, making sure to perform hand hygiene after removing your gloves.

If the patient is unable to perform his or her own colostomy care, you may need to apply or assist with application of a fresh colostomy bag. Fig. 6-5 demonstrates the basic procedure as performed by a competent patient. When assisting the patient, be sure to wear protective gloves. The unit includes two principal parts. A base portion surrounds the stoma and attaches to the body by means of a special adhesive. It protects the skin surrounding the stoma and has a rigid flange that forms a secure connection with the second part of the system, the disposable pouch. Products vary to meet individual patient needs and manufacturers' standards. Product inserts contain complete application instructions.

Sanitary supplies

Occasionally a patient requires a sanitary napkin, so be sure to know where these are kept. If a soiled napkin is to be removed, direct the patient to a bathroom or place a paper bag within reach. Dispose of the bag with the soiled napkin in the appropriate container.

Patients who suffer from poor urinary control or stress incontinence use urinary pads to protect their clothing. These supplies are similar to sanitary pads, are usually stored in the same location, and are disposed of in a similar manner. If a replacement is necessary, urinary pads are definitely preferable, but if they are not available, a sanitary napkin may serve as a temporary substitute.

TAKING A HISTORY

Radiologists depend on radiographers to assist them by obtaining accurate information about the patient's history and present condition. The answers you receive from the patient may influence how the examination is conducted. The history also helps the radiologist focus the interpretation to meet the

FIG. 6-5   APPLYING A FRESH DISPOSABLE COLOSTOMY BAG

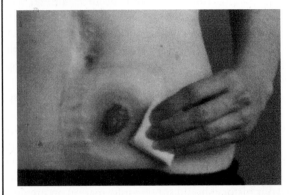

A Cleanse the peristomal area with water, and pat dry thoroughly.

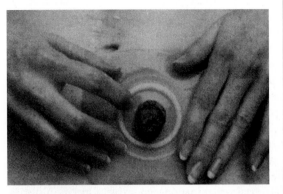

B Prepare the base portion of the unit to fit the patient according to manufacturer's directions. Center the hole over the stoma, and seal adhesive to patient's skin.

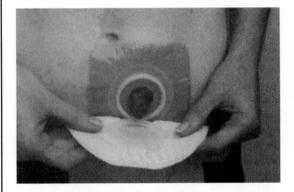

C Take care that inner surfaces of pouch are separated and pouch contains a small amount of air. Position the pouch over the base unit, starting with the lower edge.

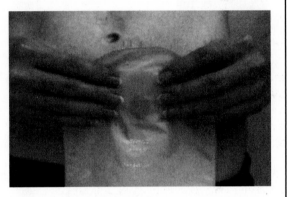

D Press the pouch firmly into place. A gentle tug will confirm proper attachment. Close the bottom of the pouch according to manufacturer's directions.

referring physician's needs. This is not a detailed medical history, but rather a thoughtful determination of why this particular radiographic study is being done.

Patients sometimes complain that they feel like products on an assembly line. The process of taking a history presents an opportunity for you to give the patient individual attention and build rapport. Your ability to gain the patient's confidence will also influence the amount of relevant information you obtain. Remember to introduce yourself, call the patient by name, and deal with immediate patient concerns as soon as possible.

Begin the history by asking a general question about the nature of the problem, such as, "Do you know why Dr. Chen wants you to have an x-ray of your chest?" Be realistic in the scope of your questions, and focus on expanding the information provided on the x-ray requisition. This is especially important when the request or order does not indicate the rationale for ordering the procedure. Most departments have policies stating that such information must be provided, but in practice the information received is often simply the admitting diagnosis, which may seem irrelevant without further explanation. The information you obtain is most useful when recorded on the forms used by your institution. This may be the paper requisition form itself or another form specific to your setting. You may also need to learn how to enter the information directly into the hospital information retrieval (computer) system.

Certain examinations require very specific histories, and the exact information required varies among radiologists. Table 6-1 provides appropriate history questions and observations pertinent to many patient complaints. You can use it to become familiar with the type of information that will be most useful in specific situations. Patients may be asked to complete a questionnaire before a study is started. For example, if intravenous iodine contrast is to be given, your history will include allergy information and any available data on the patient's renal function (see Chapter 10).

Examinations for patients with chronic conditions, or those receiving post-treatment follow-up, may require a comparison to previous diagnostic examinations. If these are not part of the current file, your history should contain information on previous relevant examinations, including when and where they were done.

TABLE 6-1

GUIDELINES FOR TAKING A HISTORY

EXAMINATION	QUESTIONS	OBSERVATIONS	EXAMPLE OF HISTORY*
Orthopedic, acute injury	How did the injury occur? when? Can you show me exactly where it hurts?	Swelling, deformity, discoloration, laceration, abrasion	Twisting injury, l. ankle, while skiing today; swelling & pain over lateral malleolus.
Orthopedic, not involving acute injury	Where does it hurt? How long has it been bothering you? Were you ever injured there? How was the injury treated? (Cast? Surgery?) Has there been any recent change?	Deformity, scars, range of motion, weight bearing	Chronic pain, r. knee 2 yrs, worse since building fence Sat. Prev Rx c̄ cortisone inj. No known injury.
Neck	Did you injure your neck? How? When? Where does it hurt? Do you have any pain, numbness, or tingling of the shoulder or arm? Which side?	Range of motion	MVA 10/12/97; lower neck pain & l. shldr pain c̄ numbness & tingling, l. hand.
Spine	Did you injure your back? How? When? Do you have pain, numbness, tingling, or weakness of the hip or leg? Which side? Any bowel or bladder problems?	Gait, range of motion	Lifting injury 2 wks ago. LBP radiating to r. hip.
Head	Were you injured? When? How? Do you have pain? Where? Did you lose consciousness? For how long? Speech, orientation, gait normal?	Speech: clarity, confusion	Severe HA, blurred vision, dizziness, & gen'l weakness, 24 hrs. No known injury. Speech slurred.

TABLE 6-1

GUIDELINES FOR TAKING A HISTORY—cont'd

EXAMINATION	QUESTIONS	OBSERVATIONS	EXAMPLE OF HISTORY*
Chest	Do you know why your doctor ordered this examination? Are you short of breath? Do you have a cough? Do you cough anything up? Do you cough up blood? Have you had a fever? Do you have any heart problems?	Respirations, cough	SOB, wheezing & r. chest pain since resp flu 4 wks ago. Moderate, nonproductive cough.
Abdomen, gastrointestinal examinations	Do you know why your doctor ordered this examination? Do you have pain? Where? Do you have nausea? Diarrhea? Have you had any other tests for this problem? (Lab tests? Ultrasound?) Do you know the results? Have you ever had abdominal surgery? When? Why?		LLQ pain, incr over past mo. of ? mass seen on US done here 10/21/02.
Urology	Do you know why your doctor ordered this examination? Do you have pain? Where? For how long? Do you have trouble passing urine? Pain? Urgency? Frequency? Have you ever had this problem before? Do you have high blood pressure?		2 prior episodes of UTI; current malaise, fever, & mid back pain.

*Can you identify the common abbreviations used by radiographers (e.g., MVA, motor vehicle accident)? See Appendix D.

In the event that a detailed history is needed, the following standard format is frequently used. Using this outline will allow you to elicit the greatest amount of data in the least amount of time and will help you avoid missing relevant information.

Onset: How did it start? What happened? When did it first trouble you? Was it sudden or a complaint that gradually got worse?

Duration: Have you ever had it before? Has it been continuous? Does it bother you all the time? How long has this attack been bothering you?

Specific location: Where does it hurt (or where is the problem)? Can you put your finger on where it hurts the most? Does it hurt anywhere else?

Quality of pain: What does it feel like? Sharp, stabbing pain? Dull ache? Throbbing pain? How severe is it? Mild, moderate, severe? (Some like to use a pain scale of 1 to 5 or 1 to 10, with 0 being no pain at all and the highest number representing the worst pain the patient can imagine.) Does it wake you up at night?

What aggravates: What seems to aggravate it? When is it worst? Is it worse after meals? At night? When you walk?

What alleviates: What has helped in the past? Does that still help? What seems to help now? Does the time of day (amount of rest, change in position, and so on) make a difference?

Tact and caution are required when obtaining a history, since anxious patients may read too much into your questions. Information regarding such serious matters as cancer, surgery, or heart attacks is best elicited in a general way rather than through blunt questions. "Do you know why your doctor ordered this examination?" is less threatening than, "Is your doctor checking for cancer?"

At this point the process of taking a history may seem complex and confusing, but this is a skill that improves with practice. Role-playing with other students, including taking turns as a critical observer, will improve your ability to take a history with sensitivity and confidence. As clinical practice provides additional knowledge and experience, you will find that your observation and history skills become increasingly accurate and pertinent.

ASSESSING CURRENT PHYSICAL STATUS

The decisions you make and the communications you initiate in the course of a radiographic procedure will be most accurate if you begin with a clear understanding of the patient's current status. In addition, the radiographer is often the first and primary observer of a significant change in the patient's current condition, and in order to accurately assess change, you must first establish a baseline for your observations.

Checking the Chart

Before you start the procedure it is important to review the requisition. Often the requisition will not have enough specific information, so this is an area in which your skill in history taking will prove valuable. When the patient is an inpatient, you will have access to the chart and can verify both the order for the procedure and the accuracy of the requisition. Note the admitting diagnosis and the most recent progress notes. This survey will help you to assess current physical status and determine whether the preparation for the examination has been done successfully. The pressures of scheduling may make such a thorough approach seem impossible, so the more familiar you become with the organization of charts and requisitions in your facility, the easier it will become to find pertinent information quickly.

Nurses' notes may also be helpful. If a recent notation reads, "Unable to stand to void," you can anticipate a need for help when transferring this patient to the x-ray table. A statement such as, "emesis × 3," during the previous 24 hours should be brought to the radiologist's attention before proceeding with a barium swallow. Medication may be needed to calm the patient's stomach long enough for the examination to take place. If such a medication has already been given, it may affect peristaltic action and therefore the interpretation the radiologist will give to a fluoroscopic study.

Some notations have special significance to the radiographer. Allergies are usually noted in red on the outside of the chart holder as well as in the history (Fig. 6-6). A patient with a previous history of allergies is sometimes referred to as an "allergenic individual" and is more likely to have an adverse reaction to contrast media. A complete account of allergies must be reported to the radiologist if the patient is to receive a contrast medium for the examination. Further assessment of allergy potential is discussed in Chapter 10.

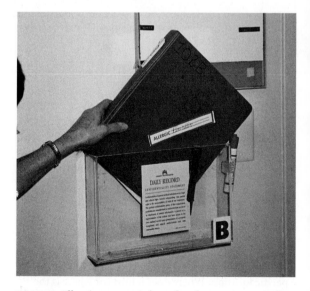

FIG. 6-6 Allergies are noted on the chart cover as well as in the history section.

Physical Evaluation

In the context of this chapter, evaluation is an ongoing process of observation, assessment, and measurement to note and evaluate changes in patient condition before, during, and after procedures in the radiographic suite. How do you know when the condition of a patient is changing for the worse? What do you look for?

The most important process in patient evaluation is sometimes called "eyeballing the patient." This skill of acute observation compares the actions and appearance of this patient with those of similar patients you have seen. You also use this skill to compare the appearance of this patient now with how he or she appeared earlier. Although this may seem intuitive, you are actually responding to subliminal changes in the overall appearance of the patient.

Skin color

One of the easiest signs to recognize is a change in skin color. Individual complexions vary, but when pale skin becomes cyanotic or olive skin takes on a waxen pallor, the change is usually quite apparent.

The term **cyanotic** denotes a bluish coloration in the skin and indicates a lack of sufficient oxygen in the tissues. This is most easily seen on the mucous membranes, such as the lips or the lining of the mouth. Nail beds may also show a bluish tinge. For some patients with heart or lung conditions this may be a chronic or usual state, but the patient who *becomes* cyanotic needs oxygen and immediate medical attention.

Any patient who looks pale and anxious and doesn't "feel well" is subject to fainting and needs to sit or lie down immediately. Do not leave the patient! A patient who loses consciousness and falls to the floor may suffer injuries far more serious than the cause of the fainting.

Skin temperature

In Chapter 3 we discussed the importance of touch as a form of communication and reassurance. Contact with your hands also allows you to make physical observations about the ongoing status of your patients. The acutely ill patient in pain may be pale, cool, and **diaphoretic,** in what is frequently called a "cold sweat." Hot, dry skin may indicate a fever, while warm, moist skin may only be a response to the weather or the room temperature. Acute anxiety can cause cool, moist skin with wet palms and shaking hands. Anxious patients may find it difficult to concentrate and may need additional instruction during the radiographic procedure. They often need more precise instructions and should receive them in writing if any follow-up care is required.

Level of consciousness

A sudden change in a patient's mental acuity may indicate a critical problem that requires immediate treatment. To recognize such a change, you must first make a baseline observation of the patient's consciousness. Four **levels of consciousness (LOCs)** are generally recognized and may be described as follows:

1. Alert and conscious
2. Drowsy but responsive
3. Unconscious but reactive to painful stimuli
4. Comatose

To establish a baseline when eyeballing the patient, note whether the patient seems alert. Observe the patient's eyes. Are they open and focused? Does the patient look at you when you speak and respond appropriately? If your observations raise questions about the patient's alertness or awareness, ask additional questions, for example, "Do you know what day it is?" or "Do you know where you are?"

Occasionally a patient will lose consciousness for no apparent reason. The only warning may be a sudden change in expression, especially if the eyes seem unfocused. The cause of such an episode may be that the patient suffers from a seizure disorder and the loss of consciousness is precipitated by the stress of the occasion. Absence (petit mal) is a seizure disorder without convulsions that can cause a brief loss of consciousness without warning.

Breathing

Changes in breathing may signal the onset of serious distress, so it is important to note how the patient is breathing. Normal breathing is quiet and calm and requires no particular attention. On the other hand, breathing that is audible, such as wheezing, gasping, or coughing, or appears to present a struggle for the patient, may require further assessment. A marked increase in the depth and rate of respiration is usually the first sign of respiratory distress.

Chronic conditions such as emphysema and cardiac insufficiency affect breathing and should be noted when assessing the patient. When these patients come to the radiology department, a chronic respiratory problem may be the presenting condition, or they may be admitted for a completely unrelated problem. For example, the emphysematous patient who needs a hernia repair or other surgery may come in for a chest evaluation before admission.

Radiographers must be alert to identify patients with **emphysema,** a form of chronic pulmonary disease that prevents patients from exhaling effectively, limiting capacity for inhaling fresh air. Patients with emphysema share several characteristics. An increased anteroposterior thoracic diameter gives them a barrel-chested appearance. This is frequently associated with an elevation of the shoulder girdle and retraction of the neck muscles—all symptomatic of costal respiration. If these patients have received instruction in positive-pressure breathing, you will observe that they purse their lips when exhaling. The emphysematous patient may have difficulty breathing, especially when stressed, and may require a low rate of oxygen administration. Recognition of the emphysematous patient is a valuable skill from a technical viewpoint, since these patients require special adjustments in exposure for chest radiography.

The anxious patient who breathes too deeply and too often (hyperventilation) may complain of feeling faint or dizzy and of tingling and numbness in the extremities. These patients have inhaled too much oxygen and exhaled too much carbon dioxide, disturbing the chemical balance of the blood. Try to persuade them to breathe more slowly or to breathe into a paper bag, which will help return their carbon dioxide level to normal.

You will recall from Chapter 4 that the inability to breathe when recumbent is called orthopnea. Patients with cardiac insufficiency, for example, will find it easier to breathe with the upper body elevated. Any sudden onset of orthopnea that is not relieved in the upright position may indicate a serious change in the patient's condition. Count the pulse rate and respirations as discussed in the section on vital signs in this chapter. Has there been a change in skin color? Is there evidence of diaphoresis or pain? If your assessment shows cause for concern, notify your supervisor or the radiologist.

If your assessment of the patient's physical status reveals abnormality of skin color, skin temperature, level of consciousness, or ability to breathe, it is important to determine whether this is a new problem. A sudden change in any of these signs is significant and may be life-threatening. Has the patient just received a contrast medium or any new medication? If so, you may be observing the first signs of an allergic reaction. Regardless of whether you can identify the cause, notify your supervisor, the radiology nurse, or the radiologist immediately when there is a change in physical status. When such changes occur, the assessment procedures in the sections that follow may be needed for further patient evaluation.

Vital signs

The following procedures used for assessment are usually referred to as the "vital signs." They involve the measurement of temperature, pulse rate, respiratory rate, and blood pressure. Radiographers do not take vital signs on most patients, and when the need does arise, it is often in response to an urgent situation. The patient in anaphylactic shock does not need a radiographer who wonders whether there is a right or wrong side to the blood pressure cuff! Sharpen your skill at taking vital signs before the need arises, and review your technique frequently. Accuracy is especially important when taking blood pressure measurements. When time allows, practice your technique by checking your coworkers and the receptionist as well. We should all be aware of our own baseline vital signs, so your practice will benefit you, the person on whom you practice, and the patient who may need your skill in an emergency. Most radiology departments have a drawer or box to keep a blood pressure cuff and gauge (sphygmomanometer), a stethoscope, and other equipment

TABLE 6-2

A QUICK REFERENCE TO NORMAL VITAL SIGNS BY AGE

AGE	TEMPERATURE (ORAL)	TEMPERATURE (RECTAL)	PULSE	RESPIRATIONS	BLOOD PRESSURE (SYSTOLIC)
Premature newborn		99.6° F (37.5° C)	140	<60	50-60
Full term newborn		99.6° F (37.5° C)	125	<60	70
6 months		99.6° F (37.5° C)	120	24-36	90
1 year		99.6° F (37.5° C)	120	22-30	96
3 years		99.6° F (37.5° C)	110	20-26	100
5 years	98.6° F (37° C)	99.6° F (37.5° C)	100	20-24	100
6 years	98.6° F (37° C)	99.6° F (37.5° C)	100	20-24	100
8 years	98.6° F (37° C)	99.6° F (37.5° C)	90	18-22	105
12 years	98.6° F (37° C)	99.6° F (37.5° C)	85-90	16-22	115
16 years	98.6° F (37° C)	99.6° F (37.5° C)	75-80	14-20	Below 120
Adult female	98.6° F (37° C)	99.6° F (37.5° C)	60-100	12-20	Below 120
Adult male	98.6° F (37° C)	99.6° F (37.5° C)	60-100	12-20	Below 120

that might be needed in an emergency. Know where this equipment is stored because even before you are proficient you may be asked to obtain it in an emergency. Table 6-2 provides a quick reference for normal vital signs according to patient age. Further discussion of normal ranges for each of the vital signs is included in the sections that follow.

Temperature. An accurate temperature reading assists in measuring the body's basic metabolic state. Although few patients will need you to take their temperature, you should be able to do so competently. In addition, this is one skill that can be useful in your own home.

Body temperatures vary during the day, being lowest in the morning and highest in the evening. Normal oral temperatures vary from 96.8° to 100.4° F (36° to 38° C). Rectal temperatures range from 0.5° to 1.0° F higher than oral temperatures; axillary temperatures range from 0.5° to 1.0° F lower. In addition, normal temperatures vary slightly from person to person. A tense, "high-strung," quick-moving individual is likely to have a higher basic temperature than the placid, slow moving person, all else being equal. What is your average temperature range?

While the Fahrenheit scale has traditionally been used to record temperature, an increasing number of hospitals have completely converted to the metric system, which means that temperatures will be recorded in Celsius units. See Box 6-2 for the formulas to convert between the Fahrenheit and Celsius scales.

Fever (pyrexia or hyperthermia) is a sign of increased body **metabolism** (energy use), usually in response to an infectious process. For adults, fever commonly refers to any temperature of 100.4° F or above when taken orally or 101.4° F taken rectally.

Temperatures may be obtained by the oral, rectal, axillary, and tympanic routes. Alert, cooperative patients usually prefer the familiar oral route.

BOX 6-2

FAHRENHEIT ⟷ CELSIUS CONVERSION

To convert from Fahrenheit to Celsius temperature: $C = (F - 32) \div 1.8$

To convert from Celsius to Fahrenheit temperature: $F = (C \times 1.8) + 32$

Examples:

1. Convert 25° C to the Fahrenheit scale.
   $F = (25 \times 1.8) + 32 = 45 + 32 = 77° F$

2. Convert normal body temperature, 98.6° F, to the Celsius scale.
   $$C = \frac{(98.6 - 32)}{1.8} = \frac{66.6}{1.8} = 37° C$$

A long-standing belief exists that the oral method is less accurate than the rectal method, but research does not confirm this. The oral route provides an accurate measure of changes in body core temperature when taken correctly with the bulb or probe of the thermometer placed well under the base of the tongue.

The oral method is not appropriate when the patient has recently had a hot or cold beverage, is receiving oxygen, or is breathing through the mouth. In these situations, the rectal or axillary method may be used. The rectal temperature is accurate and faster, while the axillary temperature is slower and somewhat less accurate. The axillary method is sometimes preferred, however, because it is less invasive. Rectal temperatures may be contraindicated in certain patients with cardiac conditions in order to avoid stimulating the vagus nerve.

Hospital patient care units use digital electronic thermometers that consist of a handheld power unit with either an oral or a rectal probe (Fig. 6-7). These instruments can be read in 1 minute or less. They emit a short beep when the highest temperature is recorded and are read from a digital display on the power unit. Disposable sleeves are used to cover the probe, avoiding the need to disinfect the thermometer after each use. Some digital thermometers incorporate the power unit, probe, and digital display in a single

small unit. This type is less sophisticated and less expensive and is not generally used by nursing service, but it may be used in the radiology department and in outpatient settings. These thermometers are also available for home use.

You are probably familiar with the use of glass thermometers, but these are no longer being used in clinical settings because of new Occupational Safety and Health Administration (OSHA) regulations that strictly limit the use of any devices containing mercury. OSHA's goal is to eliminate mercury from the workplace by 2005.

Hospitals commonly specify rectal, axillary, or tympanic routes for children under the age of 6 years and for anyone who is confused or unable to follow directions. Tympanic thermometers (Fig. 6-8) are used primarily with pediatric patients. They measure temperature at the tympanic membrane in the ear. Disposable thermometers (Fig. 6-9) are also primarily used for children. They consist of a strip of temperature-sensitive paper with adhesive backing that may be attached to the forehead.

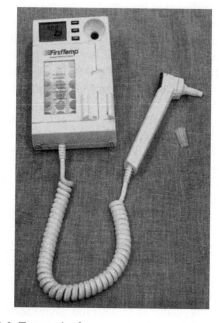

FIG. 6-8 Tympanic thermometer inserted in auditory canal.

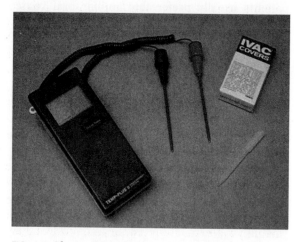

FIG. 6-7 Electronic thermometer used for oral, rectal, and axillary measurements.

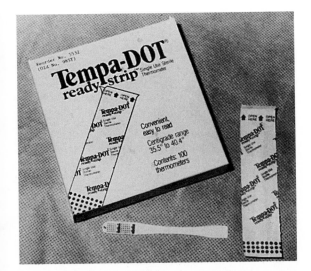

FIG. 6-9 Disposable paper strip thermometers are frequently used for children.

Patients who have unstable body temperatures can now be monitored continuously by using a special probe inserted in the external ear canal that sends an electronic signal to a digital display monitor. This system is most commonly used for comatose patients in the intensive care unit and for premature or low-birth-weight infants in the neonatal intensive care unit.

While several methods can be used to obtain accurate temperature readings, a general procedure for each common route is found in Box 6-3. Remember to tell your patient what you are about to do. When taking an oral temperature, remind the patient not to bite down and to keep his or her lips closed. Never leave a patient alone with a rectal or axillary thermometer in place.

Pulse. A pulse is the advancing pressure wave in an artery caused by the expulsion of blood when the left ventricle of the heart contracts. Since this wave occurs with each contraction, it is an easy and effective way to measure heart rate. The heart rate is measured in beats per minute.

Tachycardia (abnormally rapid pulse) occurs when the heart beats more than 100 times per minute. This may be temporary, as a result of exertion, nervousness,

or excitability, or it may be caused by a damaged heart. A rapid pulse rate may also result from interference with oxygen supply or from a large blood loss. This occurs because the heart must beat faster to circulate the remaining blood to carry as much oxygen as possible to all the cells of the body. Average normal pulse rates in adults vary between 60 and 100 beats per minute. The tense, nervous individual is more likely to be in the upper range, while athletes tend to have a slower rate.

In addition to rate, the pulse volume or quality may vary. A weak or "thready" pulse, especially if quite rapid, may indicate that the heart is not pumping enough blood.

Common pulse points are shown in Fig. 6-10. The most common site for palpation of the pulse is the radial artery at the base of either thumb. Since your own thumb has a pulse, you cannot take an accurate pulse using your thumb. Place your fingers over the artery with your thumb on the back of the wrist and compress gently but firmly. By compressing the artery against the radius, the pulse is easy to feel, especially if the patient's wrist is held palm down (Fig. 6-11). When the radial pulse rate is taken routinely, it is common to count for 15 seconds and then multiply by 4. Whenever there is an irregular rate or rhythm, count for a full 60 seconds.

If the radial pulse is weak or difficult to count, you can use the carotid artery. Place your fingers just below the angle of the mandible (Fig. 6-12). This site is easily accessible and is particularly important if a patient loses consciousness. If the pulse is not palpable at this site, the heart is not beating effectively and emergency measures are necessary (see Chapter 8).

The *dorsalis pedis* or pedal pulse is taken over the instep of the foot (Fig. 6-13). This pulse may be significant when there is a question of compromise in the peripheral circulation. For example, radiographers may be requested to check the pedal pulse during or after an arteriogram involving catheterization through the femoral artery or following the application of a cast to the lower extremity. Since inability to feel this pulse may be an important diagnostic sign, you must practice until you are certain you can detect the pulse when it is present.

BOX 6-3

TAKING A PATIENT'S TEMPERATURE

Oral Route
- Perform hand hygiene.
- Cover the oral probe with a clean plastic sleeve.
- Turn on the thermometer.
- Insert the probe under patient's tongue. Instruct patient to keep lips closed.
- Remove probe when the audible tone or flashing number indicates that the maximum temperature has been reached (about 1 minute).
- Note the temperature reading.
- Remove and discard plastic sleeve.
- Remove and discard gloves.
- Repeat hand hygiene.
- Make sure thermometer is off, and return it to storage.
- Record the temperature.

Axillary Route
- Perform hand hygiene.
- Cover the probe with a clean plastic sleeve.
- Turn on the thermometer.
- Place the probe in the axilla so that the skin folds are in direct contact with the probe. Instruct patient to hold upper arm firmly against chest wall.
- Remove probe when the audible tone or flashing number indicates that the maximum temperature has been reached (about 1 minute).
- Note the temperature reading.
- Remove and discard plastic sleeve.
- Remove and discard gloves.
- Repeat hand hygiene.
- Make sure thermometer is off, and return it to storage.
- Record the temperature.

Rectal Route
- Perform hand hygiene.
- Cover the rectal probe with a clean plastic sleeve.
- With the patient in a lateral recumbent position, cover the patient and expose the anus by raising the top fold of the buttocks.
- Slowly insert the probe past the anal sphincter. Hold the probe in place.
- When the audible tone or flashing number indicates that the maximum temperature has been reached (about 1 minute), remove probe slowly.
- Note the temperature reading.
- Remove and discard plastic sleeve.
- Remove and discard gloves.
- Repeat hand hygiene.
- Make sure thermometer is off, and return it to storage.
- Record the temperature.

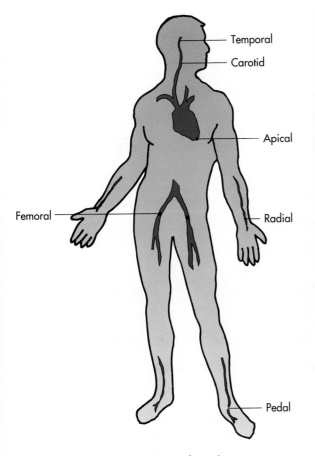

FIG. 6-10 Common pulse points.

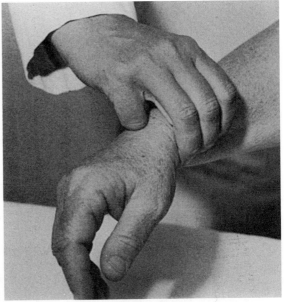

FIG. 6-11 Taking a radial pulse with patient's palm down.

If the pulse is slow or irregular, you may want to use a stethoscope to take an apical pulse. Look at the stethoscope carefully, and become familiar with its use. It may have a bell as well as a diaphragm; less expensive models may have a diaphragm only. On the bimodal stethoscope you can switch from bell to diaphragm, but for most purposes the diaphragm is preferred. Hold the earpieces of the stethoscope horizontally in front of you so that the ear tips point up slightly (Fig. 6-14). Insert the tips in your ears and then tap the diaphragm gently with your finger to be sure you can hear. Now press the diaphragm firmly over the **apex** or tip of the heart. This is normally found in the fifth anterior intercostal space at the left midclavicular line. Count the pulse for a full minute, and record the rate and any irregularities.

Compare the radial rate with the apical rate, and record both rates in the chart or on the requisition. If the apical rate is faster, the heart is not beating efficiently. If the patient also shows signs of distress, you should report to your supervisor or the radiologist.

When a patient suddenly develops an irregular pulse, complains of feeling faint, weak, or nauseated, or has a sudden onset of pain in the chest, shoulder, or jaw, a physician must be notified immediately regarding the possible onset of a heart attack.

Respirations. When a patient shows evidence of respiratory distress, a respiratory rate will help in making an assessment. To count respirations, simply note the number of inhalations per minute. This is often done while continuing to hold the wrist after the pulse has been counted, since some patients may force a change in the respiratory rate if aware that a count is being made. If you are having difficulty counting breaths, place one hand lightly on the patient's diaphragm. Compare your findings with the normal adult range of 12 to 20 breaths per minute. Slow breathing with fewer than 12 breaths per minute is called **bradypnea,** and rapid breathing

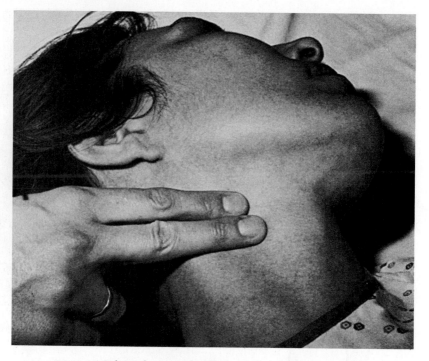

FIG. 6-12 Palpate for carotid pulse just below angle of mandible.

in excess of 20 breaths per minute is called **tachypnea.** If a patient complains of dyspnea (difficulty in breathing), or exhibits an abnormal respiratory rate, you should inform the radiologist and prepare oxygen equipment for immediate use if ordered. See Chapter 8 for information on oxygen administration.

Patients in shock or with significant blood loss have a marked increase in pulse rate and in rapid, shallow breathing as the body attempts to supply oxygen to the tissues by increasing the speed of circulation. Pleurisy or abdominal pain may also cause rapid, shallow breathing because the patient attempts to avoid pain by moving the affected area as little as possible.

Blood pressure. At any given time in the United States, about 15% of the adult population will have a significant degree of **hypertension** (abnormally high blood pressure). Of this number, approximately one fourth is unaware of their condition. Hypertension is more common in men before the age of 50 and in women after age 50. In an aging population, the incidence of hypertension gradually increases until

approximately 30% will show some elevation over normal. Essential (sometimes called primary) hypertension accounts for 85% to 90% of the diagnoses, with most of the remaining (secondary) incidence due to kidney disease or damage. Hypertension contributes to the incidence of cerebrovascular accidents (strokes) and congestive heart disease.

Abnormally low blood pressure or **hypotension** can result in a potentially life-threatening condition called **shock.** The causes for shock and their identification and treatment are discussed in Chapter 8.

Blood pressure is measured using a stethoscope and a blood pressure cuff called a **sphygmomanometer.** There are three basic types of sphygmomanometers: mercury-gravity, aneroid, and electronic. The traditional mercury-gravity instruments are available in portable, wall-mounted, and rolling floor models. These instruments are the most accurate and measure blood pressure directly in millimeters of mercury (mm Hg). Mercury-gravity manometers are currently being phased out in response to the OSHA goal to remove mercury from

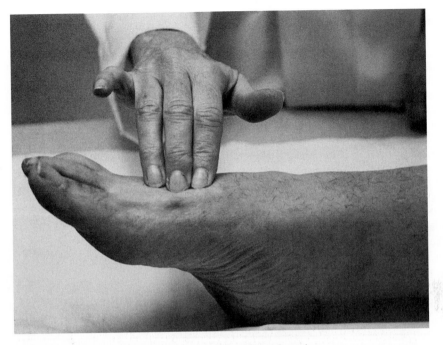

FIG. 6-13 Palpating dorsalis pedis pulse.

the workplace, so there is increasing use of small, portable aneroid instruments that use air pressure to obtain a measurement. While these manometers do not measure pressure in millimeters of mercury

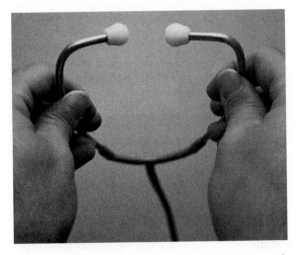

FIG. 6-14 Stethoscope ear tips point up slightly. Correctly placed ear tips improve accuracy.

directly, they provide readings in the same units. There are several designs of electronic instruments, some of which measure pressure automatically at regular intervals. You may observe potentially unstable patients who have their blood pressure repeatedly checked automatically with electronic sphygmomanometers that display a digital readout. This allows patients to be monitored closely from a remote location. In the ICU you may observe nurses using a Doppler unit to measure blood pressure when patients have an extremely weak or low pressure.

Aneroid manometers are the type most often found in the radiology department. The procedure for measuring blood pressure is detailed in Box 6-4 and is illustrated in Fig. 6-15. Since this procedure is most frequently used in an emergency, it is important to be proficient before the need arises.

A blood pressure (BP) reading is usually expressed in two figures, such as 120/78. The top figure is the **systolic** pressure and is a measure of the pumping action of the heart muscle itself. The bottom figure is

BOX 6-4

MEASURING BLOOD PRESSURE

- Perform hand hygiene and explain the procedure to the patient.
- The patient may be sitting or lying down, but the cuff should be at the level of the heart. Either arm may be used.
- Wrap the cuff snugly with the bottom edge above the antecubital space. Most cuffs are self-securing.
- Place the gauge where you can easily read the dial.
- Palpate the brachial artery pulse in the antecubital space.
- Place the stethoscope's ear tips in your ears, and press its diaphragm over the brachial artery.
- Close the valve on the bulb pump, and inflate the cuff rapidly to approximately 180 mm Hg.
- Open the valve on the pump and *slowly* release the pressure.
- Listen for the beat of the pulse while watching the gauge. Note the figure at which the pulse is first heard. Note this as the systolic reading.
- As the pressure is released, the sound increases in intensity and then, suddenly, becomes much softer. Note this point as the diastolic reading.
- Release the remaining pressure.
- If the situation permits, ask the patient to raise the arm and clench and release the fist. Lower the arm, and repeat the procedure to check the results.
- Remove the cuff, and record the results as systolic over diastolic (e.g., 140/86).
- Clean the ear tips and diaphragm of the stethoscope with alcohol, and return the equipment to its storage place.

the **diastolic*** pressure and indicates the ability of the arterial system to accept the pulse of blood forced into the system when the left ventricle contracts. If you are angry, afraid, or exercising, the top figure greatly increases. The diastolic figure may also rise, but to a lesser degree. What is a normal blood pressure? The acceptable range of blood pressure varies depending on age, weight, and physical status. As a rule of thumb, a normal systolic pressure will measure between 110 and 120 mm Hg, while the normal diastolic pressure may vary from 60 to 80 mm Hg. In other words, a consistent BP of 140/90 may be said to indicate some degree of hypertension. A diastolic pressure less than 50 mm Hg or a systolic pressure below 90 mm Hg may indicate hypotension and may also indicate shock. Hypotension is confirmed when either reading is 20% below the patient's normal baseline.

If an outpatient is to receive intravenous contrast or systemic medication, it is important to take a

blood pressure reading before the procedure begins. Hospital patients will have a reading recorded in the chart, but it is advisable to check the blood pressure if it has not been taken within 24 hours.

In order to establish a baseline or average blood pressure for an individual, three readings are customary. These may be taken over a period of time, and on some occasions are taken sitting, standing, and lying down. In an emergency, a single reading can be reported to the physician and should be compared with previously recorded results, if available. Take an additional reading as soon as possible.

COMMON LABORATORY TESTS FOR PATIENT ASSESSMENT

While radiographers are not usually responsible for monitoring laboratory test levels, it may be helpful to have a general knowledge of such values and their significance in the current condition of the patient. This information is particularly relevant when anticipating injection of contrast media for special

*A good way to remember is to think, "D is for Down."

examinations (Chapter 10). The following is a brief discussion of some of the more common tests. Normal values are shown in Table 6-3.

A complete blood count (CBC) is frequently performed as part of a diagnostic workup or a complete physical examination. The scope of a CBC may vary, depending on the laboratory and the equipment available. As many as 12 different determinations may be performed as part of a routine CBC. All CBCs include a red blood cell count,

F I G . 6 - 1 5   MEASURING BLOOD PRESSURE

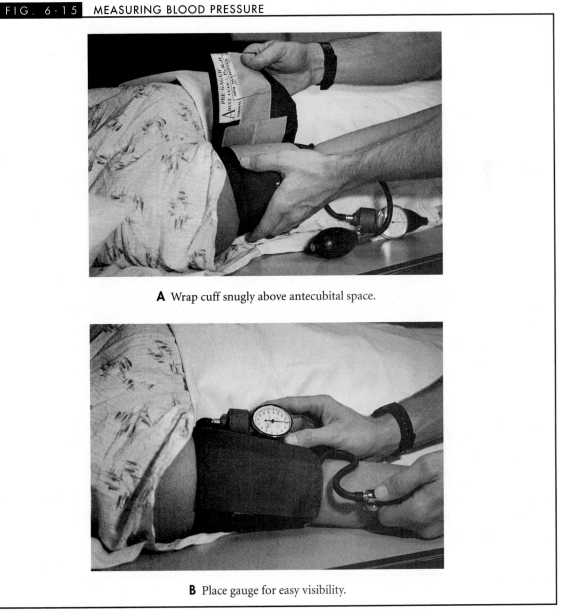

A Wrap cuff snugly above antecubital space.

B Place gauge for easy visibility.

Continued

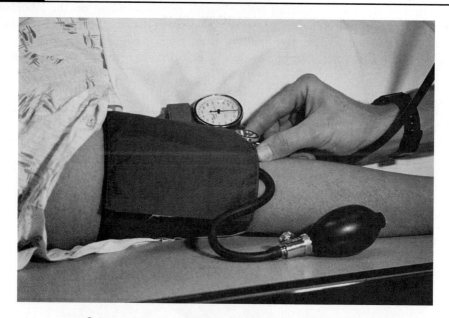

C Place stethoscope over brachial artery, and inflate cuff.

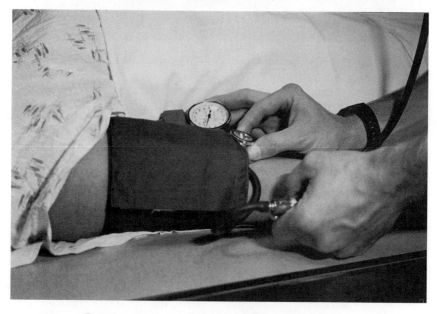

D Release pressure while listening for audible pulse.

TABLE 6-3

NORMAL VALUES FOR COMMON LABORATORY TESTS

LABORATORY TEST		NORMAL VALUE
Red blood cell count (RBC)	Men	4.2-5.4 million per ml
	Women	3.6-5.0 million per ml
	Children	4.6-4.8 million per ml
White blood cell count (WBC)		4,000-10,000 per ml
Platelet count		130,000-170,000 per ml
Hemoglobin (Hgb)	Men	13-18 g/dl
	Women	12-16 g/dl
Hematocrit (Hct)	Adults	38%-54%
	Children	30%-40%
Partial thromboplastin time (PTT)		30-45 seconds
Activated partial thromboplastin time (APTT)		21-35 seconds
Serum creatinine	Infants to 3 years	0.3-0.7 mg/dl
	Children, age 3-18	0.5-1.0 mg/dl
	Adults, 18 and over	0.6-1.3 mg/dl
Blood urea nitrogen (BUN)	Children	5-18 mg/dl
	Adults	7-18 mg/dl
	Adults over age 60	8-20 mg/dl
Serum bilirubin	Indirect	<1.1 mg/dl
	Direct	<0.5 mg/dl
	Total	0.2-1.0 mg/dl
Blood glucose	12- to 14-Hour fasting	70-100 mg/dl
Cholesterol	Total	170-240 mg/dl
	LDL	62-185 mg/dl
	HDL	29-77 mg/dl

LDL, Low-density lipoprotein; *HDL,* high-density lipoprotein.

hemoglobin concentration (Hgb), hematocrit (Hct), Red blood cell (RBC) indices, white blood cell count (WBC), WBC differential count, and platelet count. The RBC indices include mean corpuscular volume (MCV), mean corpuscular hemoglobin (MCH), mean corpuscular hemoglobin concentration (MCHC), and red cell distribution width (RDW). An evaluation of RBC morphology performed by a microscopic examination of a stained peripheral blood smear is often performed but may not be necessary unless there are significantly abnormal results in the remainder of the CBC, especially the RBC count, Hgb, and Hct. Some laboratories also report the mean platelet volume (MPV), but the diagnostic value of this test remains uncertain in routine testing.

The CBC provides specific information regarding the types and numbers of cells that make up the blood. These blood cells enable the body to transport oxygen and carbon dioxide and facilitate blood clotting and immune responses.

The red blood cell count, hemoglobin concentration, and hematocrit values all relate to the red cell component of the blood. Hemoglobin is the pigment in red blood cells that carries oxygen from the lungs to the tissues and is essential to sustain life. Carbon dioxide is produced when oxygen is utilized and is transported by red blood cells back to the lungs to be exhaled. These functions are compromised when the number of red blood cells in the circulation is decreased. This is reflected as an abnormally low RBC count, low Hgb, and/or low Hct. This information is helpful in the diagnosis and evaluation of specific disease processes affecting the blood, such as deficiency anemias, hemolytic anemias, hypoplastic bone marrows, and chronic systemic disorders such as liver, renal, and endocrine diseases. Low RBC, Hgb, and Hct values are associated with anemia, blood loss, and abnormal hydration (fluid retention), while elevated values are seen with polycythemia and dehydration (fluid loss). Dehydration is an undesirable condition when anticipating injection of contrast media because it is a predisposing factor to contrast media reaction and contrast nephropathy. The RBC count, Hgb , and Hct are the principal indicators of red blood cell abnormality, and the red blood cell indices are helpful in identifying the specific types or causes of anemias.

White blood cell counts and differential counts of the various types of white blood cells are done to detect infection or inflammation. These values are also helpful in monitoring treatment for cancer or immune deficiency diseases. The white blood cell count increases when infection or inflammation is present, providing extra cells to fight infection and perform phagocytosis. Depression of the white blood cell count is indicative of immunosuppression. A low WBC level is also seen in cases of excessive radiation exposure and in patients receiving radiation therapy or chemotherapy.

Platelets are involved in the mechanism of forming blood clots. A significant reduction in the platelet count indicates that a patient may bleed under circumstances that would normally not result in bleeding. Several laboratory measurements are used to evaluate the blood's ability to clot: the platelet count, which is part of the CBC, a platelet function test known as the Ivy bleeding time, and coagulation tests known as the prothrombin time (PT) and partial thromboplastin time (PTT). The results of these tests are used to assess risks of both hemorrhage and stroke. Sometimes an additional blood test called clot retraction time is also used to evaluate clotting potential. It is important for blood to clot

adequately so that the patient will not hemorrhage from minor injuries or invasive diagnostic or surgical procedures, so a low platelet count and/or prolonged PT and PTT indicates risk of hemorrhage. On the other hand, when blood clots too readily, clots may form within blood vessels, preventing blood flow and causing tissue necrosis. Clots lodged in cerebral vessels cause strokes; blockage of a coronary artery causes a myocardial infarction, a heart attack. Patients at risk for stroke or heart attack may be treated with anticoagulant medication such as warfarin (Coumadin). These patients are closely monitored by prothrombin time testing, and their medication dosage is determined by the test result. The importance of accurate and reliable prothrombin time measurements for these patients, coupled with variations in testing chemicals and standards across the globe, has resulted in the establishment of a standardized reporting system for prothrombin times called the international normalized ratio (INR). The prothrombin time is reported in seconds for purposes of screening for inherited or acquired coagulation factor deficiency states. The INR is reported as a numeric ratio between 2.0 and 3.0 for patients taking oral anticoagulant medications. A prolonged prothrombin time or increased INR may be a contraindication for certain invasive procedures and contrast media examinations. The prothrombin time may also affect the choice of contrast media.

Another blood test that is frequently ordered is the erythrocyte sedimentation rate (ESR or "sed rate"). This test is most commonly used to determine the presence and/or extent of infectious conditions and inflammatory processes, usually systemic in nature.

Other laboratory tests measure the presence of certain biochemicals or analytes in the blood, and a great variety of these tests is available to the physician. A few common tests of particular interest to radiographers include glucose, cholesterol, urea nitrogen, creatinine, and bilirubin.

Glucose is a form of sugar, so this test is commonly referred to as "blood sugar," but the preferred name is either serum glucose or plasma glucose. An abnormally high glucose level is called hyperglycemia, and low glucose is called hypoglycemia. Blood glucose levels are measured to diagnose and manage patients with diabetes mellitus and a group of conditions referred to as fasting hypoglycemia (see Chapter 8).

Since high cholesterol has been identified as a major risk factor for heart disease, cholesterol measurements have become quite common. A total serum cholesterol test is actually a measurement of the sum total of cholesterol incorporated in a family of cholesterol-containing substances called lipoproteins. There are two basic types of lipoproteins that are commonly assayed along with the total serum cholesterol: high-density lipoprotein (HDL) and low-density lipoprotein (LDL). LDL is sometimes called the "bad cholesterol" because elevated levels are considered to be a positive risk factor for the development of heart disease. Conversely, elevated HDL is considered a negative risk factor and HDL is often referred to as "good cholesterol." Physicians most commonly evaluate patient risk using the total serum cholesterol, LDL, and HDL levels because total serum cholesterol testing alone may be misleading.

Serum urea nitrogen, also called blood urea nitrogen (BUN), is a byproduct of protein metabolism, and creatinine is a metabolite associated with skeletal muscle mass. Both BUN and creatinine are nonprotein nitrogenous waste products that are excreted by the kidneys. When a disease process compromises kidney function, the kidneys' ability to clear these potentially toxic substances is impaired and the serum levels increase. For this reason, serum levels of both BUN and creatinine are evaluated to aid in the assessment of renal function. Abnormally high BUN levels (sometimes referred to as azotemia) may indicate impaired renal function. Elevated BUN values are also seen in cases of acute myocardial infarction, congestive heart failure, dehydration, and excessive protein intake.

Except in individuals with significantly increased skeletal muscle mass, elevated creatinine levels are rarely observed in situations other than compromised kidney function, so an elevated creatinine level is considered a more specific indication of impaired kidney function than the BUN. Creatinine assays from both serum and urine are utilized in the procedure known as creatinine clearance testing. This comparison of blood and urine creatinine values can be used to detect very early loss of kidney function, even before abnormal increases in serum levels of BUN or creatinine occur. Since some contrast media may cause kidney failure in patients with impaired renal function, BUN and creatinine levels are useful in screening patients for whom contrast media may have a toxic effect (see Chapter 10).

Serum bilirubin testing is a blood chemistry assessment that measures the amounts of waste products from the breakdown of hemoglobin. Normally these waste products are processed by the liver into conjugated bilirubin and are excreted as part of the bile via the common bile duct into the duodenum. Physiologically the bile aids in the digestion of dietary fats. Since any obstruction to the flow of bile out of the liver can result in increased amounts of conjugated bilirubin entering the peripheral circulation, increased serum levels of conjugated bilirubin may indicate early liver disease. When bilirubin levels are very high, the patient's skin and the sclera of the eyes take on a yellow color and the patient is described as jaundiced. Some imaging studies of the gallbladder and biliary system rely upon liver uptake of the contrast agent and cannot be performed when the bilirubin level is elevated (see Chapter 10). While radiographic examinations of the biliary system were once quite common, they have largely been replaced by ultrasound studies, nuclear medicine scans, and fiberoptic examinations.

ELECTRONIC PATIENT MONITORING

While acutely ill patients are usually assigned to the intensive care unit, and x-ray examinations are done using mobile units (see Chapter 11), critical patients must sometimes come to the radiology department for the use of specialized equipment. They are usually accompanied by staff from the critical care unit. Some of these patients will be monitored electronically. Patients may also be sent from the emergency department with monitors in place.

Pulse Oximeter

A common monitoring device is a pulse oximeter that is placed on a finger, toe, or earlobe, where it continuously monitors both pulse rate and blood oxygen levels (Fig. 6-16). This device is often used to observe the condition of patients who have received sedatives that may suppress respirations and is commonly used in the magnetic resonance imaging (MRI) suite for this purpose.

A photosensitive cell in the oximeter detects the difference between deoxygenated and oxygenated hemoglobin, and a digital readout displays the current status of the patient. Normal values range from 95% to 100%, and readings below 95% may indicate that tissues are receiving inadequate oxygen perfusion. Since the sensor depends on reflected light, fingernail polish must be removed before applying the oximeter to a finger. Patients with poor circulation due to chronic obstructive pulmonary disease (COPD) or coronary problems may have unreliable readings.

Arterial Catheters

One comprehensive way to monitor cardiac activity is to introduce a special arterial catheter into a large artery where it can provide continuous observation of heart rate and blood pressure. Catheter placement is a special procedure applied under sterile surgical conditions. These catheters and their placement are discussed in Chapter 11.

Electrocardiograph Monitors

A less invasive heart monitor called an electrocardiograph or ECG monitor can display and record heart rate and rhythm through the use of electrodes placed on the chest. This external monitor measures the electrical activity of the heart and displays the information graphically in the form of waves on a monitor screen. The graph may also be recorded on a paper tape. Deviations from normal are automatically recorded and may activate an auditory alarm.

Continuous ECG monitoring is standard practice in most critical care units. Patients may be brought to the imaging department while being monitored over time to detect and record cardiac irregularities. Patients from the emergency department who suffer from various acute medical or traumatic problems may also come to the radiology department while connected to an ECG monitor. ECG monitoring may be ordered during special imaging procedures or treatments to closely watch the patient's cardiac function.

When a patient is being monitored by ECG, electrodes on the patient are attached to cables that connect to an electronic display unit (Fig. 6-17). ECG electrodes are electrical contacts that can receive signals from the patient. They are incorporated into disposable adhesive patches attached to the patient's skin. It is essential that the cables and electrode patches remain secure. When a patient moves, an abnormal tracing can result, which may

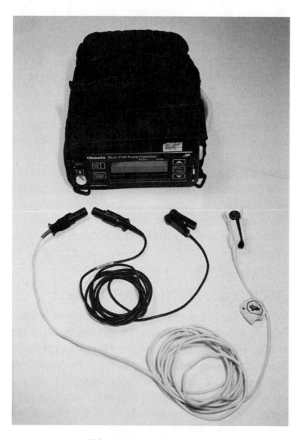

FIG. 6-16 Pulse oximeter.

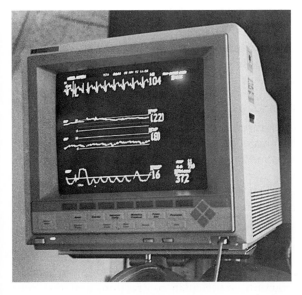

FIG. 6-17 Cardiac monitor.

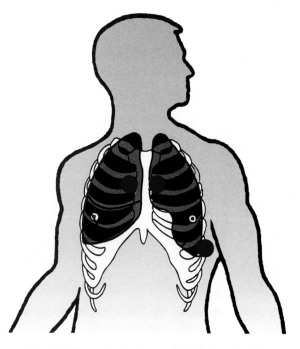

FIG. 6-18 Electrode placement for ECG monitoring.

seem to indicate an arrhythmia. If electrodes become loose or detached, a "flat-line" tracing can result that seems to indicate **asystole** (the cessation of cardiac activity). *Always check the patient and the electrodes before initiating a code.*

Three electrodes are commonly used for continuous monitoring. The two primary contacts are placed on the anterior chest, one on each side of the sternum at the level of the second intercostal space. A third is attached on the side of the chest at the level of the sixth or seventh intercostal space (Fig. 6-18). If a cable is loose, reattach it by snapping it onto the button contact on the electrode patch. If the patch falls off, cleanse the skin with a gauze pad, apply a fresh electrode patch, and attach the cable to the new patch. Supplies are usually kept in drawers in the rolling cabinet that supports the monitor.

Patients who are being monitored by ECG are sometimes temporarily disconnected from monitors when going to the radiology department. In such cases, the electrode patches may be left in place on the patient's chest so that the patient can be readily reconnected to the monitor on return to the nursing unit or emergency department. Although the patches produce minor metallic artifacts on chest radiographs (Fig. 6-19), it is not necessary to remove them unless specifically ordered by a physician. Leaving the patches in place saves time if monitoring must be resumed on an emergency basis and also saves the expense of replacing the patches.

Basic ECG rhythm recognition

While the diagnostic interpretation of electrocardiograms is a physician's responsibility, it is important that you be able to recognize a few of the configurations that may indicate a life-threatening situation. An understanding of the cardiac cycle will help you to appreciate the significance of ECG rhythm patterns. You may also find it helpful to review the basic anatomy and physiology of the heart. There are two types of myocardium (heart muscle tissue): contracting tissue and conducting tissue. Fig. 6-20 illustrates the conducting muscle tissue and its position in relation to the four chambers of the heart. The cardiac impulse is a tiny

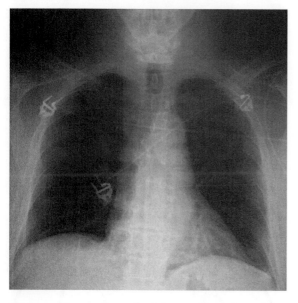

FIG. 6-19 Chest radiograph with ECG electrode artifacts.

electrical current that originates at the junction of the vena cava and the right atrium in conducting myocardium called the sinoatrial (SA) node. It spreads in circular waves over the atrial walls, causing the atria to contract. The impulse then passes through the atrioventricular (AV) node, a second area of conducting myocardium. From this node it passes through a band of conducting muscle that connects the atria to the ventricles and is called the bundle of His. The bundle of His divides into the left and right bundle branches, conducting the cardiac impulse to the left and right ventricles. The bundle branches further divide into Purkinje fibers, fine strands of conducting muscle that transmit the impulse to the contracting muscles of the ventricles.

The normal cardiac cycle includes atrial contraction, ventricular contraction, and rest. The transmission of the electrical wave causing contraction of the chamber walls is called depolarization. Each contraction is followed by repolarization, an electrical recovery period. Following

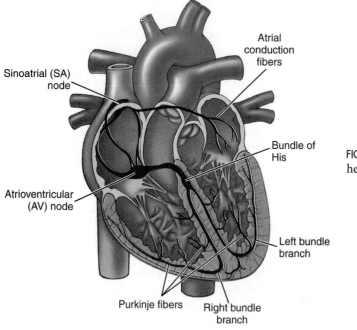

FIG. 6-20 Electrical conduction system of the heart.

ventricular repolarization, the heart rests for a moment in a state of polarization and then the cycle begins again. With normal heart function, this cycle is repeated 50 to 100 times per minute at a regular rate.

The ECG graph is centered on an isoelectric line. Deflections above and below this baseline indicate specific electrical impulses. These deflections are referred to as waves and are labeled P, Q, R, S, and T (Fig. 6-21). Together the Q, R, and S waves are called the QRS complex. The P wave indicates contraction of the atria and the beginning of depolarization. The space between the P wave and the R wave is called the P-R interval and represents the time from the beginning of the atrial contraction to the beginning of the ventricular contraction. The QRS complex represents ventricular contraction. The S-T segment indicates the time between ventricular contraction and the beginning of ventricular recovery. The T wave represents ventricular recovery (repolarization). After the T wave the tracing shows a straight line that indicates the period of heart rest. On rare occasions you may observe a small U wave following the T wave. This is an abnormal wave that indicates a low serum potassium level or other metabolic disturbance that affects the conduction of the cardiac impulse.

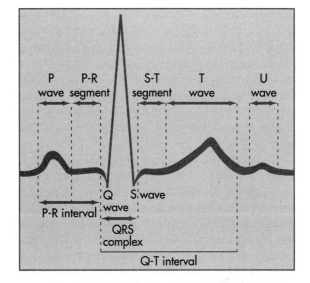

FIG. 6-21 Normal ECG waveform.

Observations of the morphology (shape), amplitude (height), and duration (graph width) of each wave are considered in relation to the baseline and to the other waves. Taken together, these findings demonstrate disturbances in heart rhythm and permit identification of abnormalities. The normal waveform is called **sinus rhythm** and is demonstrated at a normal heart rate in Fig. 6-22.

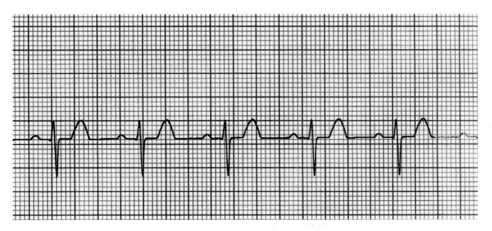

FIG. 6-22 Normal sinus rhythm, rate 80.

Sinus tachycardia (Fig. 6-23) is a rhythm in which the tracing shows a rapid heart rate without other deviations from normal. This ordinarily results from an increase in physical activity or from fear, excitement, or chemical stimulation such as too much caffeine. For patients who have a preexisting heart problem, however, this rapid rate may be a precursor to life-threatening ventricular tachycardia.

Sinus **bradycardia** with a heart rate below 60 is shown in Fig. 6-24. This slow heart rate can be perfectly normal for the healthy individual and is frequently seen in athletes who have developed a large cardiac output. In other patients this slow rate is insufficient to provide adequate oxygen to the brain and vital organs, and a pacemaker may be needed to increase and regulate the heart rate.

Premature ventricular contractions (PVCs) are irregular, early ventricular contractions that interfere with the normal rate and rhythm of the heart (Fig. 6-25). This is demonstrated on the ECG by a wide, irregular QRS complex and a loss of the P wave, which is buried in the QRS wave. PVCs can often be felt by patients who complain that "my heart flutters" or that it feels as though the heart "flops over." While an occasional PVC is not unusual and should not cause undue alarm, a run of PVCs can reduce the cardiac output by 12% to 15% if untreated.

If allowed to progress, PVCs may initiate ventricular **fibrillation,** in which the heart quivers or fibrillates and loses the ability to contract effectively (Fig. 6-26). Ventricular fibrillation is the most common cause of sudden death. A code must be called, cardiopulmonary resuscitation (CPR) initiated, and the patient defibrillated immediately if death is to be prevented (see Chapter 8).

In ventricular tachycardia (Fig. 6-27), the heart rate may be as high as 150 to 250 beats per minute. While the heart may be beating regularly, the cardiac output is too low to be effective and the patient may lose consciousness and become hypotensive. In most cases lidocaine is administered intravenously, and in some cases the patient will need to be defibrillated.

If untreated, ventricular tachycardia may progress to ventricular fibrillation.

Atrial fibrillation (Fig. 6-28) results from continuous and irregular reentry of electrical impulses back into the atria. Because these impulses are so rapid and continuous, they spur a rapid and irregular ventricular response. Atrial fibrillation in the young patient may be due to rheumatic mitral valve disease. Atrial fibrillation is more common in older patients where arteriosclerotic heart disease is the major cause. Palpitations, nausea, weakness, and fatigue may occur during an attack of atrial fibrillation. Sudden attacks tend to occur periodically before this condition becomes chronic. If the patient suffers from mitral stenosis or other left ventricular disease, cardiogenic shock or acute pulmonary edema may result (see Chapter 8). Treatment is initiated primarily to slow ventricular response and increase cardiac output. If the patient does not respond to medication, **cardioversion** may be performed. Cardioversion is an electrical stimulation of the heart to restore normal rhythm.

DIAGNOSTIC ELECTROCARDIOGRAPHY

Electrocardiography is one of the diagnostic tools commonly used in the assessment of heart disease. When an ECG tracing is done as a diagnostic procedure, a paper strip graph provides a permanent record of the test. The graph is similar to those seen on ECG monitors but is recorded using a different machine and 10 different electrode placements. The resulting test includes 12 different recordings called leads, each representing a different measurement of the electrical activity of the heart. You may encounter these graphs, or copies of them, in patients' charts. It is important to note that while the ECG is a measure of the electrical activity of the heart, a normal ECG does not necessarily indicate a completely healthy heart. Other factors, such as disease or mechanical defects of the myocardium, may be undetected by ECG.

In many hospitals today, cross training of radiographers in multiple diagnostic modalities is thought to be advantageous. The ability to perform an

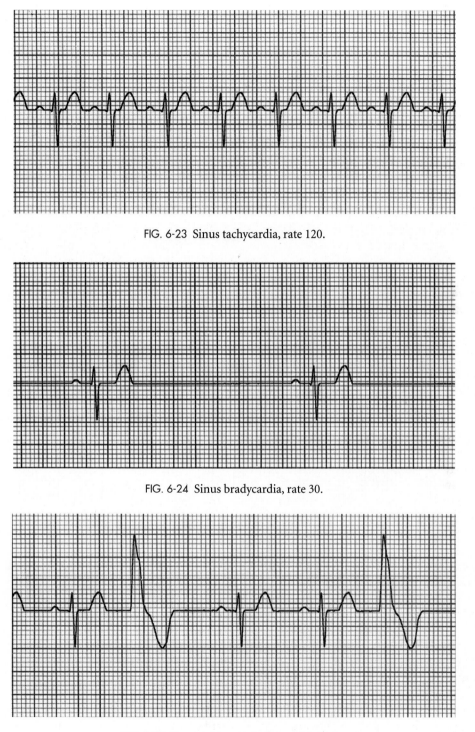

FIG. 6-23 Sinus tachycardia, rate 120.

FIG. 6-24 Sinus bradycardia, rate 30.

FIG. 6-25 Premature ventricular contractions.

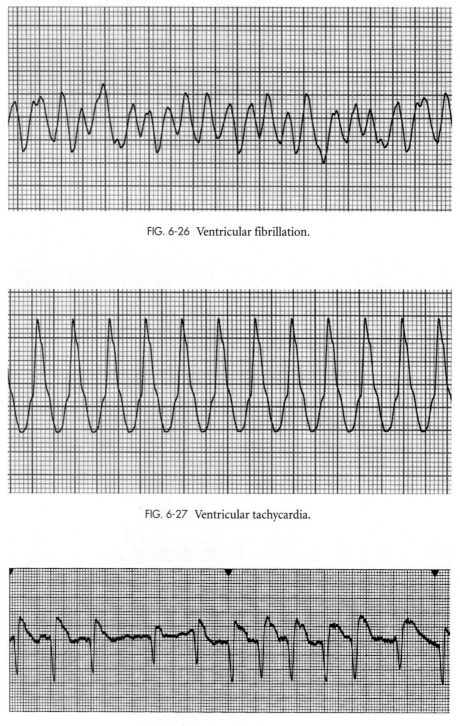

FIG. 6-26 Ventricular fibrillation.

FIG. 6-27 Ventricular tachycardia.

FIG. 6-28 Atrial fibrillation.

ECG for diagnostic purposes is one such skill. Diagnostic interpretation of ECGs requires specialized training, but learning to gather the diagnostic information is fairly simple. In smaller hospitals, cross training in this area allows for greater flexibility in staffing. It may be a requirement in an outpatient facility.

Electrocardiography Machines

The machine used for diagnostic electrocardiography is called an electrocardiograph (Fig. 6-29). Like the ECG monitor, it is attached to the patient with cables and electrodes. Electrical impulses from the patient are transmitted to the machine, where they are amplified and translated into signals that cause movement of a balanced tracing pen called a stylus. The pattern of these electrical impulses is traced by the stylus on graph paper. The resulting tracing

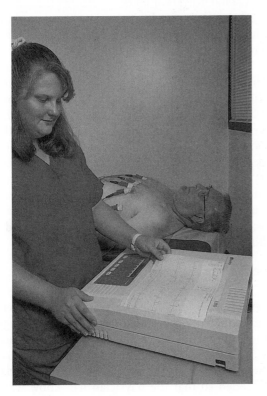

FIG. 6-29 Electrocardiograph machine.

is called an **electrocardiogram,** abbreviated **ECG** or **EKG.**

Electrocardiography machines vary depending on age, manufacturer, and level of technical sophistication. An operator's manual should accompany the machine. The radiographer who performs ECGs should be familiar with the features of the equipment and the guidelines provided in the manual. While the equipment may seem intimidating at first, an orientation will be provided.

The least sophisticated machines are single-channel machines that record one lead at a time. The operator selects the lead to be recorded and starts and stops the recording manually. Modern machines have 10 lead wires, one for each extremity and 6 for the chest. Some older machines may have only 1 chest lead wire, and the single chest electrode must be moved from one location to the next to record each of the 6 chest leads. The operator may need to enter a code to identify each lead, but most modern electrocardiographs do this automatically. The standard marking codes are listed in Table 6-4.

Multichannel machines record 3 or 6 leads at once. These machines have 10 lead wires, and all are connected to the patient before the recording begins. A three-channel electrocardiogram is illustrated in Fig. 6-30.

Some machines, both single-channel and multi-channel, are equipped with automatic sequencing capability. Once started, these units proceed automatically from one lead to the next without input from the operator. These machines also identify each lead and place a standardization mark on the tracing. Machines with automatic sequencing usually have a manual option that permits longer tracings when needed.

Interpretive electrocardiographs incorporate a computer that analyzes the tracing as it is made and prints the ECG interpretation and the specific reason(s) for the interpretation on the tracing. Patient data is entered into the computer before recording, and this data is also printed on the ECG.

Telephone transmission equipment is available for sending ECGs to remote locations for interpretation.

TABLE 6-4		
STANDARD ELECTROCARDIOGRAPH LEAD CODES		
LEADS	ELECTRODES CONNECTED	MARKING CODE
Standard Limb Leads		
Lead I	LA and RA	.
Lead II	LL and RA	..
Lead III	LL and LA	...
Augmented Limb Leads		
AVR	RA and LA-LL	–
AVL	LA and RA-LL	– –
AVF	LL and RA-LA	– – –
Precordial (Chest) Leads		
V_1	C and LA-RA-LL	– .
V_2	C and LA-RA-LL	– ..
V_3	C and LA-RA-LL	– ...
V_4	C and LA-RA-LL	– ....
V_5	C and LA-RA-LL	– .....
V_6	C and LA-RA-LL	– ......

LA, Left arm; *RA*, right arm; *LL*, left leg; *C*, chest.

Electrocardiograph Paper and Standardization

ECG paper is divided into squares to facilitate measurement of the waves, intervals, and segments. Each square measures 1 mm in each dimension, and every fifth square in each dimension is indicated with a bold line (Fig. 6-31). The bold lines form large squares that are 5 mm by 5 mm in size.

International agreements have established standards for ECGs to ensure that tracings read anywhere in the world will be interpreted in the same way. When the machine is properly calibrated, 1 millivolt (mV) of electrical potential difference will cause the stylus to move vertically 10 mm. This standard ensures that voltage will be interpreted accurately when reading the graph.

To check the calibration of the machine, the standardization button is depressed using a quick, pecking motion of the finger. Depression of the standardization button produces a 1-mV signal that makes a standardization mark on the tracing. The mark should be 10 mm high, approximately 2 mm wide, and rectangular in shape. The operation manual for the machine will provide instruction for making adjustments when the standard is not accurate.

Most machines have three standard (STD) position settings, ½ STD, 1 STD, and 2 STD, but the 1 STD setting is usually used. If the amplitude of the QRS complex is so great that it causes the stylus to move off the paper, the ½ STD setting should be used. When recording at the ½ STD setting, 1 mV causes the stylus to deflect only 5 mm. If the amplitude of the QRS complex is very low, the 2 STD setting may be used to increase the readability of the tracing. At the 2 STD setting, the standard mark will be the height of four large squares (20 mm). Fig. 6-32 shows standardization marks for each STD setting.

A standardization mark is usually placed at the beginning of the first lead recording. Some machines will do this automatically. Some physicians prefer standardization on each of the 12 leads.

The speed of the paper feed must also be standardized for the tracing to be interpreted accurately. The universal recording speed is 25 mm per second. When the patient's heart rate is very rapid or when certain parts of the complex are too close together for accurate assessment, it may be desirable to adjust the machine so that the paper runs at double speed, 50 mm per second. This change in settings will extend the recording to twice its normal length and must be noted on the tracing. The difference in recording between normal and double speed is illustrated in Fig. 6-33.

Electrocardiography Leads

As stated earlier, a standard ECG study includes 12 separate recordings called leads. Each lead represents cardiac activity as recorded from a different angle. To obtain these various leads, electrodes are placed in 10 locations, 1 on each arm and each leg and 6 on the chest. The tracing for each lead must be marked or coded so that the physician will know which angle is represented. The 12 leads are categorized as

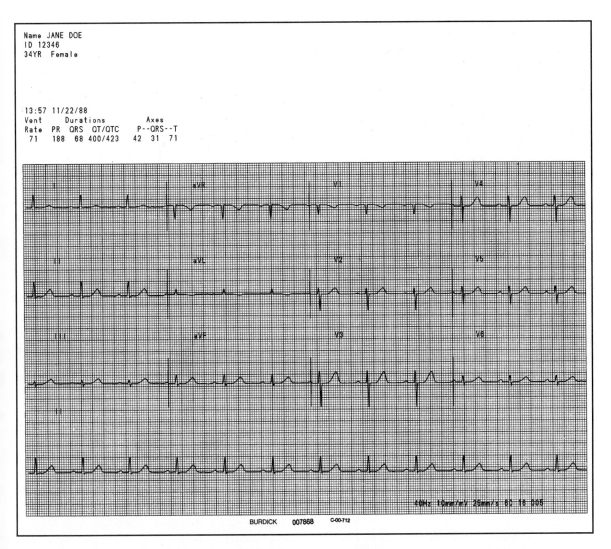

FIG. 6-30 Three-channel ECG.

standard (limb) leads, augmented (AV) leads, and precordial (chest) leads.

There are three limb or standard leads, sometimes referred to as bipolar leads, and designated by roman numerals I, II, and III. Each uses two limb electrodes to record the electric activity (Fig. 6-34). Lead I records the electrical potential (voltage) between the right arm and the left arm. Lead II records the voltage between the right arm and the left leg. Lead III records the voltage between the left arm and the left leg. The right leg provides an electrical ground. Normal recordings of leads I, II, and III are illustrated in Fig. 6-35.

The three augmented leads are termed AVR, AVL, and AVF. The "AV" portion of these terms stands for augmented voltage. R indicates the right arm, L stands for left arm, and F stands for foot, indicating the left leg. Each of these leads records the voltage from one limb electrode to the midpoint between two others (Fig. 6-36). Lead AVR records the voltage

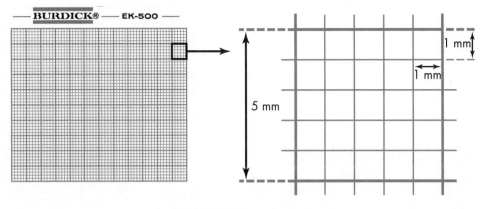

FIG. 6-31 ECG graph paper.

measured from the midpoint between the left arm and left leg to the right arm, while lead AVL records the voltage measured from the midpoint between the right arm and left leg to the left arm. Lead AVF records voltage measured from the midpoint between the right arm and the left arm to the left leg. Again, the right leg serves as a ground. Normal recordings of the augmented leads are seen in Fig. 6-37.

The six precordial or chest leads are designated V_1 through V_6, each representing a specific location on the chest (Fig. 6-38). These leads indicate the voltage between the chest wall and a point within the heart. Normal recordings of leads V_1 through V_6 are seen in Fig. 6-39. Fig. 6-40 demonstrates the progression of the signal from the SA node region to the left ventricle.

Preparation for Electrocardiography

At the time of scheduling, patients should be informed of what to expect and instructed not to

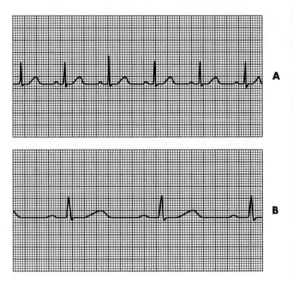

FIG. 6-33 Paper run speed. **A,** Normal recording speed is 25 mm per second. **B,** Double speed is 50 mm per second.

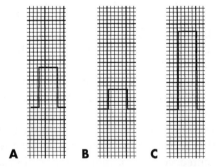

FIG. 6-32 ECG standardization marks. **A,** 1 STD. Normal standardization mark is 10 mm high. **B,** ½ STD. One-half standardization mark is 5 mm high. **C,** 2 STD. Double standardization mark is 20 mm high.

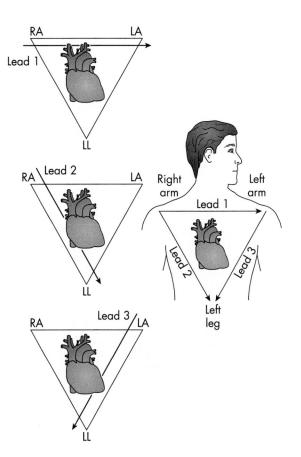

FIG. 6-34 Standard limb leads record activity of the heart from three angles.

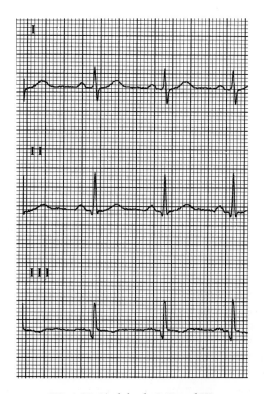

FIG. 6-35 Limb leads, I, II, and III.

apply any lotion or oil to the arms, legs, or chest. They should be advised that they will need to expose their arms, legs, and chest for the application of the electrodes so that they can dress for convenience in this regard. Patients who have never had an ECG may assume from the name of the test that electricity will be applied to their bodies. Explain that the test is painless and that only electricity *from* their bodies is being measured. Some facilities provide patient brochures that answer common questions and list instructions.

The room should be quiet and warm with a table for the patient to lie on. The table should be padded and wide enough for the patient to

relax comfortably with both arms and legs fully supported. If the table has metal parts, there must be insulation between these parts and the patient. Small pillows under the patient's head and knees will add comfort and make it easier for the patient to lie still for the duration of the test. It is most convenient to position the table so that the operator is on the patient's left side. The ECG machine should be placed as far from other electrical equipment as possible. The power cord should point away from the patient and should not pass under the table.

The patient should disrobe to the waist and wear a gown. Shoes and stockings must be removed and the lower legs exposed. The patient is instructed to lie supine with the legs separated from each other. Any tight clothing should be loosened. Arrange the gown so that the chest is accessible for electrode placement but modestly covered for the patient's

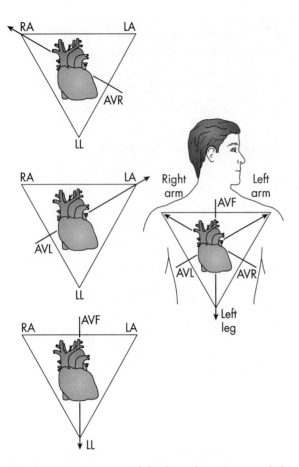

FIG. 6-36 For augmented leads, voltage is recorded between one point and the midpoint of two others.

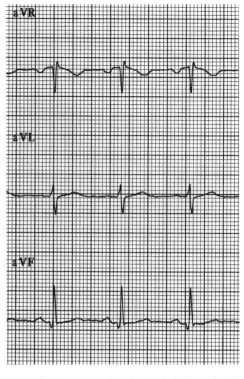

FIG. 6-37 Augmented leads, AVR, AVL, and AVF.

comfort. For the best test results, the patient should rest in this position for about 10 minutes before the start of the test. Some physicians may want you to record any medications that the patient is taking. Explain that the patient should remain in a relaxed position and must not move during the recording of the ECG. Talking during recording is not usually a problem, as long as the patient remains still and relaxed.

Turn on the machine's power switch, and allow it to warm up. The operation manual will state the time needed for this process.

The next step is to place the electrodes on the patient. The electrodes are attached to the patient's

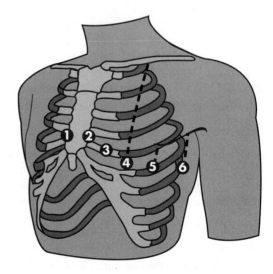

FIG. 6-38 Placement locations for chest leads.

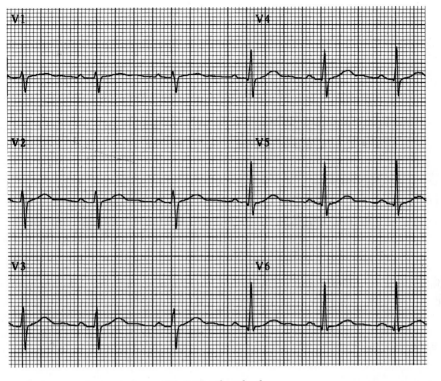

FIG. 6-39 Chest leads.

skin and have an attachment for the cable ends. Disposable adhesive electrodes are most commonly used. The skin in the areas where electrodes are applied must be clean, dry, and oil-free. If the patient did not have an opportunity to prepare for the examination, you may have to remove oil or lotion from the skin before applying the electrodes. This can be accomplished by rubbing the area briskly with an alcohol pad and wiping it with a tissue. Since skin does not conduct electricity well, an electrolyte compound is incorporated into disposable electrodes to enhance the electrical contact and ensure a reliable tracing.

Attach an adhesive electrode firmly to the fleshy, outer surface of each upper arm and to the inner surface of the calf of each leg. Attach six electrodes

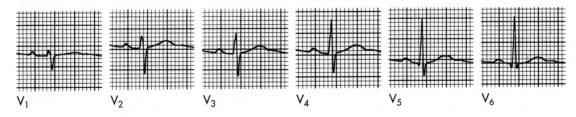

FIG. 6-40 Sequence of heartbeats from each of the precordial leads demonstrates progression of electrical signal from the SA node to the left ventricle.

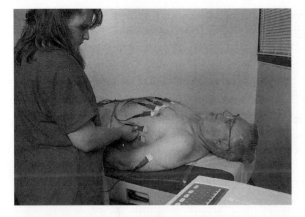

FIG. 6-41 Patient with electrodes in place for ECG recording.

to the chest according to the diagram in Fig. 6-38. The patient in Fig. 6-41 has electrodes properly placed.

The next step is to attach the patient cable to the patient electrodes. The patient cable is a branching cable used to connect the electrodes to the machine. The cable has 10 branches called lead wires, and each is labeled for the specific electrode to which it should be attached. Take care to attach the lead wires to the correct electrodes, as improper connections will result in an inaccurate tracing. When the electrodes are all connected, arrange the cords so that they lie on the patient's body. This practice reduces interference and avoids the possibility that the weight of a hanging cable will loosen a connection.

Obtaining the Tracing

The procedure for making the tracing will vary, depending on the equipment. If you have an electrocardiograph with automated controls, activate the automatic start button and monitor the electrocardiograph while it records all 12 leads. The machine will standardize and code the tracing.

If you have a machine that is manually controlled, set the lead selector control to STD, turn on the recorder control, and activate RUN. The stylus will create a flat line. Use the position control knob to center the baseline on the graph paper. Check the

standardization by pressing the standardization button as previously described. The stylus should rise the height of two large squares on the tracing paper (10 mm).

Turn the lead selector control to lead I, and code the lead unless your machine does this automatically. Run at least 8 to 10 inches of clean, high-quality tracing with no artifacts. Switch to lead II and then to lead III, repeating the same steps. Run at least 4 to 6 inches of high-quality recording for leads AVR, AVL, and AVF. Continue recording to obtain 4 to 6 inches of high-quality tracing for leads V_1 through V_6. When all of the chest leads are complete, slowly turn the lead selector control back to STD, one setting at a time. Turning too rapidly may damage the gears of the dial. Run a straight baseline, and then turn off the record switch.

When the ECG is complete, turn off the machine, disconnect the lead wires, and remove the electrodes. It is a good practice to double-check that the leads were properly connected as you disconnect them. Assist the patient off the table and to the dressing room. Discard disposable electrodes, return all equipment to its proper place, and perform hand hygiene.

Artifacts

ECG artifacts are irregularities in the tracing that do not represent the electrical activity of heart impulses and that interfere with the appearance of the ECG. The operator must monitor all ECG recordings for artifacts. When they occur, the recording should be stopped and the problem corrected. Any leads affected by artifacts should be repeated.

The artifacts most commonly seen are muscle artifact, alternating current artifact, wandering baseline, and interrupted baseline.

Muscle artifact (Fig. 6-42) causes a fuzzy, irregular baseline due to muscle contraction. Muscle artifact is most commonly seen when anxiety or discomfort causes the patient to tense muscles. If the patient is chilly, shivering may cause this artifact. Muscle artifact can usually be avoided by providing reassurance, encouraging the patient to relax and let the muscles go limp, and by ensuring the patient's warmth and comfort. Sometimes muscle artifact occurs as a result of tremors due to nervous system disorders

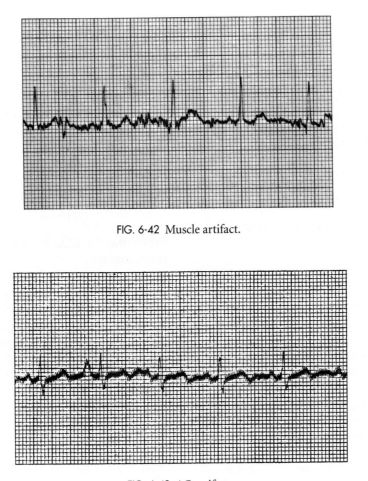

FIG. 6-42 Muscle artifact.

FIG. 6-43 AC artifact.

such as Parkinson's disease. In these cases, it may be helpful to have the patient place the hands under the body. If the operator has the freedom do so, placing gentle pressure on the patient's shoulders may be reassuring and help the patient to relax. The operator must be understanding and try to record when the tremor is at a minimum.

Alternating current (AC) artifact (Fig. 6-43) is caused by electrical interference. AC artifact appears as tiny spiked vertical lines that are very close together and are consistent throughout the tracing. Newer electrocardiographs are electrically shielded, and this artifact is seldom seen with modern equipment unless the patient is affected by current leaking from an electric appliance on his or her body, such as a TENS unit.* With older equipment, electrical interference may be caused by other electrical equipment in the room, fluorescent light fixtures, improper grounding of the electrocardiograph, or wiring in the structure of the room. When AC artifacts appear, turn off all electrical appliances and fluorescent lights in the room and make sure the

---

*TENS stands for transcutaneous electrical nerve stimulation. The unit consists of a pad containing electrodes and attached by wires to a battery power source. TENS units provide mild electrical pulses to a limited area of the body as a treatment for pain.

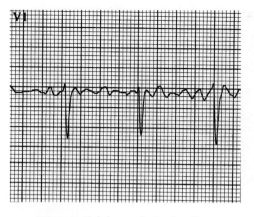

FIG. 6-44 Subtle wandering baseline.

machine is connected to a properly grounded outlet. Check to be certain that the lead wires follow the body contour and do not dangle from the table, as they are more likely to be influenced by current from other sources when this occurs. If these measures do not solve the problem, try moving the patient table to another location at a greater distance from the walls.

Subtle wandering baseline (Fig. 6-44) is an indication of poor electrical contact. This artifact is seen when electrodes are not in firm contact with the skin, when the contacts between the electrodes and the lead wires are loose, or when oily skin has not been properly cleansed. It is important to identify and correct this artifact because it can sometimes lead to a mistaken diagnosis.

Major wandering baseline (Fig. 6-45) is caused by patient movement or by electrical interference from activity within the room. People moving about near the patient may cause this artifact.

Interrupted baseline (Fig. 6-46) is an artifact that occurs when there is an intermittent interruption of electrical transmission caused by detachment of a lead wire or by a broken wire. When a broken wire is determined to be the cause, the patient cable must be repaired or replaced.

Preparing the ECG for Interpretation and Storage

The ECG recording is part of the patient's permanent record and must include the patient's name and an identifying number such as the birth date or file number. Data should also include the patient's age and sex, the testing date, and any variations from the usual STD or machine speed. With computerized machines the operator enters patient data into the computer and the machine prints the identification on the tracing automatically.

ECG paper is delicate and subject to damage when folded or scratched. Paper clips and staples must not be used to secure ECGs. If clear tape is used, it must be a high-quality tape that will not

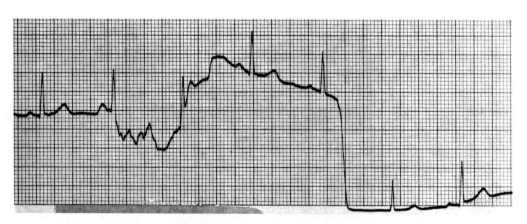

FIG. 6-45 Major wandering baseline.

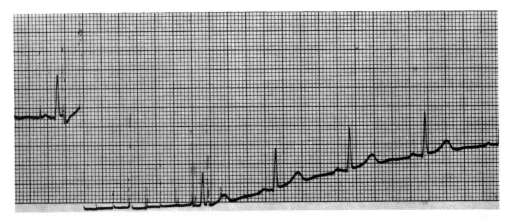

FIG. 6-46 Interrupted baseline.

deteriorate or yellow with age. There are four basic types of graph paper: chem/thermal, wax-coated, plain paper, and glossy paper. Tape should not be used on chem/thermal paper because chemicals in the adhesive will darken the tracing.

Depending on the format of the ECG, your facility's protocol may require that it be photocopied and/or mounted in a special mounting folder. Convenient mounts are commercially available that display the entire study on a single surface. When mounting, the tracing is edited to eliminate excess recording and portions that contain artifacts, retaining the best portion of each lead. Take care to match each lead to its correct location in the mount and to mount all leads right side up.

When correctly identified, edited, and prepared, the ECG is presented to the physician for interpretation, together with the patient's chart and any previous ECG studies for comparison.

Exercise Tolerance Testing

An exercise tolerance test, also called an ECG stress test, is a special diagnostic ECG study that compares resting tracings with those obtained under the stress of physical exercise. Stress tests are used to detect and/or evaluate cardiac ischemia. The ECG is monitored and recorded while the patient performs exercise. The exercise is usually performed on a treadmill, but a stationary bicycle or a simple set of stairsteps is sometimes used. The patient's blood pressure and pulse are also monitored during the exercise. Resting ECGs are usually performed both before and after the stress portion of the test.

Exercise tolerance testing is performed only in facilities that have trained staff and special equipment to respond to a cardiac emergency, which could arise during the test. Various protocols are used for stress testing. If your duties involve assisting with exercise tolerance ECG tests, you will be instructed in the specific protocols observed in your facility, including the procedure for patient instruction and preparation.

ELECTROENCEPHALOGRAPHY

Another physiological monitoring and recording device is the electroencephalograph (EEG). This is not commonly seen in the radiology department. The EEG machine is similar in function and design to the ECG unit, but the cables are attached to electrodes on the patient's scalp to record or monitor the electrical activity of the brain. This device is commonly used to evaluate patients with convulsive disorders, but it can also help the physician diagnose other conditions that affect brain activity. An EEG can display cessation of electrical activity in the brain, providing one of the criteria used to determine legal death, especially in situations involving organ donation.

Most monitoring devices are applied in a critical care setting, and special training is necessary both to apply and to monitor these electronic instruments. They are useful in providing rapid and accurate information but are also subject to error when connections become loose, are placed incorrectly, or when the patient moves. Chapter 11 provides more information about some of the highly sophisticated patient monitoring systems used in the intensive care unit.

CONCLUSION

Your assessment skills are invaluable tools for making the right clinical decisions and taking the right actions. Sharpening these skills will help you develop confidence as a radiographer and will increase your patients' confidence in you.

If you are in doubt about the change in a patient's status, you have resources available to help you, such as the chart, the nursing staff, your supervisor, and the physician.

Think of yourself both as an extension of the radiologist and as a patient advocate. Look for changes in patients' mental and physical status, and be ready to take steps to avoid emergencies. Listen to your patients, and meet their needs to the best of your ability.

REVIEW QUESTIONS

1. When a patient who is brought to the radiology department with an IV running requests a drink of water, it is important to:
   A. offer a glass of cool water with a straw
   B. refuse the request
   C. record the I&O
   D. check the chart for fluid orders
   E. none of the above
2. When an outpatient is referred for examination, which of the following data must be obtained for the radiologist?
   A. the procedure requested
   B. pertinent history
   C. pertinent information about current physical status
   D. all of the above
   E. none of the above
3. Your initial assessment of patient status should include:
   A. checking I&O
   B. evaluating skin temperature by touch
   C. evaluating LOC
   D. both A and B
   E. both B and C
4. A blood pressure reading:
   A. depends on age, weight, and physical status
   B. should be taken before IV contrast or systemic medication is given
   C. shows hypertension in 35% of adults
   D. both A and B
   E. both B and C
5. A serum bilirubin test is used to measure:
   A. blood oxygen levels
   B. nitrogen in blood
   C. blood glucose status when fasting
   D. conjugated hemoglobin content in blood
   E. total serum cholesterol

CRITICAL THINKING EXERCISES

1. Mrs. Morgan, a missionary wife, has just returned from overseas with a fever of unknown origin (FUO) and has been referred for a chest x-ray. What can you think of that might be causing Mrs. Morgan's fever? How would you use the history guidelines in this chapter to obtain relevant information for the radiologist?
2. A 16-year-old male, Larry Doyle, was hunting when he was attacked by a swarm of yellow jackets. While running away, he fell and severely twisted his ankle. He has been admitted to the emergency department to rule out a fractured ankle. The numerous stings have caused swelling over much of his exposed hands and arms. Would it be important to monitor Larry's vital signs? Why or why not? What problems might you encounter? How might his pulse and respirations be affected by anxiety and pain?

3. Any sudden change in vital signs can be extremely important. Hector Garcia has been given an antibiotic for a urinary tract infection. This is the second occurrence of infection in 6 weeks, and he has now been referred for an excretory urogram. While waiting for the initial film to be checked, he complains of feeling short of breath and has a poorly defined discomfort in his chest. What might cause these symptoms? What should you do?

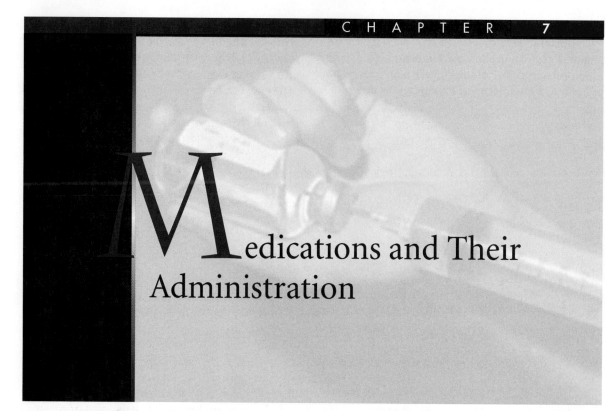

Medications and Their Administration

At the conclusion of this chapter, the student will be able to:

- Define the term standing order.
- Explain the meaning of adverse effects.
- Give an example of a trade name and a generic name of a medication typically seen in the radiology department.
- Demonstrate how to look up a medication in a comprehensive drug reference book.
- State the five rights of medication administration.
- Demonstrate the steps used in the administration of oral medication.

- List five routes of medication administration.
- Identify the veins suitable for intravenous (IV) injections.
- Demonstrate the steps taken to discontinue an IV infusion.
- State the average rate of flow for IV fluids expressed in drops per minute.
- Identify the sites used for intramuscular injections.

allergen	infiltration
ampule	intradermal
anesthetic	intramuscular
angina pectoris	intravenous infusion
antidote	metabolize
buccal	parenteral
cathartic	potent
diluent	standing order
edema	subcutaneous
extravasation	sublingual
generic	synergistic
hematoma	topical
hydrostatic pressure	toxic

THE RADIOGRAPHER'S ROLE

THE CURRENT EMPHASIS on acute care and shorter hospital stays has increased the percentage of patients who arrive at the radiology department with complex monitors and arterial lines in place. Some patients may have medication pumps that deliver measured amounts of drugs at regular intervals. If a pump is set up for self-administration of pain medication, the patient can administer the agent as needed for pain relief. **Intravenous infusions** are very common. They deliver fluids and medications into a vein at a slow and constant rate by gravity flow. Radiographers may need to monitor these systems while patients are in their care, but the nursing service is responsible for the initiation of most routine medication administration. Patients who must not miss a dose in their prescribed medical regimen will have their medications brought to them by a nurse.

Radiographers become more involved in medication administration when medications are given for radiographic procedures. Examples include radiopaque drugs injected or ingested to provide radiographic contrast, **anesthetic** agents (drugs that cause insensibility to pain) injected before the insertion of arterial catheters, and sedation to calm the patient or relieve pain during invasive procedures and magnetic resonance imaging (MRI) examinations.

When there is a sudden change in a patient's status or when emergencies occur in the radiology suite, the radiographer must be able to quickly locate medications. One example might be a severe allergic reaction to a contrast medium. An acute angina attack, a sudden asthmatic episode, or an insulin reaction are other typical emergencies seen by radiographers where prompt administration of medication may be essential. The radiographer will be responsible for checking the allergic history of patients, preparing medication for administration, verifying patient identification, assisting the physician, and monitoring the patient after the medication has been given. If state regulations and hospital policies permit, radiographers might be expected to administer and chart the medication or contrast medium.

If medications are given in the radiology department, a physician selects the drug, determines the route of administration, and prescribes the exact dosage. *No medication should ever be given without a physician's order and supervision.* Orders may be written or verbal and may sometimes be in the form of a standing order. Verbal orders given in the radiology department should be written or countersigned by the physician before leaving the area. This area of patient care has a high potential for medicolegal problems. For your own protection, you must be familiar with the rules governing medication administration in your state as well as in your institution.

A **standing order** consists of written directions for a specific medication or procedure, signed by a physician and used only under the specific conditions stated in the order. Such orders are found in a Policy and Procedures Manual or Standing Orders book available for immediate reference in the radiology department. For example, many radiology departments have standing orders to administer a **cathartic** (strong laxative) preparation before certain radiographic examinations. In this case the standing order would state which examinations require the advance cathartic preparation, the name and amount of the drug, the time to be administered, and any patient conditions that would preclude implementation of the order. It would be signed by the radiologist and would be reviewed and countersigned on a regular basis. A sample of the patient instruction sheet might also be included.

Although a comprehensive knowledge of drugs is not essential for a radiographer, you must become familiar with the names, dosages, and routes of administration for medications used in imaging departments. If this seems intimidating, be reassured that only a limited number of drugs, with a few standard dosages of each, are used with any regularity. Knowledge of these medications greatly facilitates the task of assisting the physician and aids in determining whether departmental stocks of medications and medication supplies are adequate and up to date. It also enables the alert radiographer to prevent errors by questioning and double-checking any medication orders or records that seem unusual or inappropriate.

Any drug may produce side effects in certain patients. Radiographers use this knowledge to anticipate possible adverse drug reactions and to recognize and report signs and symptoms of side effects as they occur. This awareness is very important, since radiographers are often the first to observe the onset of medication responses that could have serious consequences. For information on responding to drug reactions, see Chapter 8.

MEDICATION NOMENCLATURE AND INFORMATION RESOURCES

The terms *drugs* and *medications* are often used interchangeably in the health care field. Medications are substances prescribed for treatment and produce therapeutically useful effects. Drugs, the more general term, denotes substances used in diagnosis, treatment, or disease prevention, or as a component of a medication. In common usage, this term is also applied to chemicals such as narcotics or hallucinogens that affect the central nervous system (CNS), causing behavioral changes and possible addiction. Drugs may replace a missing substance in the body such as estrogen or insulin. Some medications, such as digitalis, are made from plants; others, such as heparin, come from animal sources. Others, such as penicillin, are produced by microorganisms. Many

drugs today are manufactured from synthetic materials. Drug synthesis and the rapidly expanding application of genetic engineering promise vast possibilities for the future.

Each medication has a **generic** name that identifies its chemical family. If the drug consists principally of one chemical, it may also be referred to by its chemical name. For example, acetylsalicylic acid is the chemical name for the generic drug, aspirin. Manufacturers give their products brand names that are also called proprietary or trade names. The same generic substance may be manufactured by several different companies and given a different trade name by each. For example, a synthetic antibacterial containing trimethoprim and sulfamethoxazole is produced by Roche under the name Bactrim and by GlaxoSmithKline as Septra. The generic and trade names of some drugs are used interchangeably. For instance, the generic term *epinephrine* is used just as frequently as the trade name Adrenalin for this common emergency drug. Since medications may be ordered by either generic or trade names, you should be familiar with both terms. When the radiologist calls for epinephrine, the knowledgeable radiographer will reach for Adrenalin without having to read the small print on each container in the emergency drug box.

Setting the standards for control of drugs is part of the role of the U.S. Food and Drug Administration (FDA). This includes strict rules concerning efficacy, purity, potency, safety, and toxicity of both prescriptive and nonprescriptive (over-the-counter or OTC) medications.

The study of drugs is an ongoing process, since new medications are constantly added to the medical repertoire. In addition, no single textbook can provide information for all contingencies. For these reasons, the radiographer should be acquainted with other methods of obtaining medication facts on a continuing basis. One useful resource is the information sheet enclosed in each drug package. The FDA requires that all drug packages include the following data: trade name, generic name, chemical composition, chemical strength, usual dose, indications, contraindications, and reported side effects. Package inserts from frequently used drugs may be kept on file in the imaging department to avoid opening a package when this information is needed. If you collect and study inserts from the drugs used most frequently, you will soon develop a useful information base for medications important in your clinical setting.

Another useful medication reference is the *Physicians' Desk Reference* (PDR). This book, which is published annually, lists drugs alphabetically by their generic names, by their trade names, and according to their uses. A separate section indexes the products made by each manufacturer. In the product description you will find information similar to that found in the package inserts. The radiology department library usually includes a PDR, and the radiographer should become familiar with its use. *Mosby's GenRx* is another comprehensive medication reference. It comes with a password providing Internet access to the most current medication information updates. Changes in the pharmaceutical industry, including the introduction of so-called designer drugs, have increased the speed at which medications are developed, approved, and marketed. As a result, medication references quickly become outdated, so it is more important than ever that medication information sources be current. In-service classes and college courses may also provide useful medication information. This is especially important if your state law and job description permit you to administer medications and contrast media.

MEDICATION PROPERTIES
Pharmacokinetics

Pharmacokinetics is the study of how drugs enter the body, are absorbed, reach their site of action, are **metabolized** (physically and chemically changed), and exit the body. These processes are important, because they affect the ways in which individuals respond to medications. Individual response can vary greatly depending on age, physical condition, sex, weight, or immune status.

Absorption

Absorption is the process by which a drug enters the systemic circulation in order to provide a desired effect. Oral medications are absorbed through the mucosal lining of the gastrointestinal tract. Other medications are injected and absorbed through the muscle or fat layers. When medications are injected directly into a vein or artery, no absorption is needed.

Distribution

Distribution is the means by which a drug travels from the site of absorption to the site of action, usually through the bloodstream. This process depends on adequate circulation. Drugs act more quickly in organs with an abundant blood supply, such as the liver, heart, brain, and kidneys.

Metabolism

Metabolism is the process by which the body transforms drugs into an inactive form that can be excreted from the body. Most drug metabolism occurs in the liver, where enzymatic action transforms a drug into metabolites that can be excreted via the intestinal tract or the kidneys.

Excretion

Excretion refers to the elimination of drugs from the body after they have been metabolized. Drugs may be excreted by way of the kidneys, intestines, lungs, or exocrine glands. The kidneys are the chief organs of excretion, but the route depends largely on the chemical makeup of the drug. Portions of some drugs may escape metabolism and be excreted unchanged in the urine. Volatile substances such as alcohol and certain anesthetics are excreted through the lungs. For this reason, postoperative patients are encouraged to cough and breathe deeply to help clear their bodies of the anesthetic agent. Other drugs are metabolized in the liver, excreted into the bile, and then routed through the intestines for elimination. Some medications are metabolized in the liver, and their metabolites are transported by the bloodstream to the kidneys for excretion. If kidney function is impaired or if the patient is dehydrated, drugs can be retained in the body and a **toxic** (poisonous) effect can occur if patients on medications have insufficient fluid intake.

Pharmacodynamics

Pharmacodynamics is the study of the effects of drugs on the normal physiological functions of the body. The most common mechanism of drug action is the binding of drugs to the receptor sites on a cell. After a drug reaches its site of action, it exerts its effects on the cell's receptor sites. The drugs and receptors fit together much like a lock and key. The action of a drug on specific cells is called the therapeutic effect, and it results in anticipated outcomes such as diuresis, increased cardiac output, or relief from pain. When receptors and drugs lock together, the therapeutic effects occur. Each cell in the body contains specific, unique receptors. For example, diphenhydramine (Benadryl) blocks the receptor sites of histamine cells and reduces the itching and swelling caused by an allergic reaction. A drug that produces such a specific action and promotes the desired result is referred to as an *agonist*. A drug that attaches itself to the receptor, preventing the agonist from acting, is called an *antagonist*.

MEDICATION EFFECTS

As stated in the previous section, medications are administered for a predictable physiological response called the therapeutic effect. In addition to the desired outcome, side effects may occur, which may or may not be harmless. If the side effects are severe enough to outweigh the benefits of the medication, the physician may choose to discontinue the drug.

Toxic effects develop when a drug accumulates in the body because of inadequate excretion, impaired metabolism, overdose, or drug sensitivity. Elderly patients are more likely to have poor cardiac, renal, or hepatic function. These conditions increase the possibility that toxic effects might occur. The specific drug that treats a toxic effect is called an **antidote.**

An *idiosyncratic* reaction occurs when a patient overreacts or underreacts to a drug or has an unusual reaction. For example, some individuals become very agitated, rather than sedated, when phenobarbital is administered.

An *allergic* reaction occurs when a patient has been sensitized to the initial dose of a medication and develops an allergic response to the **allergen** (substance to which a sensitivity has been established) and related drugs. Drug allergies may be slight or severe, and the extent of the reaction is unpredictable.

Knowledge of some of the more common medications helps you evaluate changes in the condition of patients in your care. Reference to the medication record in the patient's chart may help you determine whether a change in status is caused by medication or by deterioration in the patient's condition. For example, if the patient is taking an anticholinergic medication such as atropine, this may cause a dry mouth. This side effect has nothing to do with the patient's state of hydration. Opiates may slow the respiratory rate, and vasodilators may cause the blood pressure to drop. Such effects are the usual consequence of the specific medication and are taken into account when the drug is prescribed.

Adverse side effects are not a normal consequence of most prescribed medications. They may range from mild nausea, flushing, or diarrhea to critical situations including cardiac arrest or other life-threatening states. Hives, respiratory distress, or abrupt changes in blood pressures are all symptoms demanding a physician's immediate intervention. See Chapter 8 for information on responding to allergic reactions and other changes in a patient's condition that may occur as adverse effects of medications.

In addition to toxic effects, there are many occasions when drugs taken together have a **synergistic** (additive) effect that may go far beyond the desired outcome. For example, a patient who is taking a prescribed medication for high blood pressure and then takes an OTC diuretic may become hypotensive and feel weak and faint. Since many drugs interact when taken together, the physician who orders a new drug should have the patient's chart and should question the patient about taking OTC medications or drugs prescribed by other physicians.

FREQUENTLY USED MEDICATIONS

The medications listed in the text that follows are used regularly in many radiology and special imaging departments. These general descriptions illustrate how such medications are used but are not meant to be exclusive. The specific drugs used at your institution may be different while meeting the same needs. See Table 7-1 for a more extensive list of medications that you may encounter.

Medications Used to Treat Allergic Reactions

Diphenhydramine (Benadryl) is the most frequently used antihistamine. It also has sedative and anticholinergic (drying) side effects. It can be given orally before the injection of iodinated contrast media to patients who are at risk of having an allergic reaction. For adults, the usual oral dose is 25 to 50 mg, and for children weighing over 20 pounds, the dosage is 12.5 to 25 mg. Benadryl may also be given intramuscularly (IM) or intravenously (IV) if the patient has an allergic reaction. The dosage is 10 to 50 mg, IV or IM, and may be increased to 100 mg as necessary. The maximum safe dosage in a 24-hour period is 400 mg intramuscularly or intravenously. Cortisone is also prescribed for these purposes.

For patients with an acute allergic reaction, epinephrine (Adrenalin) is administered subcutaneously (SC), IM, or IV. To control angioedema, shock, or respiratory distress, the physician administers a small dose of Adrenalin (0.2 to 1 ml of 1:1000 solution) and increases the dosage if required.

When patients with a severe or incapacitating allergic response do not appear to respond to the treatment just described, methylprednisolone (Solu-Medrol) may be administered intravenously. This is a corticosteroid that acts as an antiinflammatory agent, preventing or reducing **edema** (swelling) of the tracheobronchial tree. This treatment minimizes the possibility of respiratory arrest. Solu-Medrol is provided in a two-compartment vial with the diluting fluid and soluble powder separated by a plunger/stopper. The directions for mixing are provided, but you should become familiar with the preparation of this and all common medications before the need arises.

Antimicrobials

This category includes disinfectants such as alcohol and Betadine, an iodine compound commonly used in radiology departments for skin preparations before sterile injection procedures.

The antimicrobial category also includes *antibiotics,* which are medications given to treat wound infections and infectious diseases. Antibiotics can be subclassified as antibacterial, antifungal, and so on, according to the type of organisms against which they are most effective. Some antibiotics treat a very narrow range of microorganisms. Bactrim, for instance, is used to treat specific infections of the urinary tract. Others are referred to as "broad-spectrum" antibiotics and are effective against a wide variety of pathogens.

The use of some medications has come full circle. As new medications like vancomycin came into use, many of the earlier antibiotics were no longer used. Since an increasing number of infectious organisms have become resistant to the modern antibiotics once used to treat them, some of the old reliable treatments, such as penicillin, have been revived.

Anticonvulsants

Anticonvulsant medications are prescribed for patients with chronic seizure disorders (see Chapter 8). Preventive doses taken regularly allow seizure-prone individuals to continue the activities of daily living. When seizures are prolonged or follow closely, intravenous administration of medications such as diazepam (Valium) or fosphenytoin (Cerebyx) may be necessary. Diazepam is available on the crash cart or in the emergency drug box. Physicians commonly order an initial dose of 5 to 10 mg of diazepam IV. The dose may be repeated at 10- to 15-minute intervals up to a total dose of 30 mg.

Antiarrhythmics

A wide variety of medications is used to treat chronic cardiac arrhythmias. For acute attacks of ventricular tachycardia or ventricular fibrillation, however, lidocaine is the drug of choice. It is available on the crash cart and is administered as an IV infusion in a solution of dextrose and water.

Analgesics

Analgesics are drugs that can relieve pain without causing loss of consciousness. As a group, opioids

TABLE 7-1

A CATEGORIZED TABLE OF SOME COMMON MEDICATIONS

CATEGORY	EFFECT	EXAMPLE	COMMON SIDE EFFECTS
Adrenergics (vasoconstrictors)	Stimulate the sympathetic nervous system, causing constriction of smooth muscle lining of the respiratory tract	Epinephrine (Adrenalin), ephedrine, isoproterenol (Isuprel), metaraminol bitartrate (Aramine), phenylephrine hydrochloride (Neo-Synephrine)	Dry mouth
Adrenergic blocking agents	Block the production of epinephrine in the body, causing dilation of blood vessels and decreased cardiac output; used as antihypertensive	Methyldopa (Aldomet), clonidine (Catapres), prazosin (Minipress)	Fatigue, light-headedness
Analgesics	Relieve pain	Acetaminophen (Tylenol) Aspirin Codeine, meperidine (Demerol), methadone, morphine, phenacetin	Negligible Anticoagulant Respiratory depression
Anesthetics	Promote loss of feeling or sensation	General: thiopental sodium (Pentothal), halothane (Fluothane), nitrous oxide Local: lidocaine (Xylocaine)	Nausea
Antiarrhythmics	Prevent or relieve cardiac arrhythmias (dysrhythmias)	Quinidine, verapamil, propanalol, lidocaine	Bradycardia, congestive heart failure
Anticholinergics	Depress the parasympathetic nervous system and act as antispasmodics of smooth muscle tissue; decrease contractions, saliva, bronchial mucus, digestive secretions, and perspiration; used as preparation for surgery and endoscopy to suppress secretions	Atropine, belladonna, propanthelone bromide (Pro-Banthine), scopolamine (hyoscine)	Dry mouth

TABLE 7-1

A CATEGORIZED TABLE OF SOME COMMON MEDICATIONS—cont'd

CATEGORY	EFFECT	EXAMPLE	COMMON SIDE EFFECTS
Anticoagulants	Inhibit the clotting mechanism of the blood; used to keep intravenous (IV) lines and arterial catheters open during diagnostic procedures	Heparin, warfarin (Coumadin)	Bruising, spontaneous bleeding
Anticonvulsants	Inhibit convulsions	Phenytoin (Dilantin)	Rash, slurred speech
		Carbamazepine (Tegretol)	Rash, itch, sun sensitivity
		Lorazepam (Ativan)	Sedation, dizziness, weakness, unsteadiness
Antidepressants	Relieve or prevent depression	Amitriptyline (Elavil), imipramine (Tofranil)	Drowsiness, dizziness, weight gain
		Fluoxetine (Prozac)	Nervousness, diarrhea
Antiemetics	Relieve or prevent vomiting	Trimethobenzamide hydrochloride (Tigan), prochlorperazine (Compazine)	Drowsiness, dry mouth, blurred vision
Antifungals	Treat or prevent fungal infections	Systematic: griseofulvin Topical: Tinactin	Negligible
Antihistamines	Relieve the symptoms of allergic reactions	Diphenhydramine (Benadryl), chlorpheniramine maleate (Chlor-Trimeton)	Drowsiness
Antimicrobials	Suppress the growth of microorganisms	Internal: Penicillin, tetracyclines, sulfadiazine, erythromycin, cephalosporins (Keflex, Keflin)	Diarrhea, yeast infections
		External: Sulfonamides, thimersol (Merthiolate), Betadine	Allergic reactions
Antiperistaltics	Slow peristalsis of the gastrointestinal tract	Tincture of opium (Paregoric), loperamide (Imodium)	Constipation
Antipsychotics	Treat psychoses, schizophrenia	Haloperidol (Haldol)	Nausea, decreased sweating, dry mouth, stiffness
		Fluphenazine (Prolixin)	Constipation, shaking

Continued

TABLE 7-1

A CATEGORIZED TABLE OF SOME COMMON MEDICATIONS—cont'd

CATEGORY	EFFECT	EXAMPLE	COMMON SIDE EFFECTS
Antipyretics	Reduce fever	Aspirin	Bruising
		Acetaminophen (Tylenol)	Negligible
Antitussives	Reduce coughing	Dextromethorphan (Romilar)	Negligible
		Codeine	Nausea
Antivirals	Prevent or treat viral diseases	Acyclovir (Zovirax), amantadine, zidovudine (AZT)	Nausea, vomiting, diarrhea, and headache.
Barbiturates	Depress the central nervous system, respirations, and blood pressure; induce sleep	Pentobarbital sodium (Nembutal), secobarbital (Seconal), phenobarbital	Nausea, itching, constipation
Bronchodilators	Dilate smooth muscle; used to treat asthmatic attacks and some allergic reactions	Theophylline (Theo-Dur), aminophylline	Insomnia, decreased appetite, irritability
		Albuterol (Ventolin)	Hypertension, angina, vomiting, vertigo
Cardiac depressants	Restrain or slow heart activity	Quinidine, procainamide (Pronestyl)	Nausea, diarrhea, heartburn
Cardiac stimulants	Strengthen and tone the heart; increase cardiac output	Digitalis, gitalin (Gitaligin), lanatoside C (Cedilanid)	Weakness, blurred vision
Cathartics	Stimulate peristalsis; promote defecation	Bisacodyl (Dulcolax), castor oil, magnesium citrate	Dehydration, weight loss, abdominal cramping
Diuretics	Stimulate the flow of urine	Chlorothiazide (Diuril), furosemide (Lasix), acetazolamide (Diamox)	Potassium depletion, diarrhea, cramps, fatigue, metallic taste
Emetics	Induce vomiting	Ipecac	Potential dehydration
Hypoglycemics	Lower blood sugar level	Insulin	Cold sweat, anxiety, headache, confusion
		Chlorpropamide (Diabinese), tolbutamide (Orinase)	
		Metformin (Glucophage)	Risk of severe acidosis in cases of kidney failure. Contraindicated with iodine contrast media until normal kidney function has been validated

TABLE 7-1

A CATEGORIZED TABLE OF SOME COMMON MEDICATIONS—cont'd

CATEGORY	EFFECT	EXAMPLE	COMMON SIDE EFFECTS
Opioids (narcotics)	Analgesic sedatives with a potential for addiction; classified as controlled substances under the Harrison Act	Morphine, meperidine (Demerol), codeine	Respiratory depression
Opioid antagonists	Prevent or counteract respiratory depression and depressive effects of morphine and related drugs	Naloxone hydrochloride (Narcan), nalorphine (Nalline), naltrexone (Trexan)	Nausea, vomiting, tachycardia, hypertension
Radioactive isotopes	Radioactive forms of elements used for diagnosis and treatment	Iodine-131, cobalt-60	
Sedatives	Depress and relax the central nervous system and reduce mental activity	Barbiturates, paraldehyde, chloral hydrate	Clumsiness, dizziness, drowsiness
Skeletal muscle relaxants	Relax skeletal and striated muscle tissue	Succinylcholine (Anectine)	Respiratory depression
Stimulants	Stimulate the central nervous system	Caffeine, sodium benzoate, amphetamines (Benzedrine, Dexedrine)	Insomnia, restlessness
Tranquilizers	Reduce anxiety	Minor: diazepam (Valium), chlordiazepoxide (Librium) Major: chlorpromazine (Thorazine), trifluoperazine (Stelazine)	Drowsiness, decreased coordination, slurred speech
Vasodilators	Relax the walls of blood vessels, permitting a greater flow of blood	Isosorbide dinitrate (Sorbitrate), Nitroglycerin Hydralazine (Apresoline)	Dizziness, headache, flushing, tachycardia Headache, hypotension Headache, anorexia, vomiting, diarrhea, palpitations

are the most effective analgesics. The term opioid describes any drug, natural or synthetic, whose actions are similar to those of morphine. The *opioid* family, whose name derives from opium, includes morphine, codeine, and meperidine (Demerol); *opiate* is the more specific term applied only to natural opium derivatives. The term *narcotic* means "sleep-inducing" and was once used as a synonym for analgesic, but this word can no longer be used with precision because it has come to stand for too many different things. It denotes not only those analgesic CNS depressants that may lead to physical dependence, but also to cocaine, marijuana, and LSD, which are legally classed with opiates as narcotics.

Controlled substances are drugs with a high potential for abuse and misuse and therefore are kept in a locked container. Stocks of these medications must be counted daily, and when any medication is given it must be listed on forms that include the date, the patient's name, the dose, and the name and title of the person administering the medication. Use of these drugs is monitored by the U.S. Drug Enforcement Administration (DEA) and can be prescribed only by individuals who hold a DEA license.

Opioids act by depressing the central nervous system, relieving pain, and producing drowsiness. Excessive doses can result in depressed respirations, coma, and possible death. Among the most frequently prescribed are morphine sulfate (MS) and meperidine (Demerol). These injectable medications are given in a dosage of 10 to 30 mg of morphine or 50 to 100 mg of Demerol. Fentanyl (Sublimaze), another highly **potent** (powerful) opioid analgesic, is given to patients who are sensitive to other analgesics or to those who are not responding to such medications with adequate pain relief. The physician determines the dosage of this medication based on age, weight, use of other drugs, and the procedure involved. The action of Sublimaze is almost immediate and lasts 30 to 60 minutes after intravenous administration. It is supplied at a strength of 50 micrograms per milliliter (mcg/ml), and the usual dose is 1 to 2 ml. Respiratory depression peaks 5 to 10 minutes after injection and may last for several hours, depending on the dosage.

Patients who have received any CNS depressant must be monitored closely. Respiratory depression is a life-threatening side effect, so narcotic antagonist medication and resuscitation equipment should be immediately available. Since patients may be some distance from the radiographer, a pulse oximeter is attached to the patient's finger, toe, or earlobe. A digital readout of the pulse and blood oxygen saturation can be viewed from the control room or console area. If the oxygen saturation drops below 95%, the patient is asked to respond and take a few deep breaths and is then observed closely. If the oxygen saturation continues to drop or the patient does not respond adequately, a physician is notified immediately.

Analgesics may be given to help the patient cope with painful procedures or to lessen a pre-existing pain during the procedure. While the pain might be the reason for the examination, it might also be caused by an unrelated problem that produces enough discomfort to prevent compliance. For example, a patient may have painful arthritis of the cervical spine that makes it extremely difficult to lie still throughout an MRI of the abdomen.

Analgesics with a low potential for side effects (aspirin, ibuprofen, acetaminophen, and naproxen sodium) are frequently used to alleviate discomfort. Although these drugs are analgesics, they are not controlled substances. Self-medication with OTC analgesics is very common, especially in the elderly. Children should never be given OTC medications in the radiology department without a physician's order. As a general rule, even at home, children should be given analgesics other than acetaminophen (Tylenol) only under the direct instruction of a physician.

Sedatives and Tranquilizers

Sedatives or tranquilizers exert a quieting effect, often inducing sleep. They are not analgesics but may provide relief from pain by promoting muscle relaxation. Tranquilizers reduce anxiety and mental tension more effectively than sedatives and often provide some sedation as well. At low doses tranquilizers do not impair mental acuity, but as the dosage increases, patients tend to feel drowsy and their speech may become slow and slurred. Some patients experience a brief loss of inhibition, similar to the effect of alcohol, which causes them to talk and act inappropriately. Individuals taking tranquilizers may have slowed reaction time and should not drive or operate machinery. Diazepam (Valium) is a tranquilizer commonly prescribed as premedication for various interventional diagnostic procedures.

Phenobarbital and other barbiturates are sedatives and were formerly used as preoperative medications. Their use for this purpose has been largely supplanted by diazepam. Phenobarbital is still used with other medications to treat patients with seizures.

Both diazepam and midazolam (Versed) have a tranquilizing effect and may be given with morphine to anxious and uncomfortable patients. The premedication dosage of Valium for anxiety ranges from 2 to 20 mg given IM or IV. The physician may administer larger doses as needed to achieve relaxation. Very large doses are sometimes given to control grand mal seizures. When Valium is injected IV, it is administered slowly, taking at least 1 minute for each 5 mg (1 ml) given. Avoid using small veins of the hand and wrist, since Valium irritates blood vessels and may cause phlebitis and damage to the vein. When Valium extravasates (infiltrates into surrounding tissues), it can be very painful, causing irritation and swelling.

Versed is sometimes given when a previous administration of an analgesic or Valium has not relaxed the patient or relieved pain. The initial dose of Versed in this instance is 1 mg and can be increased to a usual maximum of 10 mg at the physician's discretion.

Antagonists

The most common antagonists encountered by radiographers are those formulated to counteract the effects of sedatives and analgesics.

Valium and Versed are benzodiazepine drugs that may be given to produce relaxation and/or sedation, as previously described. An overdose produces respiratory depression and loss of psychomotor function as a toxic effect. Flumazenil (Romazicon) is a medication developed to counteract the effect of these drugs. Romazicon can antagonize the sedation and the impairment of recall and psychomotor

function produced by benzodiazepines. Patients who receive Romazicon should be monitored for resedation, respiratory depression, or other residual effects for up to 2 hours based on the dosage and duration of the benzodiazepine used. For the reversal of conscious sedation by benzodiazepines, the recommended initial dose of Romazicon is 0.2 mg (2 ml) administered IV over 15 seconds. If the desired level of consciousness is not obtained after waiting an additional 45 seconds, additional doses may be given to a maximum of 1 mg (10 ml) until the desired effect is achieved. To minimize the possibility of pain or inflammation, Romazicon should be administered through a freely flowing IV line into a large vein. The use of Romazicon is associated with seizures in some patients who have been taking benzodiazepines over a long period of time.

Naloxone (Narcan) counteracts the effects of opiates such as morphine and prevents or reverses respiratory depression, sedation, and hypotension. A rapid reversal of opiate depression can cause nausea, vomiting, tachycardia, and nervousness. Although Narcan can be administered SC or IM, the most rapid onset of action is obtained with a dilution of Narcan in saline or 5% dextrose in water administered intravenously. To reverse respiratory depression, 0.1 to 0.2 mg Narcan should be administered IV at 2- to 3-minute intervals until adequate ventilation is achieved.

Local Anesthetics

Lidocaine (Xylocaine) is a local anesthetic injected to eliminate sensation in a specific area before a painful procedure. You may have received such an injection before having dental work or when having stitches placed to close a wound. Xylocaine is provided in a variety of strengths and is available with or without epinephrine. The addition of epinephrine causes constriction of adjacent blood vessels and localizes the anesthetic effect to the immediate area. If your department stocks more than one type, be sure you understand which one the physician requires.

Succinylcholine Chloride

When working in a trauma unit or emergency department, the radiographer may occasionally come in contact with patients who have received succinylcholine chloride (Anectine), a skeletal muscle relaxant that may be given to facilitate insertion of an endotracheal airway or to initiate diagnostic studies and treatment for patients who are combative because of shock, fear, or intoxication. Since all muscles are temporarily paralyzed, artificial respiration is necessary, and patients are monitored closely until the effects of the medication wear off. Succinylcholine does not cause the patient to become unconscious, and since the period of paralysis is very short, these patients are frequently agitated or combative as the paralysis dissipates.

General Precautions

Some of the drugs discussed in the previous sections can cause respiratory depression, and any of them could cause an allergic reaction in a sensitive individual. Know where the resuscitation equipment and oxygen are kept, and be familiar with the code routine of your institution (see Chapter 8).

This discussion has touched on some of the medications frequently used by radiographers. You must become thoroughly familiar with the protocols of your institution. Your card file with the package inserts serves as a handy resource to help you stay current in your knowledge of the dosage, actions, and side effects of these drugs.

MEDICATION ADMINISTRATION

The information in this section provides a basis for assisting the physician in medication administration, but it is not a substitute for directions from the physician. In preparation for medication administration, the first step is to check the order. If you have questions about dosage or method of administration, check with the physician or your supervisor. Second, verify the medication and check the expiration date. Third, check for allergies in the chart or obtain an allergy history from the patient. Last but not least, remember to perform hand hygiene before preparing the medication. When preparing medications, the memory device shown in Box 7-1 will help you to avoid errors.

BOX 7-1

SIX RIGHTS OF MEDICATION ADMINISTRATION

The right dose
Of the right medication
To the right patient
At the right time
By the right route
With the right documentation

Dosage

The usual dose or dosage range for each medication is included in the information on the package insert and is also available in the PDR and *Mosby's GenRx.* Physicians are not required to prescribe the usual dose and may specify a different dose for very good reasons, but when an order specifies a much higher dose than usual, be sure to verify the accuracy of the order before proceeding.

Some textbooks provide formulas for calculating pediatric drug dosage based on the child's age and the usual adult dose. No formula is provided here because of the risk of serious error. Some drugs are not approved for pediatric use. Others require a higher or lower dose than such formulas would indicate. When a medication or contrast medium is approved for pediatric use, the recommended pediatric dose according to the child's age and/or weight will be stated in the package insert and in medication references.

The metric system, with which you are already familiar, is usually used for measuring patient weight when calculating dosage and is also used for measuring medications. To convert a patient's weight from pounds to the kilogram (kg) units used in the metric system, divide the weight in pounds by 2.2, the number of pounds in a kilogram.

$$\text{Pounds (lb)} \div 2.2 = \text{Kilograms (kg)}$$

Example: What is the metric weight of a child weighing 46 lb.?

$$46 \text{ lb} \div 2.2 \text{ lb/kg} = 20.91 \text{ kg}$$

Liquid medications are measured in units from liters (L, slightly more than a quart) down to milliliters (ml), which are thousandths of a liter. One milliliter is equal to 1 cubic centimeter (cc), and 1 ounce equals 30 ml.

Since liquid agents are often diluted for use, the strength is expressed as a ratio of the amount of the drug to the total volume of solution. For example, 1:1000 indicates a dilution of 1 part drug to 1000 parts of water or other solvent.

If the active ingredient is a solid, it is measured by weight in grams (g), milligrams (mg), or micrograms (mcg or μg). The strength of solids dissolved in a liquid is designated in terms of weight per volume, often mg/ml. You will often need to determine how much liquid will provide a given dose of a solid:

$$Dose/strength = Volume$$

Example: If the drug is supplied in a strength of 4 mg/ml, and you want to administer 10 mg, you will need 2.5 ml:

$$\frac{10\,mg}{4\,mg/ml} = 2.5\,ml$$

Conversely, you may need to know how much of a solid is delivered in a given volume of liquid:

$$Strength \times Volume = Dose$$

Example: If 2 ml of solution is given and the strength is 4 mg/ml, the dose would be 8 mg:

$$4\,mg/ml \times 2\,ml = 8\,mg$$

Practice these calculations so that you can do them quickly and flawlessly whenever you are required to prepare a parenteral medication.

Routes of Administration
Enteral route—oral, sublingual, rectal, and nasogastric tube

The enteral route applies to sublingual, rectal, and oral sites of drug application and to medications administered via nasogastric tube. Drugs placed under the tongue (**sublingual**) or inside the cheek (**buccal**) can be absorbed into the blood through the oral mucosa and are immediately available without having to be digested and absorbed through the stomach or bowel. When coronary arteries are unable to supply the heart muscle with sufficient nutrients and oxygen, a crushing pain called **angina pectoris** results. If nitroglycerin is administered sublingually, it is absorbed directly into the bloodstream, dilating the coronary arteries. This helps relieve the pain by improving circulation to the heart muscle. Patients with angina should have their medication with them at all times, including during x-ray procedures. An emergency supply of nitroglycerin is usually stocked in the radiology department.

When a patient is severely nauseated or unable to swallow, medications can be administered by rectum. Various forms of suppositories and enemas are available for this purpose. The rectal administration of suppositories and enemas is discussed in Chapter 9. While medication can be absorbed directly through the rectal mucosa, portions may be expelled prematurely, making dosage unreliable. An effective alternative for these patients is to administer medications and liquid nutrition through a nasogastric tube. The use of a nasogastric tube is effective, and the dosage is easily controlled. Nasogastric tubes are discussed in Chapter 11.

The oral route of medication administration is the easiest and most familiar. When medication is taken orally, it must dissolve in the stomach and then pass into the small intestine, where the majority of the absorption takes place. Some oral medications are irritating to the stomach and are provided in an enteric or coated form that allows the tablet to pass through the stomach before dissolving. These medications should not be chewed or broken, since this would negate the benefit of the enteric coating. Oral medications are supplied in a variety of other forms, including tablets, capsules, granules, and liquids. Some tablets are chewable, but almost all medication should be swallowed with varying amounts of liquid, usually water. Liquid medications are usually taken with water as well. Granules are mixed with a specified amount of liquid. Follow the directions on the package insert.

One way to minimize errors when administering drugs is to establish a set routine and follow it unfailingly. The steps in Box 7-2 serve as a guide to establishing a procedure for the administration of oral medications.

PROCEDURE FOR ORAL MEDICATION ADMINISTRATION

- Perform hand hygiene.
- Obtain the proper medication, and read the label.
- Prepare the medication tray with a medicine cup and a glass of water (if appropriate). Read the label again.
- Show the physician the label, and pour the correct amount of medication directly into the medicine cup. When pouring liquids, hold the label against the palm of your hand so that it will stay clean and legible.
- If the physician requests that you administer the medication, check the patient's identification, stay with the patient while the medication is swallowed, and offer water if permitted.
- Return the tray, and discard the remaining water and medicine cup.
- Repeat hand hygiene.
- Chart the medication.

Medication inhalation

Some lung conditions are treated with inhalation therapy. Liquid medications are vaporized and administered by an inhaler or nebulizer and inhaled by the patient. For example, albuterol is administered with a metered dose inhaler for asthma control. Respiratory therapists apply these treatments and also instruct patients in proper techniques for self-administration of these medications at home. The inhalation route is also used for the administration of radioactive gases for nuclear medicine lung perfusion studies.

Topical route

The **topical** route of administration refers to the application of medication to the surface of the skin. Some topical medications are applied for a local effect, such as when calamine lotion is used to relieve the itch of poison ivy. Other topical medications are used for a systemic effect, and this type of administration is also termed *transdermal*. These medications are applied to the skin in a paste form or on small adhesive disks and are absorbed through the skin into the bloodstream. One such topical drug, nifedipine, is used by patients with heart conditions to increase vascular dilation. Other examples include the transdermal nicotine patches used to treat symptoms of nicotine withdrawal when quitting smoking and adhesive scopolamine disks to treat vertigo and to prevent motion sickness.

Parenteral injections

Although patients may prefer to take medications orally, some drugs cause irritation of the gastrointestinal tract, cannot be absorbed by this route, or must be given by a route that will produce a very rapid response. By using the **parenteral** route, medications can be injected directly into the body. Parenteral injections may be given in several ways and are classified as intradermal, subcutaneous, intravenous, or intramuscular, according to the injection method used (Fig. 7-1).

Parenteral equipment. The equipment needed for each type of parenteral injection is summarized in Table 7-2. Hypodermic needles are supplied in various diameters and lengths. The gauge of a needle indicates its diameter, and the gauge increases as the diameter of the bore decreases. An 18-gauge needle is larger around than a 22-gauge needle and delivers a given volume of fluid more rapidly. A 22-gauge needle can be used for much smaller veins since it makes a smaller hole and excessive bleeding or **hematoma** (collection of blood in tissues) is less likely when it is removed. The length of hypodermic needles is measured in inches and may vary from $1/2$ inch, used for accessing IV line ports and for intradermal injections, to $4^{1}/_{2}$ inches, needed for intrathecal (spinal canal) injections. A $2^{1}/_{2}$-inch length is typical for IV needles, and the usual gauge ranges from 18 to 22 for adults.

As stated in Chapter 5, the widespread incidence of bloodborne infection has placed increasing emphasis on the prevention of accidental needlesticks. New Occupational Safety and Health Administration (OSHA) regulations require the use of

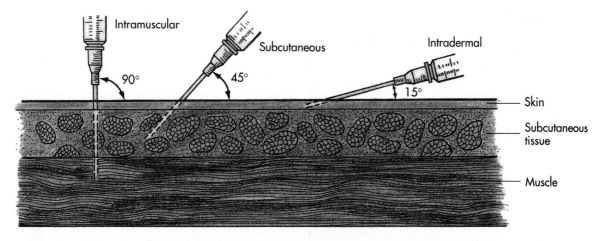

FIG. 7-1 Methods of parenteral injection.

engineering controls to decrease the risk to health care workers from contaminated needlesticks and have led to the development of new devices. These engineering controls include two types of devices: needleless systems for accessing established IV lines and sharps with a built-in safety feature or mechanism that effectively reduces the risk of an exposure incident. These new sharps are called Sharps With Engineered Sharps Injury Protection, or SESIPs for short. Examples of SESIPs and other equipment for parenteral injection are illustrated in Fig. 7-2.

Injectors have also been designed that can deliver a measured amount of medication through the skin by the use of a high-pressure jet. These injectors are said to be less painful, protect against accidental needlesticks, and have the advantage of being reusable for up to a week without resterilization. Jet injectors are considerably larger than disposable syringes and are currently much more expensive to use. They are most practical for diabetics who require frequent administration of insulin and for use in mass immunization programs.

Disposable plastic syringes are supplied in individual sterile paper wraps, sometimes with a needle attached. Syringes are composed of a barrel with a measurement scale on the outside and a plunger

TABLE 7-2

EQUIPMENT FOR PARENTERAL INJECTIONS

	INTRADERMAL	SUBCUTANEOUS	INTRAMUSCULAR	INTRAVENOUS
Dose volume	<1 ml	<2 ml	<5 ml	<1 liter
Needle type	SESIP hypodermic	SESIP hypodermic	SESIP hypodermic	SESIP butterfly needle or IV catheter
Needle length	5/8 inch	5/8 inch	1 inch	1 1/2 inch
Needle gauge	26 ga	23-25 ga	22 ga	18-20 ga

SESIP, Sharps With Engineered Sharps Injury Protection; *IV,* intravenous; *ga,* gauge.

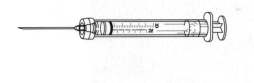

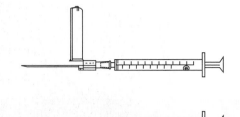

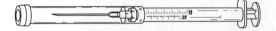

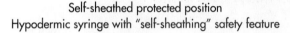

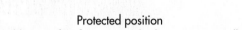

Self-sheathed protected position
Hypodermic syringe with "self-sheathing" safety feature

Protected position
"Add-on" safety feature attached to syringe needle

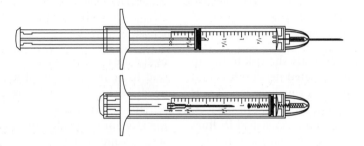

Retracted protected position
Hypodermic syringe with "Retractable technology" safety feature

FIG. 7-2 Examples of new Sharps with Engineered Sharps Injury Protection (SESIPs).

to force the contents through the needle. The plunger tip is usually made of latex.

In recent years an increasing number of individuals have become sensitized to latex. This has caused a return to the use of glass syringes for such patients. Glass syringes (Fig. 7-3) are not disposable and are sterilized before each use. Since the plunger is ground to fit the barrel precisely, both barrel and plunger may be marked with code numbers that must match in order for the syringe to work. When you open the wrap, you will need to assemble the two parts. To avoid contaminating the syringe, pick up the plunger by the handle only and insert it into the barrel. Needles are supplied separately.

After selecting a needle suitable for the administration, twist the hub of the needle firmly onto the syringe and fill the syringe in the same manner as the disposable syringe. After use, discard the needle into the sharps container. The barrel and plunger must be separated and placed in a container with disinfectant until they can be sterilized.

Parenteral routes. Intravenous administration is the parenteral route that offers the most immediate results in terms of effect. As the medication is dispersed through the bloodstream, the latent time until it reaches the site of action is very short. This extremely important route is covered in detail later in this chapter.

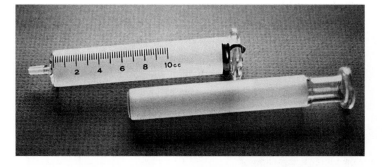

FIG. 7-3 Glass syringe.

Intradermal injections (between the layers of the skin) were formerly given to test patient sensitivity to contrast media. Experience has proved that a complete history is a more accurate predictor of allergic reactions than the intradermal "skin test," and most radiographers are not likely to perform this procedure. The anterior surface of the forearm is a typical site for intradermal injections. Only very small quantities may be injected intradermally, so a tuberculin syringe is used; it is finely calibrated and comes with a very small (26-gauge) needle. The tuberculin skin test introduced in Chapter 5 involves an intradermal injection to the anterior forearm.

Subcutaneous (under the skin) medications are injected at a 45-degree angle using a ⅝-inch needle with a size 23 to 25 gauge. Syringes used for subcutaneous injections are usually 2 ml or smaller in size, since it is painful to inject a large quantity beneath the skin. The most convenient areas for subcutaneous injections are on the upper arm and on the outer aspect of the thigh.

Intramuscular (into the muscle) injections are sometimes given in larger amounts. The syringe may be larger than that for subcutaneous injection (up to 5 ml), and the needle size is also larger, usually 22 gauge. The injection is given into the deltoid muscle of the upper arm (Fig. 7-4), the gluteal muscles in the hip area (Fig. 7-5), or the vastus lateralis muscle of the lateral thigh (Fig. 7-6). For children under 5 years of age, the vastus lateralis site is preferred to the gluteus site. Since the gluteus maximus muscle only develops fully through walking and running, a danger of damage to the sciatic nerve

exists when injections are given into this area before the muscle is sufficiently developed. Injections are not usually given into the anterior thigh because this site is extremely painful and the discomfort may persist for several days.

Intra-arterial administration involves percutaneous access to the artery by a needle, frequently followed by catheter placement to permit injection at a specific anatomical site. Intra-arterial injections are performed by physicians, and radiographers are most likely to encounter this route of administration in the angiography suite. This procedure is performed under conditions of surgical asepsis and is described more fully in Chapter 12.

The intrathecal or intraspinal method of administration is used when a contrast medium is to be injected through a spinal needle directly into the subarachnoid space. Myelography is the most common imaging procedure that requires the intrathecal method. The procedure is called a lumbar puncture and is performed by a physician using surgical asepsis. This procedure is described more fully in Chapter 10.

Preparation for parenteral administration. To prepare for parenteral injections, specifically intradermal, subcutaneous, and intramuscular injections, the radiographer assembles the proper syringe and needle and an alcohol wipe for cleansing the skin. Next, the medication is obtained and the label is read carefully. The medication label states the name of the medication and its strength and also gives an expiration date past which the drug should not be used. Be sure to keep the container until the medication is charted. When medications are not used frequently

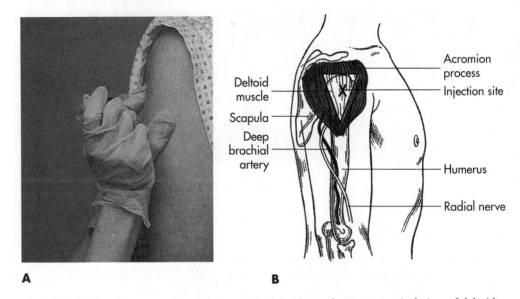

FIG. 7-4 **A,** Site of intramuscular injection into deltoid muscle. **B,** Anatomical view of deltoid muscle injection site.

(as in an emergency kit or on a crash cart), they should be checked often. Out-of-date supplies should be discarded and replaced. *Never borrow medication or equipment from the crash cart!* If supplies have been used for an emergency, they should be replaced as soon as possible.

A common rule of thumb is to read the label three times before administration: when selecting the container, while preparing the dose, and again just before injection. *This is essential to be absolutely certain that you have the correct drug and the proper strength and that the expiration date has not been exceeded.* Draw up the medication into the syringe from the ampule or vial, or select the appropriate prefilled syringe unit. Follow the procedure outlined in Box 7-3.

Ampules are glass containers with narrow necks that are opened by breaking the glass. Although ampules are now used infrequently, you may encounter them in the radiology department as part of a sterile tray. When a drug is supplied in ampule form, a filtration needle is used to fill the syringe from the ampule to prevent the possibility of drawing up minute particles of glass. A small file is used to

nick the neck of the ampule. The top then snaps off easily. Use a small gauze sponge to protect your fingers when opening the ampule, since the glass may break unevenly and cut your hand (Fig. 7-7). Next, securely attach the needle to the syringe and remove the needle cover, taking care not to contaminate the needle. Place the needle tip in the ampule below the solution level and withdraw the required amount of the medication into the syringe. Hold the syringe to the light to check for air bubbles. If bubbles appear, hold the syringe with the needle pointing up, and tap the side of the syringe. As the bubbles rise, they can be ejected with gentle pressure on the plunger. The removal of air is essential to accurate dosage measurement and may also affect patient safety. Now, read the label again. The ampule is retained until after the drug has been administered and charted. Before the drug is administered, replace the filtration needle with an injection needle and show the physician the ampule and the syringe while stating aloud what has been done. After administration, the medication is charted and the ampule, together with any remaining medication, is discarded. Perform hand hygiene.

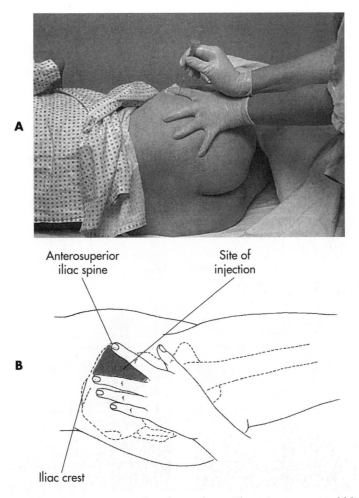

Anterosuperior
iliac spine

Site of
injection

A

B

Iliac crest

FIG. 7-5 **A,** Injection site into ventrogluteal muscle avoids major nerves and blood vessels. **B,** Anatomical view of ventrogluteal muscle injection site.

If the medication is supplied in a vial, there are several variations in the preparation procedure. First, pull off the vial's protective cap, exposing the rubber stopper and taking care not to contaminate it. *Do not remove the outer retaining ring.* This ring is essential to prevent the rubber stopper from being forcibly ejected when drawing up the medication. Since this is a closed system, you must inject a volume of air equal to the amount of fluid you wish to remove. Remove the needle cover, and pull down the plunger of the syringe to the desired reading.

Insert the needle or needleless cannula through the stopper, and inject the air into the bottle. Invert the bottle, and make sure the needle tip or cannula is below the fluid level. Then, pull down the plunger to the desired reading and check for bubbles. If there are any, dislodge them, inject them into the vial, and withdraw the plunger again until the dosage is correct. Then, remove the needle or disconnect the syringe from the cannula, replace the needle cover, and proceed as previously described (Fig. 7-8).

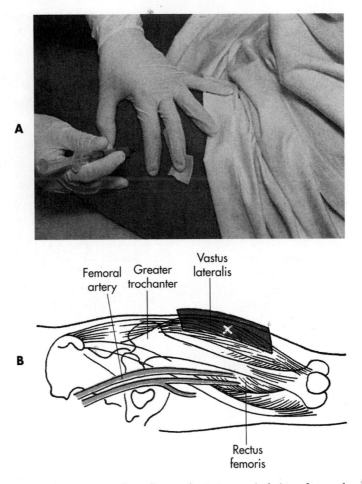

FIG. 7-6 **A,** Injection site into vastus lateralis muscle. **B,** Anatomical view of vastus lateralis muscle injection site.

The vial was originally designed as a multiple-dose container, but the frequency of contamination is so great that multiple use is now restricted to use for the same patient on the same day. Vials of local anesthetic are sometimes used repeatedly for the same patient during a radiographic procedure. When using a vial after the first time, clean the stopper with an alcohol wipe. (Alcohol is not needed for the first injection because the stopper is sterile when the vial is opened.) When the procedure is completed, discard the vial and any remaining medication. Some vials are not meant for multiple use and are so marked. For medications dispensed in relatively small quantities (10 ml or less), vials have largely been replaced by preloaded syringes that are discarded after use.

Intravenous Route

IV fluids and medications are administered to meet specific needs. Patients respond rapidly to medication administration via this route. The IV injection is used for delivering most emergency medications when an immediate response is critical.

Dehydrated patients may need fluid and electrolyte replacement. The most common replacement fluids are normal saline or a 5% solution of dextrose in

PARENTERAL INJECTION PROCEDURE

- Explain to the patient what you are about to do.
- Select the appropriate site.
- Don clean gloves.
- Cleanse the selected area with the alcohol pledget.
- Hold the skin taut with your nondominant hand.
- Insert the needle at the correct angle, and pull back slightly on the plunger.
- If no blood is present, inject the medication.
- Withdraw the needle quickly, and wipe the injection site.
- See to the patient's comfort.
- Remove your gloves, and perform hand hygiene.
- Chart the medication.
- Discard the container, and any remaining medication.

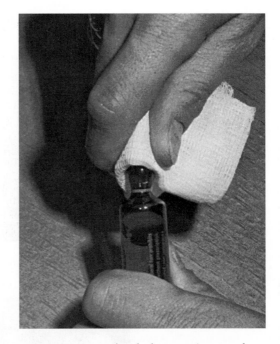

FIG. 7-7 Protect hand when opening ampule.

water (D5W). These solutions are usually stocked in radiology departments. If you are starting or replacing IV fluids, be certain that the solution is correct. Less common solutions, or those containing medication, may need to be replaced by the nursing service. The IV route may be used to administer medications, parenteral nutrition, or chemotherapy. This is also the route used to inject contrast media for radiographic examinations of the urinary tract and for some computed tomography (CT) studies, and to provide sedation during invasive procedures and MRI examinations. (See Chapter 10 for discussion of contrast radiography, Chapter 11 for a discussion of central venous catheters and arterial lines, and Chapter 12 for CT and MRI procedures that may involve injections.)

Venipuncture may be accomplished with a hypodermic needle, a butterfly set, or an IV catheter (Angiocath). The use of hypodermic needles is generally restricted to phlebotomy for obtaining laboratory samples and for single, small injections. A butterfly set is preferable to a conventional hypodermic needle for most IV injections and is often used for direct injections with a syringe. This apparatus consists of a needle with plastic projections that

may be taped to the patient's skin after the needle is in place (Fig. 7-9). This prevents movement of the needle in the vein. Attached to the needle is a short length of tubing with a hub that attaches to a syringe. The syringe is filled from a vial or ampule and is then attached to the tubing. Before the butterfly needle is inserted into the vein, the tubing is filled with liquid from the syringe to avoid injecting air into the vein.

IV catheters are frequently used instead of butterfly sets when repeated or continuous IV injections or infusions will be administered. The IV catheter is a two-part system consisting of a needle that fits inside a flexible plastic catheter. The catheter hub may have wing-shaped plastic projections similar to the butterfly set to aid in holding the needle during venipuncture. The needle portion is solid rather than hollow and serves as a stylet to prevent blood flow through the catheter. This combination unit is inserted into the vein, and the catheter is advanced by slipping it forward over the needle. The catheter is then secured with tape, the needle is withdrawn, and

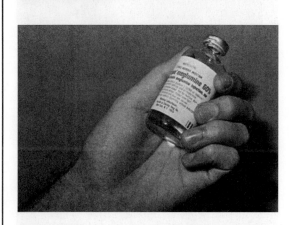

A Check label for drug name, correct strength, and expiration date.

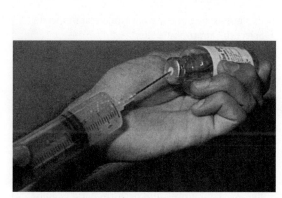

B Pull back on plunger to desired dose reading. Inject air into air space in vial.

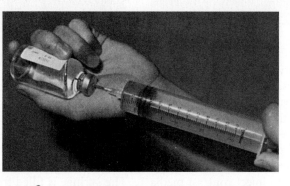

C Tip vial downward to withdraw solution.

the catheter is connected to the supply system. IV fluid, medication, or a contrast medium can then be administered by syringe through an injection port on IV tubing from a hanging bottle or bag.

An intermittent injection port (sometimes called a saline lock) is a small adapter with a diaphragm that is attached to an IV catheter when more than one injection is anticipated.

One of the engineering controls mentioned previously to minimize hazards posed by needlesticks is the use of "needleless" systems such as the Baxter InterLink IV Access System (Fig. 7-10). These systems facilitate blood draws and IV medication administration without the use of needles once an injection port or IV line has been established. An important feature of the system is a self-healing rubber substance used for medication vial caps, intermittent injection ports, and access ports on IV tubing. These caps and ports can be repeatedly penetrated by blunt plastic cannulas without damaging their integrity. The blunt cannulas are used to draw up medications and to access established IV lines for blood draws and medication administration. The use of a needleless system greatly reduces needle use and its attendant hazards in the health care setting.

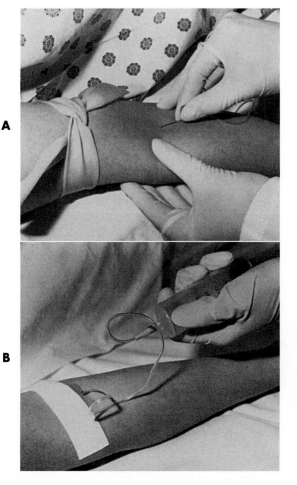

FIG. 7-9 Butterfly set facilitates direct IV injection. **A,** Needle projections provide grip for venipuncture. **B,** Tubing provides needle stability during injection.

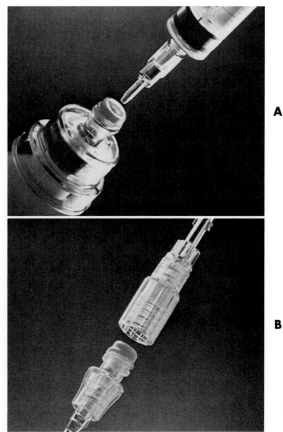

FIG. 7-10 Example of needleless IV access system. **A,** Needle-free safety is facilitated with Baxter InterLink System Vial Adapter, shown here fitted to top of multiple-dose vial. The special adapter, which fits any standard 20-mm neck vial, equips it to accept blunt InterLink Cannula. **B,** When added security is desired, InterLink Threaded Luer Lok Cannula securely connects to Inter-Link Injection Site without taping. This Luer locking feature provides a secure, sterile, and leak-free connection between IV devices that minimizes contamination through touch.

When a procedure requires the IV infusion of a large volume of fluid, an IV pole and infusion set are needed. Setting up fluid administration equipment is not complicated but is another skill that improves with practice. IV solutions are provided in bottles and plastic bags (Fig. 7-11). The bags have a cap over the sterile port through which the drip chamber of the IV tubing is inserted. The drip chamber is removed from its wrappings and inserted into the sterile port. Care must be taken not to contaminate either component.

Solutions supplied in bottles have a removable cap and sometimes a rubber diaphragm covering a rubber stopper. The cap is removed, and the diaphragm is pulled off without touching the stopper. The drip chamber is then inserted through the stopper, taking care that the clamp on the IV tubing

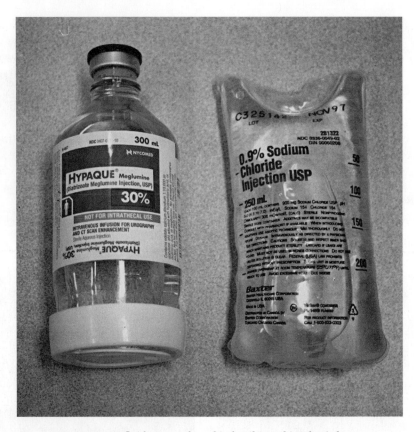

FIG. 7-11 IV fluids are packaged in bottles and in plastic bags.

is closed. Now the bottle or bag may be inverted and hung on the IV pole. When it is in place, the cover at the other end of the IV tubing is removed, the clamp is opened, and the fluid is allowed to run into a basin until the tubing is free of bubbles. The clamp is then closed and the tip covered to keep it sterile. The procedure is illustrated in Fig. 7-12.

Starting an IV line. The veins most often used for initiating IV lines are found in the anterior forearm, the posterior hand, the radial aspect of the wrist, and the antecubital space (Fig. 7-13). Usually the antecubital veins on each arm are large enough and near enough to the surface to be easily seen. Although they may be the easiest to locate and to puncture, there are drawbacks to their use. Easy access to these veins is important in emergencies and for routine blood draws. Overuse, however, may cause these veins to become scarred or sclerotic, causing serious problems for patients receiving long-term care. When antecubital IV lines remain in place for some time, they become uncomfortable and inhibit the patient's ability to flex the elbow. Flexion at the elbow may crimp the catheter, preventing IV flow. For these reasons the nursing service tends to use antecubital veins as a last resort. In imaging departments, the IV line is usually placed only for the duration of the procedure, and the use of antecubital veins is acceptable when necessary. A vein of adequate size is essential when a bolus of contrast will be delivered at a rapid rate. For children this usually requires an antecubital site. When placing an IV line in an antecubital vein, a flexible IV catheter must be used and the elbow should be restrained in extension by attaching it to an arm board. Flexion of the elbow with a needle or catheter in an antecubital vein can rupture the vein, causing **extravasation** (leakage into surrounding tissue), hematoma, and scarring.

To select a vein, first secure the tourniquet proximal to the intended site. Instruct the patient to open and close the hand a few times and then hold a tight fist. These measures restrict circulation and enlarge the veins, making them easier to identify and to penetrate accurately. The ideal vein can be readily seen and palpated. It is at least twice the diameter of

the needle or catheter you plan to use, and the vein appears not to bend or curve for a distance at least equal to the length of the needle or catheter. If a suitable vein is not immediately apparent, let the arm hang down for a few seconds, then gently slap the skin over the area where the vein should appear. This may increase the likelihood that the vein will stand out well. If a suitable vein is still not apparent, remove the tourniquet and begin again with the other arm. Fig. 7-14 shows the step-by-step procedure for initiating an IV line using an IV catheter.

FIG. 7-12   IV INFUSION SETUP

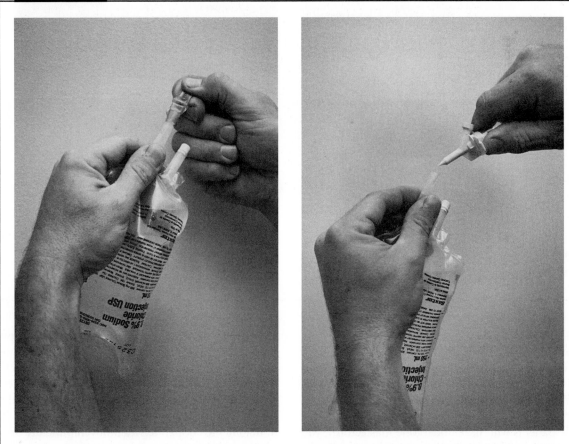

A Remove protective cover from access port. Avoid contamination.

B With tubing clamped off, insert drip chamber firmly into access port.

Continued

FIG. 7-12 IV INFUSION SETUP—cont'd

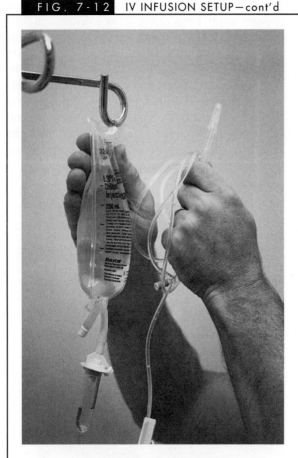

C Invert bag or bottle, and suspend from pole.

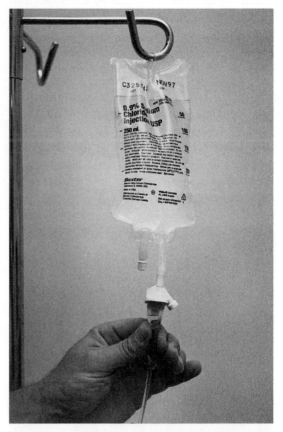

D Pinch drip chamber to draw fluid into chamber. Fill chamber about half full. Unclamp to fill tubing and reclamp. Setup is ready for attachment to IV catheter.

As you practice with classmates, suitable veins may appear readily. In the clinical setting, however, it is often more difficult. Obese patients may have veins that are too deep to be seen or palpated, and elderly patients may have veins that are easily seen but roll under the skin or are too crooked to be suitable. For patients who have undergone mastectomy, you should select a vein on the extremity opposite the side of the mastectomy site, since these patients often suffer from lymphedema, which causes boggy tissue and may obstruct the vein.

Patients who have had extensive IV therapy, especially chemotherapy, may have scarred and sclerotic veins that preclude a routine approach. Infants and children also present challenges. Their small veins are more difficult to see and feel, and the situation is often complicated by the child's refusal or inability to cooperate. Attempt venipuncture only when you have a reasonable expectation of success, and seek more experienced help whenever you are in doubt. The range of situations in which you feel competent will increase considerably with experience.

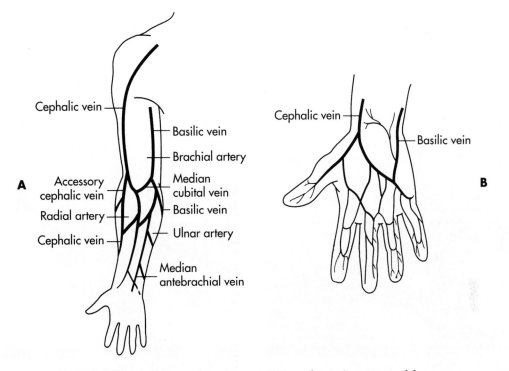

FIG. 7-13 Veins used for venipuncture. **A,** Veins of anterior aspect of forearm.
B, Superficial veins of dorsal aspect of hand.

If a particular patient's situation is beyond your skill level, or if you have attempted venipuncture twice on a patient unsuccessfully, consult another team member. Most hospitals have an IV therapy department with specially trained and highly experienced nurses who will assist you with difficult situations. Some hospital policies state that all IV lines for chemotherapy patients and children under a certain age must be started by IV therapy personnel.

IV medication administration. Once the IV line has been established, many IV medications are administered through an intermittent injection port or through access ports on IV infusion tubing. Before injecting through IV lines, check to be sure that the medications involved are compatible. Chapter 10 addresses the subject of compatibility between contrast media and common medications. After checking the patient identification and the medication label, draw up the correct dosage into a syringe. Cleanse the port with alcohol, and inject the medication through the port. When an intermittent injection port is used, a small amount of flush solution is injected through the port to prevent blood from coagulating inside the catheter and to remove any residual medication that may not mix compatibly with the current injection. The system is flushed immediately after it is established and again after each use using sterile saline solution. Physicians may order the use of heparin solution as a flush for some patients.

Sometimes medications will be administered through the IV line using the "piggyback" method. This involves connecting a bag or bottle of medication via its own IV tubing to an existing IV line. The amount of medication may be considerable, or it may need to be dispersed in a large quantity of

diluent (diluting liquid). In this case the piggyback line is filled and clamped before being attached to the IV line; the IV line is then clamped, and the piggyback line is opened.

Extravasation. Occasionally IV fluids or medications may leak or be accidentally injected into the tissues surrounding a vein. This extravasation, also called **infiltration,** may be painful and dangerous.

FIG. 7-14 VENIPUNCTURE USING IV CATHETER

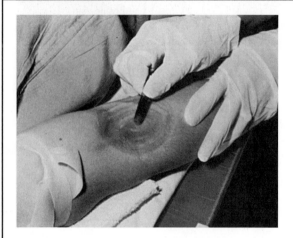

A After securing tourniquet and selecting vein, cleanse skin according to protocol for your institution.

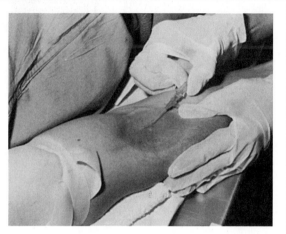

B Wearing gloves, hold catheter at an acute angle to skin and insert into vein. Advance catheter over stylet until hub is against skin. Blood return into catheter and hub indicates successful placement.

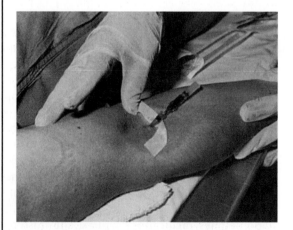

C Secure hub in place with tape.

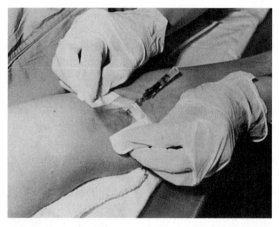

D If IV line will remain in place after procedure, treat site with antiseptic ointment and cover with protective film. Add a label with date, time, catheter gauge, and your initials.

FIG. 7-14 VENIPUNCTURE USING IV CATHETER—cont'd

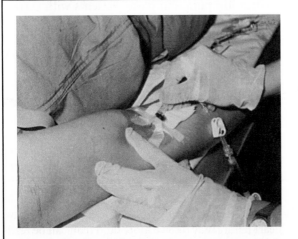

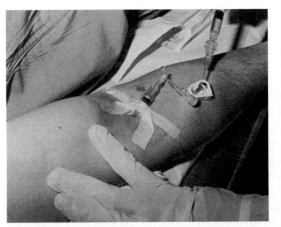

E Holding pressure on vein near tip of catheter, remove stylet and connect to delivery system to catheter. In this illustration, intermittent injection port with attached flush syringe is secured to catheter.

F If intermittent injection port is used, flush catheter and discard syringe.

The patient is likely to complain of discomfort, and you may observe swelling at the site. The following precautions help minimize the possibility of extravasation:

- Check for backflow of blood to be certain that the catheter is properly situated before injecting.
- Immobilize the catheter at the injection site.
- Stop the injection immediately if the patient complains of discomfort at the injection site, if you note swelling around the injection site, or if any resistance to injection is felt.

When extravasation does occur, you must remove the needle and attend to this problem before proceeding with an injection at another site. Assure the patient that the pain is only temporary. Maintain pressure on the vein until bleeding has stopped completely to avoid the additional complication of a hematoma at the site of the extravasation. After the bleeding has stopped, apply a cold pack to the affected area to help alleviate the pain. This will also cause constriction of the blood vessels in the area and help to keep the infiltration localized. If cold packs are not readily available, a terry towel can be wrapped around ice cubes, or ice in a plastic bag can be applied. A dry towel may be wrapped around the bag to protect the skin and hold the bag in place. Replace the cold pack with another as soon as it melts. Ice packs are applied to the extravasation site for 20 to 60 minutes and repeated three times a day until swelling is diminished. An incident report must be completed for any extravasation involving a potentially irritating medication or contrast medium. Advise outpatients to consult their physicians or to report to the emergency department if inflammation or discomfort persists.

At one time hot packs were recommended for the treatment of all IV infiltrations because the increased circulation that results with heat helps the body to absorb the extravasated fluid more rapidly. Research now confirms that the safest and most effective treatment for infiltration of contrast media and other irritating substances is the application of cold packs, which tends to limit the area of involvement.

Discontinuing an IV line. When you must discontinue an IV line, you will need a sterile adhesive bandage,

bandage scissors, and cotton balls or gauze sponges. Perform hand hygiene, and inform the patient of what is to be done. Wearing protective gloves, close the drip control and gently remove the adhesive tape holding the catheter. If it is necessary to cut the tape, take care not to cut the catheter, which may be doubled back under the tape. With the site where the catheter enters the vein exposed, remove the catheter with a long, smooth pull and apply pressure to the site with a cotton ball or sponge. Maintain the pressure for one minute or until the bleeding stops, and then cover the site with the sterile adhesive bandage.

One reason for using a sterile cotton ball or sponge rather than an alcohol wipe is that the adhesive bandage is more likely to stick when dry pressure is used. Otherwise, you must wait until the alcohol has dried completely.

With the patient in a safe, comfortable position, dispose of the equipment in the proper container, remove your gloves, and repeat hand hygiene.

Precautions. Most needles and syringes are provided in sterile wraps, used once, and then discarded. One common on-the-job injury is an accidental skin puncture by a contaminated needle. As discussed in Chapter 5, Standard Precautions are essential for your safety as well as that of the patient. For this reason we strongly urge you to use caution and apply the following rules when dealing with parenteral equipment:

- Wear gloves when dealing with any object contaminated by blood or when inserting or removing an IV line.
- Dispose of all syringes and needles directly into a puncture-proof container without recapping.
- Use safety-designed needles and needleless devices whenever possible.
- Always follow established rules of aseptic technique.
- Read the label three times: before drawing up the medication, after drawing it up, and with the physician before administration.
- Check patient identification before administration.
- Monitor the patient carefully for side effects.

Monitoring IV fluids. Patients who are receiving IV administration of fluids may come to the radiology

department with a standard IV set, or possibly a medication pump, in place. Patients with certain kidney diseases or cardiac problems will need to have their fluid intake closely monitored. For these patients especially, you must know how fast the IV set is supposed to run, not just how fast it was running when the patient entered the radiology department. Since these patients are almost always accompanied by their charts, check the orders. If in doubt, call the nurse in charge of the patient.

Most patients easily tolerate 15 to 20 drops per minute from a standard IV set. At this rate the patient receives approximately 60 ml per hour. If an IV infusion runs too fast, a patient with a condition such as chronic obstructive pulmonary disease or congestive heart failure may receive more fluid than can be readily assimilated, causing fluid to accumulate in the lungs (pulmonary edema). Since an IV set may also contain medication, the patient could suffer a toxic effect or an overdose. On the other hand, slow IV administration might cause inadequate medication dosage or prevent a contrast medium from being visualized effectively. The drip rate is controlled by a clamp below the drip meter (Fig. 7-15) that can be opened or closed to control the rate of flow. Practice using this control in the laboratory before confronting it in the clinical area. If you have changed the flow rate for any reason and are concerned about regulating it correctly, be sure to notify the nursing service when the patient is returned to their care.

You may encounter an IV dripping slowly with a microdrip set (Fig. 7-16). The small size of the drops allows continuous flow at a reduced volume. This system was once used extensively to keep an IV line open for medication administration and is still used on occasion, especially for pediatric patients, but intermittent injection ports have largely replaced "keep open" IV lines.

When checking an IV set, remember to check the height of the bottle or bag. It should always be 18 to 20 inches above the level of the vein. If the bottle is inadvertently placed lower than the vein, blood will flow back into the catheter or tubing and may clot, causing the fluid to stop flowing. This frequently necessitates restarting the IV line at a new site. On the other hand, an IV solution that is too high may

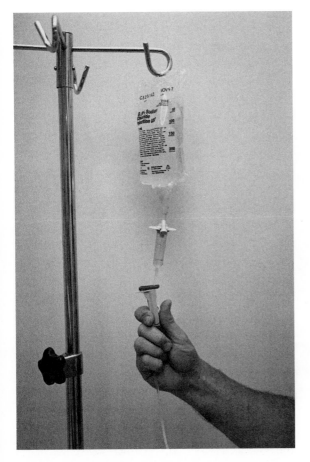

FIG. 7-15 IV flow control. Practice improves precise regulation of drip rate.

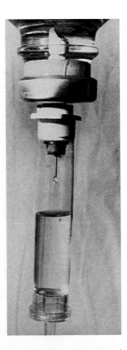

FIG. 7-16 Microdrip chamber.

cause fluid to infiltrate into the surrounding tissues because of the increased **hydrostatic pressure.**

Always remember to check the area around the injection site. If it is cool, swollen, and boggy, the IV solution may have infiltrated. In the case of infiltration, turn off the IV set and treat the area for extravasation as previously described.

Medication pumps (Fig. 7-17) are used for various reasons, including patient-controlled pain medication, parenteral nutrition, and continuous medication administration. If your clinical area deals frequently with patients on medication pumps, and especially if your work involves IV injections through lines governed by pumps, you must understand the operation of the specific pumps used in your facility. Medication pumps can be plugged into an electrical outlet, but most pumps also have batteries that allow operation during transport. An alarm system is part of the pump and will emit a warning sound when the solution supply is low, when flow is interrupted, or when the battery power is weak. The ability to handle pumps competently is most easily acquired by hands-on practice under the direction of experienced personnel.

When a hanging supply of IV fluid is running low or when the pump alarm signals an interruption in flow, you may be strongly tempted to work rapidly, complete the procedure, and return the patient promptly to the nursing service rather than cope with changes in the IV system. All too often this results in a nonfunctioning or "blown" IV line. For some patients, starting a new IV line presents no particular problem. Unfortunately, patients who are hospitalized and receiving IV fluid or medication usually have the fewest suitable veins. This is particularly true of pediatric patients, whose tiny veins are fragile and

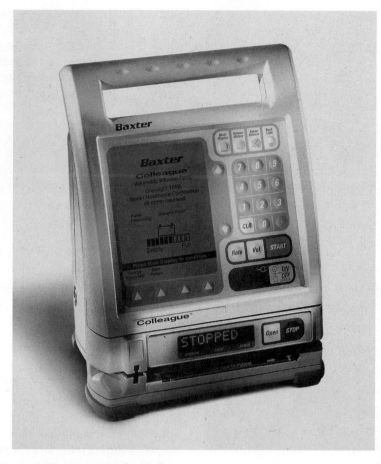

FIG. 7-17 IV pumps regulate infusions and permit self-administration of IV medications.

difficult to access. Patients receiving chemotherapy or parenteral nutrition are also likely to present difficulties when a new site is needed. You can avoid some of these problems by following these suggestions:

- Call in advance, and inform the medication nurse if the procedure will be lengthy.
- Whenever possible, plug in the pump rather than relying on battery power.
- Watch IV fluid levels, and allow time for replacement before the IV fluid is exhausted.
- If an IV set does run out, or if the alarm sounds despite precautions, call the nursing service immediately rather than waiting until the patient is returned to the nursing unit.

CHARTING MEDICATIONS

When a medication is given by a physician or by a radiographer under the physician's supervision, it is always recorded in the patient's chart. The notation is made in the appropriate section of the chart and includes the time of day, the name of the drug, the dosage, and the route of administration. A typical entry in the medication record might read: 10:50 AM, Benadryl, 50 mg, PO. Each entry must include the identification of the person who charted it. Initials alone are not considered adequate identification. If the medication record calls for initials, there is another place in the chart, often on the same page, where each set of initials is identified with the signer's full name. For legal reasons, the radiographer who charts medication must use the exact procedure established by the institution.

If an emergency prevents the charting of medications at the time they are given, the radiographer should make a written notation of the time, drug, and dosage so that accurate information will be available when the charting is completed. If this is not done, the pressure of the situation may lead to confusion of the facts. The time, sequence, and dosage of several medications may be forgotten or charted incorrectly. Any medication prescribed or administered by a physician should be charted by the physician; if charted by the radiographer, the physician should countersign it. The legal significance of complete accountability in such situations cannot be overemphasized.

The administration of contrast media is sometimes charted as a medication. More often, it is implied by the general charting of the examination and confirmed by a specific statement in the radiologist's report. If the latter method is employed, special notation may be required when there is a variation from the usual medium or dosage for a specific examination.

Physicians enter an account of the procedure and any medications given in the progress notes. The radiographer is responsible for checking that the drug, time, dose, and route of administration are clearly expressed. This avoids the possibility of duplication and provides guidelines for the nursing staff if follow-up care is needed. In hospitals using problem-oriented medical recording (POMR), the radiographer may chart directly on progress notes; in other situations, charting may be on the nurses' notes. Some hospitals have a medication administration sheet on which all medications must be charted. Charting routines vary. Familiarize yourself with the routine of your specific clinical area.

CONCLUSION

The radiographer is called upon to play an important role in the administration of medications. Knowledge of common medications and their proper administration will enable you to fulfill this role. Oral, topical, or parenteral medications may be administered in the radiology department, and each administration requires specialized knowledge and equipment. Intravenous access systems are used extensively in hospitals and are the most frequent route of medication administration in imaging departments. The establishment of these systems, as well as their use and monitoring, requires that the radiographer have a high degree of knowledge, skill, and awareness. Supervised clinical practice and familiarity with state regulations and institutional procedures are required to implement this knowledge.

The charting of medication and the monitoring of patients are significant aspects of medication administration and must not be overlooked. The radiographer must recognize the potential harm and legal complications that could result from medication administration errors and strive for error-free performance.

REVIEW QUESTIONS

1. Medications given in imaging departments are most often administered via the route that provides the most rapid response. This is the:
   A. subcutaneous route
   B. intradermal route
   C. intramuscular route
   D. intravenous route
   E. intrathecal route
2. A common side effect of an anticholinergic drug is:
   A. nausea
   B. dry mouth
   C. bruising or spontaneous bleeding
   D. constipation
   E. insomnia
3. A parenteral administration involving 5 ml of Benadryl may be given IV or:
   A. intradermally
   B. subcutaneously
   C. intramuscularly
   D. intra-arterially
   E. any of the above

4. The average flow rate for infusion of IV fluids is:
   A. 5 to 10 drops per minute
   B. 15 to 20 drops per minute
   C. 40 to 50 drops per minute
   D. 60 drops per minute
   E. 100 drops per hour
5. Which of the following are parenteral routes of administration?
   A. intravenous
   B. enteral
   C. intramuscular
   D. all of the above
   E. A and C only

CRITICAL THINKING EXERCISES

1. Mrs. Short is a patient with moderately controlled epilepsy who complains of upper abdominal pain. She has remained NPO in preparation for this examination and did not take her medicine last night or this morning. As she enters the dressing room she falls heavily to the floor in a major motor (grand mal) seizure. "Here, give her this medicine," her husband orders. "She takes it by mouth." Which routes of administration are most appropriate for such patients? Should you administer medicine from her purse? Why or why not? What risks are involved in giving oral medication to unconscious patients?

2. Mrs. Erbele, a 50-year-old woman who lives alone, fell from a step stool in her basement. She was unable to stand and remained on the floor until found by her daughter 48 hours later. She has been admitted to the emergency department with dehydration and a possible hip fracture. An IV of D5W is running at 60 ml per hour when she is brought to the radiology department. In an attempt to assist as you and another radiographer transfer her to the x-ray table, she rolls onto one side. As you position her, you note that her IV has stopped dripping. What could have caused this? What should be checked first? What actions should you take? Should you discontinue the IV?

3. Matt Wren, age 5, was discharged from the hospital after a short stay for treatment of burns to his arms and chest suffered in a fall into a bonfire. Today he has been sent for chest x-rays due to the persistence of a severe cough. He is crying and extremely agitated. His mother states that he is so apprehensive about any medical treatment that his physician has prescribed phenobarbital to calm him. She states that she gave him a dose an hour ago and asks whether you think another dose is needed to calm him before the examination. What are the implications of this situation? What should you do? What should you tell the mother? Should you tell anyone else?

Dealing With Acute Situations

At the conclusion of this chapter, the student will be able to:

- List criteria for trauma centers to be designated as Level I, Level II, or Level III.
- Define triage.
- State the code routine used by a specific clinical site and describe the anticipated events when a code is initiated.
- Demonstrate the abdominal thrust (Heimlich) maneuver.
- Discuss the procedures for assisting patients during attacks of asthma, epistaxis, angina, nausea, or syncope.
- List the four levels of consciousness.

- List precautions to be taken in handling patients with possible fractures of the spine, ribs, or extremities.
- Contrast diabetic coma and insulin reaction or hypoglycemia.
- Discuss seizure disorders, including safety precautions and observations to be recorded.
- Recognize the signs of both physical and psychological shock.
- Explain the differences between syncope and vertigo.

anoxia	ischemic
cannula	pleural effusion
cardiac arrest	pneumonia
cardiac tamponade	pneumothorax
concussion	respiratory arrest
defibrillator	STAT
dehiscence	stridor
epistaxis	tracheostomy
erythema	tremor
evisceration	triage
hemorrhage	urticaria
hemothorax	ventilator

THE DICTIONARY DEFINES AN EMERGENCY as a serious, unexpected event that demands immediate attention. Sudden deterioration in the status of any patient under your care is an acute situation requiring an appropriate response. Whether such a situation leads to a more serious problem may depend on your ability to act quickly and efficiently. Seen from this perspective, no patient problem can be considered trivial. You will experience many acute situations over the years, and you must be prepared to minimize the possibility of further injury or complication.

EMERGENCY DEPARTMENT

The emergency department (ED) of most hospitals serves a variety of clients. Individuals with health insurance may use urgent care or surgical centers for minor emergencies. For the poor and uninsured, however, the emergency department often serves the additional function of family physician. Many such admissions to the ED present valid problems, even if they are not emergencies. This can rapidly overload both staff and facilities, especially in an urban setting. Establishing priorities and functioning effectively under such circumstances can demand intense application of your patient care and assessment skills. In addition to the material on trauma units in the following paragraphs, you will find information about the use of radiography in trauma units in Chapter 11.

TRAUMA UNITS

Many hospitals have specialized facilities designated as trauma units, which are usually part of the emergency department. There are three designated levels of trauma facilities:

- Level I trauma centers are able to care for all levels of injuries. These facilities are usually found in large institutions. They are staffed around the clock with physicians, surgeons, and support personnel who are highly trained in the care and treatment of traumatic injuries. Level I hospitals have access to transfer facilities, such as helicopter rescue units that permit the most seriously injured to reach the center in a relatively short time. A Level I hospital must be able to provide emergency radiography, fluoroscopy, computed tomography (CT), and magnetic resonance imaging (MRI) procedures around the clock. There must also be access to nuclear medicine studies, angiography, and sonography. Facilities for neurological care must also be available.
- Level II trauma centers are the next level of trauma care. An emergency department physician is on 24-hour duty, as are emergency trained nurses and radiology staff. Surgical radiographic and fluoroscopic procedures must be available, as well as the ability to perform angiography, CT, and MRI procedures. Patients will be transferred to Level I facilities only if necessary.
- Level III trauma centers are smaller community hospitals that usually have an ED physician and radiographer on call at night. Trauma patients with life-threatening conditions will be transported to a Level I or Level II hospital as needed.

Trauma units are designed to cope with massive, life-threatening injuries. Many units have the resources to accept patients who have been airlifted directly to the unit from a considerable distance. Trauma physicians receive highly specialized training in the diagnosis and treatment of traumatic injuries. Although the composition may vary slightly, the staff usually consists of one or more physicians who are emergency department specialists, trauma nurses, an anesthetist or respiratory therapist, radiographer(s), phlebotomist, and one individual (usually a nurse) to act as record keeper.

Research has proven that victims of massive trauma who survive the initial injury have a greater chance of recovery if their condition can be stabilized within the first "golden" hour after the accident. For this reason, every minute is precious, and trauma teams work under great pressure. The care of highly trained personnel and the immediate availability of equipment for diagnosis and treatment have greatly improved the potential for saving lives.

The transport team, usually made up of qualified emergency medical technicians (EMTs, sometimes called paramedics), delivers the patient as soon as an airway has been established, bleeding has been controlled, and the patient has been immobilized. The first assessments made by the physician at the trauma center involve evaluation of cardiac status, respiratory status, and the possibility of vertebral fracture. Trauma patients are transported on a rigid backboard and are not removed from it until spinal fracture has been ruled out. The danger of paralysis is so great that this ranks directly after **respiratory arrest** (cessation of breathing) and **cardiac arrest** (cessation of heartbeat) in terms of priority.

The radiographic protocols usually state that chest, pelvis, and lateral cervical spine images should be taken on all trauma patients. The cassettes for these radiographs should be available in each mobile unit to avoid delays. In addition to mobile x-ray, and possibly C-arm fluoroscopic units, many trauma areas also have a CT scanner and a small surgical suite immediately adjacent to them. Many emergency facilities also include an emergency x-ray room.

If accident victims must be taken to the imaging department, their conditions have usually been stabilized. They have been thoroughly examined by a physician, blood loss has been controlled, an airway has been established, intravenous (IV) fluids have been started if necessary, and medication for pain or blood pressure control has been given. When radiographs are taken on the way to the operating room, cast room, or intensive care unit (ICU), a nurse usually accompanies the patient.

Emergency patients are subject to sudden changes in condition and may go into physical or psychological shock. Treatment for shock is discussed later in this chapter. Once the acute phase of an accident is over, many patients who were full of fortitude experience a delayed emotional reaction. This may consist of uncontrollable crying or a compulsive urge to tell everyone about the accident. They may even have a physical reaction, such as fainting, trembling, or violent nausea. Your most positive action is to be available, offer nonverbal support, and watch carefully for any signs of a deteriorating physical condition. Your ability to speak calmly and work competently under pressure is reassuring.

When accident victims are brought to x-ray dressed in street clothes, it is sometimes necessary to remove garments before the radiographic examination. Avoid cutting or tearing clothing whenever possible. Keep all the patient's personal possessions in one place. One easy system is to place everything in a plastic bag clearly identified with the patient's name. The bag is then placed on the stretcher or wheelchair with the patient. Check the procedure in your clinical area, and be consistent in using it.

MULTIPLE EMERGENCIES

Ordinarily the radiographer will encounter only one emergency at a time. Occasionally, however, a single accident will have multiple victims, or several acute situations may develop simultaneously. In these cases, you must assess priorities. If you see that it may be difficult for you to cope alone, do not hesitate to call for assistance before the situation places lives in jeopardy.

Although patients are usually admitted to the radiology department on a scheduled or first-come, first-served basis, exceptions must obviously be made for emergencies. An order designated **STAT** (from the Latin *statim*) is to be done at once and indicates that the patient's well-being may be seriously jeopardized by any delay. When more than one patient from the emergency department requires examination at the same time, the radiographer may need to determine which patient's status is the most urgent. Generally the highest priority is assigned to patients whose vital signs are unstable and whose immediate care depends on the results of the examination, such as those in severe respiratory distress. With two cases of apparently equal urgency, start with the patient who can be examined in the shortest time, since this decision will result in the shortest total waiting period.

DISASTER RESPONSE

On rare occasions a major incident such as a plane crash, train wreck, tornado, or earthquake will require that many victims be cared for at the same time. These events are properly termed disasters. Every general hospital is required to have a carefully designed and written "disaster plan," and each member of the health care team must be familiar with the plan and his or her role in it. Disaster drills are regularly scheduled exercises that prepare the hospital staff to function effectively if the disaster plan must be implemented. A major disaster may involve all emergency services in the community, so your hospital may coordinate its drills with those of other agencies. The radiographer must be familiar with the plan for the institution and participate actively in the practice drills.

The process of identifying the victims, performing initial examinations, and assigning priorities for further care is called **triage.** A triage station is set up in a large area, such as a lobby. The triage officer, usually an emergency care physician, directs triage activity. Simplified methods of patient identification and record keeping are used to minimize the time required for paperwork. Usually patients are assigned numbers, which are written on tags and attached to their wrists or ankles. These numbers are used to identify the radiographs and any required records.

Although disaster plans differ among hospitals, certain elements are usually similar. A single person is responsible for the overall implementation of the plan. This person is notified immediately of the nature and scope of the disaster and evaluates the need for additional personnel, coordinating activities with other institutions and governmental agencies as needed. A special communications network, established in advance, is used to notify all needed personnel who are not on duty. This system usually consists of a series of telephone calls, with each person called contacting three or four others before leaving home for the hospital. This method provides rapid notification to many people without jamming the hospital telephone lines. As the health care team assembles, a group leader in each department will assign personnel to specific activities. In such a situation you may be expected to perform services other than radiography, such as caring for less severely injured victims, answering the phone, or keeping records.

After the disaster is under control and normal procedures are reestablished, it is important to conduct a situational debriefing. While this may appear bureaucratic, it provides the opportunity to summarize events and evaluate activities that could have been handled more efficiently. The intense demand that accompanies a disaster allows individuals to function far above their usual level. Often this is followed by a poststituational stress that can last for some time. Debriefing provides the opportunity to express fear, doubts, and grief and can help avoid a prolonged reaction to such events.

Natural disasters, motor vehicle accidents, or any other catastrophic events can be seen in the modern trauma unit 365 days a year. Unfortunately, emergencies can also occur inside a health care facility. A staff member can suffer a serious fall, a client can suffer a cardiac event in the waiting room, or the condition of a patient on the x-ray table can suddenly deteriorate. Before we discuss specific conditions, you should first learn how to obtain assistance in an acute situation. The process of obtaining help will vary depending on your situation. When other team members are nearby, use a loud, firm voice to call for a specific person by name, for example, "Dr. Logan, please come to Room 3 immediately." Your control over the situation is reassuring to the patient and will be more effective than a distressed cry for "Help!"

EMERGENCY CALL SYSTEMS

When working alone, or when qualified assistance is not immediately available, use the emergency call system. Each hospital has a procedure to call for emergency help, and several specific codes are usually available depending on the situation. The fire code mentioned in Chapter 4 is one example. Other codes may be used to announce the arrival of trauma patients in the emergency department or to cope with a situation that demands security personnel. If you need to summon help for the patient undergoing cardiopulmonary arrest, there is also a special code for this emergency. Most hospitals have a designated group of health care workers who respond to this type of code. This code team usually consists of one or more physicians, several nurses, a respiratory therapist, and an electrocardiographer. If a code is called in the diagnostic imaging department, your role may be to record the treatment and medications given, document time, take specimens to the laboratory, or answer the phone. Know your role and be completely familiar with whatever

system is used. Practice going through each code procedure until you feel comfortable and able to function professionally, even under these stressful circumstances.

Emergency Carts

Emergency carts, or "crash carts," are rolling, multidrawered cabinets that are kept in strategic locations throughout the hospital (Fig. 8-1). The code team usually brings the cart from the location nearest the patient. These carts vary somewhat, but each has certain essential items such as airways, artificial ventilation equipment, emergency medications and the equipment for administering them, a board to slip under the patient when giving external cardiac massage, a blood pressure cuff, a stethoscope, and a defibrillator that can also serve as a cardiac monitor. Box 8-1 lists equipment commonly found on the emergency cart. The cart should be inspected

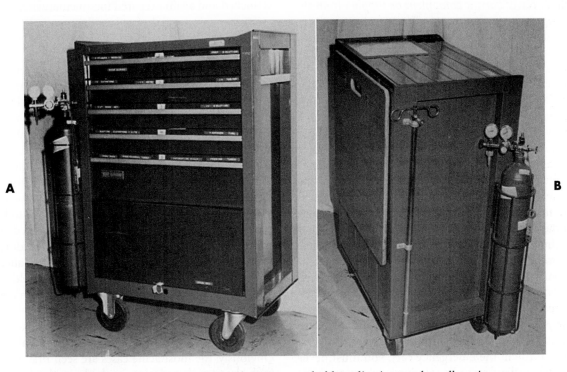

FIG. 8-1 Emergency cart. **A,** Front view. Drawers hold medications and small equipment. **B,** Additional equipment attached to back and sides: backboard for performing CPR, IV pole, and oxygen tank.

BOX 8-1

EQUIPMENT COMMONLY FOUND ON THE CODE CHART

Backboard	Sterile and nonsterile gloves
Stethoscope	Cutdown tray
Blood pressure cuff	Suction bottle
Ambu bag	Hemostat
Laryngoscope	Scissors
Endotracheal tubes	Needles, syringes
Tongue blades	IV solutions and tubing
Suction catheters	IV cannulas
Tracheostomy tubes	Blood collection tubes
Flashlight	Drugs according to institutional protocol
Protective gowns, eyewear, masks	Pen, paper, checklist for cart contents

daily and should have a list of contents to ensure that emergency supplies are available for instant use. Some hospitals seal the cart after supplies are replenished. *Never borrow equipment or supplies from the emergency set for routine use.* This practice results in the absence of lifesaving items when they are most needed.

Table 8-1 lists medications typically found on an emergency cart and can help you become familiar with common emergency drugs and their actions. It is extremely important to learn both the proprietary (trade) and generic names. If a drug should be requested by trade name, and the emergency stock is the generic equivalent by a different manufacturer, you must be able to quickly identify the correct medication by the generic name. This table is not meant to be a substitute for thorough knowledge of the contents of the emergency cart in your clinical setting.

Some emergency carts contain bags of intravenous solutions to which potent medications, such as lidocaine, have been added. These medicated IV solutions should be stored in a different part of the cart where they can be more easily differentiated from routine IV fluids. Since items may be stored incorrectly in the emergency cart, you must never select a medication or IV solution solely on the basis of its location. Always double-check the labels on any medications or solutions as you remove them

from the cart. Don't allow the urgency of the moment to interfere with the use of correct procedures.

After an emergency cart has been used, it must be restocked and again prepared for an emergency.

PATIENT EVALUATION

Patients come to the imaging department in widely varying states of health. As you use the skills learned in Chapter 6, you will be able to evaluate patients and observe changes in their clinical signs and conditions. Individuals suffering from prolonged illness or trauma, or those who are weakened by extensive preparation for examination, may suffer a sudden, life-threatening change in status. Patients with a history of chronic cardiac or pulmonary disease are at greater risk when an invasive procedure is to be performed. Before any patient is injected with a contrast medium or subjected to an invasive procedure, a thorough history of previous cardiac events, allergies, chronic diseases, and medications should be taken. Baseline vital signs must also be taken and recorded.

Patients in the emergency department are classified as nonurgent, urgent, or acute (life threatening). Obviously, the most acute cases are seen first. Even with the specialized care available in the United States today, trauma is the most common cause of death for individuals under 40. Deciding the

TABLE 8-1

EMERGENCY CART MEDICATIONS

AGENT	ACTION
Adrenalin (epinephrine)	Increases cardiac output, constricts blood vessels, raises blood pressure, relaxes bronchioles, aids respiration
Aminophylline	Reverses bronchospasm
Atropine	Respiratory/circulatory stimulant; dries secretions
Benadryl	Antihistamine
Caffeine sodium benzoate	Diuretic; cardiac/respiratory stimulant
Calcium chloride	Combats tetany
Decadron (dexamethasone)	Antiinflammatory
Digoxin (digitalis)	Increases cardiac output
Dilantin (phenytoin)	Anticonvulsant
Glucagon	Increases blood sugar
Heparin	Inhibits blood coagulation
Inderal (propranolol)	Cardiac antidysrhythmic
Isoptin (verapamil)	Cardiac antidysrhythmic
Isuprel (isoproterenol)	Relieves bronchospasm
Lasix (furosemide)	Diuretic
Levophed (norepinephrine, levarterenol)	Raises blood pressure
Narcan (naloxone)	Opioid antagonist
Nitrostat (nitroglycerin)	Vasodilator, relaxes walls of blood vessels, increases circulation
Sodium bicarbonate	Combats acidosis
Solu-Medrol (methylprednisolone)	Antiinflammatory
Sterile water	Diluent
Theophylline	Stimulant respiratory system, mild diuretic
Valium (diazepam)	Tranquilizer, antiseizure agent
Xylocaine (lidocaine)	Anesthetic, antidysrhythmic

order in which patients receive treatment is ultimately the emergency department physician's responsibility.

Families of trauma victims can be distraught and demanding when they perceive that others are being cared for first. On these occasions, your role is to reassure and explain to concerned individuals how priorities are set in such emergency situations.

OXYGEN AND SUCTION

As a radiographer you will encounter many patients who need supplemental oxygen. Since the need for oxygen and/or suction can be sudden and dramatic, you should be familiar with the mechanics of both

wall-mounted and mobile systems. The administration of oxygen is noninvasive, and until a physician can evaluate the patient, it is appropriate to provide a low flow rate of oxygen to any patient who experiences acute anxiety accompanied by a rapid heart rate and shortness of breath. Oxygen is prescribed for patients with a wide range of illnesses and in any case of trauma that impairs oxygen uptake.

Oxygen Administration

Oxygen (O_2) can be administered by various means. A nasal **cannula** (tubing) is the simplest and most frequently used device for longer-term oxygen administration (Fig. 8-2). Always make certain that the oxygen is flowing through the cannula before

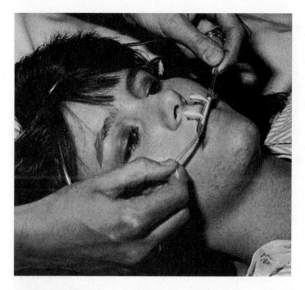

FIG. 8-2 Nasal cannula for oxygen administration.

placing it on the patient. The oxygen should be delivered at a rate of 4 liters per minute (L/min) or less, since higher rates dry out the nasal mucosa.

An oxygen mask is used to provide both oxygen and humidity. It is shaped to conform to the patient's face and is held in place by an elastic strap. The simple face mask (Fig. 8-3) is used primarily for

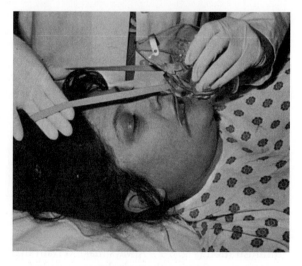

FIG. 8-3 Oxygen mask.

short-term therapy because it is somewhat uncomfortable and the patient is unable to eat or drink when it is in place. It fits loosely and delivers oxygen concentrations that can vary from 30% to 50%, depending on the fit and the oxygen flow rate. Attach the mask to the oxygen supply, and adjust the flowmeter to deliver 3 to 5 L/min. Place the mask over the nose and mouth, and slip the elastic band over the patient's head.

High-flow masks are designed to administer high concentrations of oxygen. A nonrebreathing mask, for example, has an attached reservoir bag that fills with 100% oxygen and a valve to prevent exhaled gas from being breathed again. This mask can supply 100% oxygen to the patient if used properly. Partial rebreathing masks that can deliver oxygen at 60% to 90% are also available, as is the Venturi mask, which delivers a controlled oxygen concentration of 24% to 55%. To meet a patient's specific needs, a physician may prescribe such specialized masks.

An oxygen tent is used when a higher rate of humidity and oxygen is needed than is available in the normal air. Tents are used most frequently in the pediatric department because they are more acceptable to children. If you are required to x-ray a patient in a tent, check with the nursing staff before turning off the oxygen, and complete the procedure in as brief a period as practical. Be sure to replace the tent and side rail. Ensure that the mist and oxygen are adjusted to the required levels before leaving the area.

Most patients on long-term oxygen therapy are able to function adequately with the aid of portable oxygen and a nasal cannula. Others, who must have a higher continuous rate of oxygen flow, require a **tracheostomy** (an artificial opening into the trachea) that is connected to the oxygen supply. An artificial airway may then be inserted into the trachea and mechanical ventilation initiated. A **ventilator** powered by compressed air administers a controlled respiratory rate, inspiratory volume, and oxygen content. When a radiograph is needed on a patient with an artificial airway, care must be taken not to disconnect or kink the tubing while positioning the patient. An alarm on the ventilator alerts the staff to sudden changes in respiration. If the alarm sounds

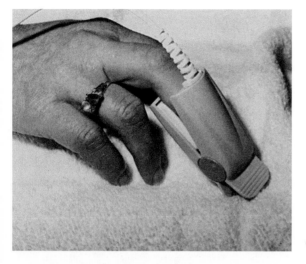

FIG. 8-4 Pulse oximeter probe in place on finger.

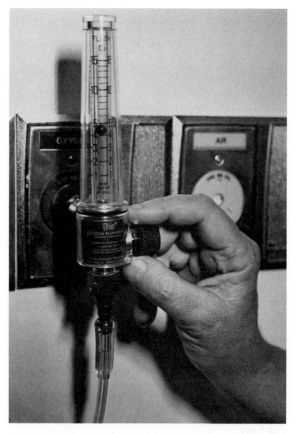

FIG. 8-5 Oxygen flowmeter at wall outlet.

while positioning the patient, do not turn off the alarm. The nursing staff will monitor the procedure and help position the patient as necessary. Chapter 11 provides further discussion on radiography of patients receiving mechanical ventilation.

A pulse oximeter (Fig. 8-4) may be in use for patients who have recently been removed from a ventilator or whose oxygen level may be compromised. Take care not to disturb the wires leading to the monitor when you move the patient.

In most imaging departments and acute care units, oxygen is available from a wall or ceiling outlet. An oxygen flow gauge for a wall unit is shown in Fig. 8-5. The dial on the side is used to adjust the flow rate, which is indicated by the level of the ball shown near the center of the gauge.

During transport, or in areas where oxygen is not otherwise available, portable oxygen units are used. You must be familiar with the operation of these units and with the procedure for ensuring that they will be immediately available when needed. The oxygen tank has an on-off valve that usually has a dial indicating how much gas remains (Fig. 8-6). A separate valve adjusts the rate of oxygen flow, and an associated flowmeter shows the delivery rate in units of liters per minute. *Both valves must be turned on to provide oxygen to the patient.* When

transferring a patient, you may need to switch the oxygen supply from the wall outlet to the portable unit. First, note the flow rate. Open the main valve on the portable oxygen tank and adjust the flow to the correct rate. Then, disconnect the tubing from the wall unit and connect it to the portable tank. Shut off the wall supply.

The oxygen flow rate for many patients is 3 to 5 L/min. Severely compromised patients, such as trauma victims in shock, may receive oxygen at a much higher rate. Patients with emphysema or chronic obstructive pulmonary disease (COPD) receive oxygen at a slower rate, less than 3 L/min. These patients must not receive a higher rate of flow, since the level of carbon dioxide in the blood controls their rate of respiration. If too much oxygen is

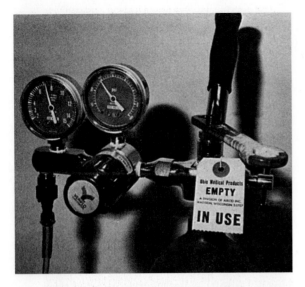

FIG. 8-6 Portable oxygen tank controls.

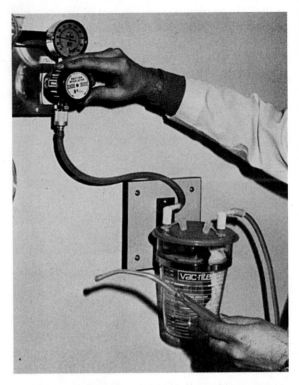

FIG. 8-7 Wall-mounted suction apparatus ready for use.

administered, their respiratory rate may become too slow for adequate ventilation. If you are caring for a patient who is already receiving oxygen, note the rate of flow and check periodically that it is correctly maintained.

Suction

Mechanical suction is used when a patient is unable to clear the mouth and throat of secretions, blood, or vomitus. Most hospitals today have a wall-mounted suction apparatus (Fig. 8-7), but some areas of the imaging department may still rely on moveable machines. If suction procedures were not part of your orientation, you must assume responsibility for understanding and operating this equipment. If you are responsible for ensuring that the suction system is operational, check that:

- The pump is working
- The receptacle is connected to the pump
- An adequate length of tubing connects the suction catheter to the receptacle
- An assortment of disposable suction catheters is on hand

Be alert to the need for suction whenever a patient becomes nauseated, is bleeding from the mouth or nose, or is unable to swallow and cope with

secretions because of a low level of consciousness. If a patient does begin to aspirate mucus or vomitus, turn the patient immediately to the lateral recumbent position, don gloves and a face mask or goggles, and attempt to clear the airway manually. Remember to stand to one side when clearing an airway, since the sudden violent expulsion of the obstructing material may spray your face. If a reflex cough does not clear the airway at this point, suction is needed.

It is unusual for a radiographer to work alone with an unconscious patient who is likely to aspirate. Such patients are usually accompanied by a nurse or physician, and your role is to assist in the procedure. Unwrap the suction tip attached to the suction apparatus, and turn on the suction. At this point the nurse proceeds with suctioning while you hold the patient in position. When the emergency is over, be sure that you have cleaned or replaced the receptacle and replaced the disposable tip and tubing so that the suction unit will be ready for use when needed.

If you must suction the patient yourself, use your emergency call button or call for help while you unwrap the catheter and turn on the suction. After you have cleared the patient's mouth, pull the chin down and forward while inserting the suction catheter tip over the tongue in the midline. Do not insert the catheter forcibly, since you may injure the larynx. Any suctioning beyond the pharynx should be done by a physician or someone trained in this procedure.

RESPIRATORY EMERGENCIES
Abdominal Thrust

Respiratory arrest caused by choking may occur, for example, when an older person attends a festive meal and has difficulty chewing food, such as a piece of meat. To avoid embarrassment, the person may swallow the meat whole, causing it to lodge at the larynx. The combination of alcohol, talking while eating, and poorly fitting dentures may result in a "café coronary," which is not a heart attack at all.

When any foreign body lodges in the opening of the trachea, victims become quite agitated, their faces become congested, and they may tear at their collars or clutch their throats. Since the lungs hold more air than is normally used during respiration, the reserve supply can be used to help dislodge the foreign body by using a technique called the abdominal thrust (Heimlich maneuver). Ask, "Can you speak?" If the person does not answer, tell the person what you are about to do. Place your arms around the victim's waist from behind. With your thumb on the outside of your fist, place the fist on the abdomen just below the sternum, and with the other hand grasp your wrist. Quickly and forcefully apply pressure upward against the diaphragm just below the ribs (Fig. 8-8). This will compress the lungs and will frequently expel the aspirated object. Never insert fingers into the mouth of a conscious patient in an effort to retrieve an obstructing object. Severe bite injury can occur, and the obstructing material can be forced farther into the throat during the struggle. If foreign material is visible in the mouth

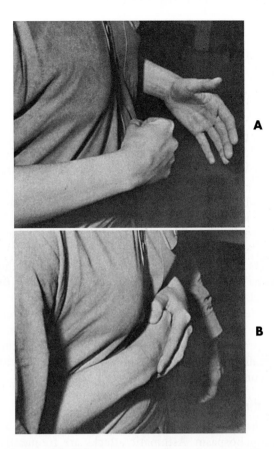

FIG. 8-8 Heimlich maneuver. **A,** Encircling victim from behind, place knuckles of your right fist over solar plexus. **B,** Grasp right wrist with left hand. Squeeze forcefully and quickly against diaphragm.

of an unconscious patient, use gloved fingers to grasp the tongue and lower jaw. Insert the index finger of the other hand at the base of the tongue, and sweep it forward to clear the obstruction. This should never be done for children if the obstruction is not clearly visible in the mouth and easily accessible.

Children more frequently aspirate foreign objects such as large wads of chewing gum, buttons, small toys, or coins that have been held in the mouth. Many of the deaths from foreign body aspiration occur in children less than 1 year of age. Consumer product safety standards regulating minimum sizes of toys and toy parts for young children have markedly decreased the incidence of fatal aspiration incidents.

Foreign body obstruction should always be suspected in children when there is a sudden onset of coughing or **stridor** (a harsh sound on inspiration). In infants, if respirations and coughing stop:

- Turn the infant prone with the head lower than the trunk.
- Support the head by firmly holding the jaw.
- Deliver up to five forceful back blows between the shoulder blades using the heel of the hand.
- While supporting the head and neck, turn the infant over, head lower than torso.
- Place the three middle fingers on the sternum just below the nipple line.
- Administer five thrusts over the sternum, taking care not to press over the liver.

In children ages 1 through 8, you may use the same Heimlich maneuver as in adults, with a series of quick subdiaphragmatic thrusts. Use good judgment in determining the amount of force, however, since young children have a relatively large and unprotected liver. The smaller the child, the greater the chance that damage to the liver could occur.

Asthma

Asthma is difficulty in breathing caused by bronchospasm. Asthmatic attacks are frequently precipitated by stress, and if the radiologic procedure is new or frightening, dyspnea may result. The usual response to respiratory distress is to administer oxygen, but this is not the treatment of choice for patients with asthma. The objective is to relieve the bronchospasm. Most chronic asthmatic individuals carry a nebulizer with a bronchodilating medication. Patients with asthma should take their medication into the examining room. For an acute episode, the treatment is an injection of epinephrine, which is ordered by the physician. Although it is frightening for both the patient and the radiographer, a single asthmatic attack is seldom fatal.

CARDIAC EMERGENCIES
Heart Attack

If a patient complains of sudden, intense chest pain, often described as a crushing pain, you should assume that the patient is having a heart attack until proven otherwise. Since the pain is caused when a portion of the heart wall becomes **ischemic** (lacking blood circulation), you must prevent further damage by minimizing patient exertion. Patients may underestimate the importance of this type of pain and assume instead that the sudden onset is "terrible heartburn" or "indigestion from that peanut butter sandwich." Pain may be referred to the left arm, jaw, or neck. These patients often become diaphoretic, have an irregular heartbeat, become pale, and may feel nauseated and short of breath. Stay with the patient, obtain help, and assist the patient to a comfortable position. If the patient has shortness of breath, raise the head and administer oxygen at 3 to 5 L/min.

Angina Pectoris

Angina occurs when the coronary arteries are unable to supply the heart with sufficient oxygen. Episodes of chest pain are precipitated by exertion or stress and are usually relieved by rest or sublingual nitroglycerin. The discomfort caused by angina varies from a vague ache to an intense crushing sensation. Frequently it is described as severe indigestion, since it often presents as pain under the sternum. As discussed in Chapter 7, patients who suffer from angina are treated with nitroglycerine. If substernal pain is not relieved with rest, inform the radiologist and be prepared to give a dose of nitroglycerine. A second dose may be ordered 3 to 4 minutes later. An emergency supply of nitroglycerin is usually stocked in the imaging department. Remember that patients with chronic angina can also suffer an acute heart attack.

Cardiac Arrest

For health care workers, one of the most anxiety-producing situations is to discover an unconscious patient or to observe a patient suddenly lose consciousness. When this occurs, it is important to initiate the "shake and shout" maneuver. Most patients who have simply fainted will respond if you call out their name and give them a gentle shake. If there is no response, feel for the carotid pulse and observe for respiration. If the patient has stopped breathing or no pulse is detected, an emergency code must be initiated to summon a specially trained medical team immediately.

Under most circumstances the code team will arrive in less than a minute after being called. Time is vital, since lack of effective circulation to the central nervous system can cause irreparable brain damage in 3 to 5 minutes. While awaiting the code team, you should proceed with cardiopulmonary resuscitation (CPR) only if you are trained and certified in this procedure.

CPR is the basic life support system used to ventilate the lungs and circulate the blood in the event of respiratory or cardiac arrest. Correct instruction in CPR is a vital part of your professional education. Your class should be given by a certified instructor, and you should take responsibility for updating your CPR card regularly. We have chosen not to provide CPR instruction here, since recommendations are updated frequently and printed materials are easily obtained from the American Heart Association or the American Red Cross. We do believe that practice on a resuscitation dummy is essential. Your local college, fire department, and hospital in-service department may also offer courses taught by certified instructors that include lectures, film, practice time, and review and testing sessions.

Even if you are certified in adult CPR, do not attempt CPR on infants or children unless you are also currently certified specifically in pediatrics. Courses for health care professionals usually include the techniques for infants and children.

Occasionally a patient who has had a laryngectomy is seen in the radiology department. These individuals have a permanent opening in the trachea (tracheostomy) and have had the larynx removed. They are unable to talk normally. They may have learned esophageal speech (the ability to swallow air and form words while belching it back), or they may use an artificial larynx. Care must be taken not to obstruct the airway. If the patient with a tracheostomy undergoes cardiopulmonary arrest, you must ventilate through the tracheostomy when doing CPR.

Once the code team has arrived, you may no longer feel needed, but a radiographer can perform several important tasks. Record keeping is essential. Write down the time the attack started and when the code team responded. As previously discussed, you may be asked to record times and amounts of medications or when defibrillation was administered. It may be necessary to obtain equipment, call for other personnel, or monitor a telephone.

When a code is initiated, your help may be needed to connect the patient to the cardiac monitor. The monitor is connected by means of electrode wires that snap onto adhesive disks attached to the patient's upper torso (see Chapter 6). The wire electrodes and adhesive pads are stored with the monitor. Learn to check the monitor and the related supplies in your area. You may need to know how to connect a patient to the monitor, print a tape of the monitor reading, and change the tape when necessary. Since cardiac monitors vary, use of this equipment should be part of your orientation and in-service instruction.

With the help of the cardiac monitor, the code team may determine that the **defibrillator** (Fig. 8-9) is needed. This machine administers an electric shock to correct an ineffectual cardiac rhythm. The defibrillator does not need to be plugged in, since it has an auxiliary battery system for use beyond the reach of electrical outlets. It must be turned on and set at the proper voltage. Two paddles attached to the machine make contact with the patient's chest. The paddle surfaces must be covered with disposable pads to protect the skin and facilitate the electrical contact. When the equipment and the team are ready, CPR is interrupted, and the word "Clear!" is used to signal caution before the shock. This is a warning to stand clear of the patient, the bed, or anything connected to the patient. A distance of 2 feet is adequate. If the first shock is not successful, defibrillation may be repeated.

The initial rhythm in sudden cardiac arrest is usually ventricular tachycardia, followed by ventricular fibrillation. Ventricular fibrillation will convert to asystole (the heart will stop beating) within just a few minutes. Rapid defibrillation greatly increases the probability of a successful outcome. Approximately 30% of the victims of ventricular fibrillation can survive following early CPR if defibrillation

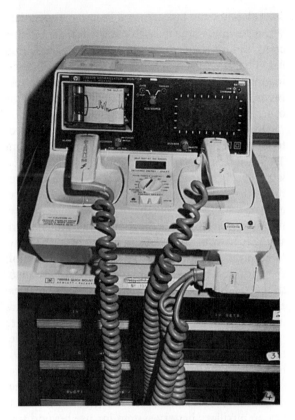

FIG. 8-9 Defibrillator.

takes place within 4 to 5 minutes. Even with early CPR, fewer than 10% of victims will survive if defibrillation cannot be initiated earlier than 10 minutes after collapse.

One recent development in treating cardiac arrest is the use of automatic external defibrillators (AEDs). These devices are very effective when used by personnel with only a limited amount of training and are easier to learn to use than a conventional defibrillator. Some of these defibrillators are completely automatic and have the ability to analyze cardiac rhythm, identify ventricular tachycardia and fibrillation, and automatically deliver a shock. A semiautomatic version also exists in which the operator presses a button to start rhythm analysis. If the AED identifies ventricular fibrillation, the need for shock is indicated, and the operator will press the shock control.

The use of AEDs has been reduced to four simple steps:

1. Turn on the power.
2. Attach the adhesive pads to the victim's chest.
3. Turn on rhythm analysis.
4. Press the shock control to deliver the shock, if indicated.

While different brands and models have a variety of features, including different monitors, paper strip readouts, and operating instructions, application of the device is simple. If your institution uses AEDs, periodic instruction will be provided. Your participation in both CPR and AED classes can help you to be prepared and effective in cardiac emergencies.

TRAUMA
Head Injuries

Patients who have received a blow to the head may have sustained serious injury, even when there are no external signs of trauma. Damage may occur with or without a skull fracture. The brain is soft, has a rich blood supply, and is suspended in cerebrospinal fluid within the skull. A severe blow to the head causes the brain to bounce from side to side, resulting in injury on the side opposite the blow. This is usually called a contrecoup injury. A minimal amount of damage, characterized by "seeing stars" or very brief loss of consciousness, is called a **concussion.** If bleeding or swelling occurs inside the skull, a rise in intracranial pressure (ICP) may cause seizures, loss of consciousness, or respiratory arrest. Incidentally, similar symptoms may also occur in patients with increased ICP due to brain tumors.

As mentioned in Chapter 6, four levels of consciousness (LOCs) are generally recognized and are described as follows:

• Alert and conscious
• Drowsy, but responsive
• Unconscious, but reactive to painful stimuli
• Comatose

The Glasgow Coma Scale is a numerical scale that can be used to objectively assess changes in a patient's level of consciousness over time (Table 8-2). The patient who is alert and oriented when admitted, but then becomes increasingly incoherent, drowsy, and

TABLE 8-2

GLASGOW COMA SCALE

ACTION	RESPONSE	SCORE
Eyes open	Spontaneously	4
	To speech	3
	To pain	2
	None	1
Verbal response	Oriented	5
	Confused	4
	Inappropriate words	3
	Incomprehensible sounds	2
	None	1
Motor response	Obeys commands	6
	Localized pain	5
	Flexion withdrawal	4
	Abnormal flexion	3
	Abnormal extension	2
	Flaccid	1
Highest Possible Score		15

stuporous, may be showing signs of increased ICP. The earliest signs of increasing pressure may be irritability and lethargy, frequently associated with a slowing pulse and slow respirations. Notify the attending physician immediately if you suspect a change in level of consciousness. Remember that the unconscious patient must have side rails in place, should not be left alone, and must be constantly monitored to maintain an airway.

Some trauma patients are under the influence of alcohol. Their condition may vary from inappropriate jocularity to an alcoholic stupor, or they may be argumentative or verbally abusive. It is easy to assume that the unconscious intoxicated patient has only "passed out" because of a high level of blood alcohol, but these patients are just as subject to sudden changes in condition as nonintoxicated persons. Be especially alert to LOC changes in these patients, because the effects of alcohol may obscure important symptoms. Patients taking pain medications, or those who are insulin dependent and have gone too long without insulin, may exhibit similar signs and symptoms.

Spinal Injuries

Every trauma patient should be considered to have a potential spinal injury and should be evaluated by the ED physician before being moved. Even slight movement of a spinal fracture may cause pressure on the spinal cord, resulting in paralysis or death. For this reason, exposures should be made without moving the patient whenever possible. When a change of position is required, as for a lateral lumbar radiograph, use a "log rolling" approach, which keeps the body in one plane. This two-person procedure avoids twisting or bending the spine (Fig. 8-10).

Patients with possible cervical spine fractures are immobilized with cervical collars and other radiolucent devices. These must remain in place during initial radiographic examinations and until a physician has determined that it is safe for them to be removed. A cross-table lateral radiograph of the cervical spine is taken and evaluated before moving the patient from the backboard.

Chest Injuries

Motor vehicle accidents and falls are two of the most common causes of chest injuries seen in the imaging department. Deaths due to crushing or penetrating wounds of the thorax comprise a significant number of the trauma deaths each year. Fractured ribs are intensely painful and can be life threatening if a lung or blood vessel is punctured. If a **hemothorax** (blood in the pleural space) or **pneumothorax** (air in the pleural space) results, the lung can collapse, greatly reducing the available surface for oxygen exchange.

The treatment for either pneumothorax or hemothorax involves a thoracotomy, in which a surgical opening is made through the chest wall and a tube is inserted between the visceral pleura and the parietal pleura. This tubing is connected to a water seal chest drainage system that helps the lung expand by removing fluid or air from the pleural space (Fig. 8-11). The chest drainage unit is set or hung below the level of the bed. While the tubing is long enough to allow the patient a certain amount of movement, the unit is below our usual level of vision. It is essential to be aware of a chest drainage

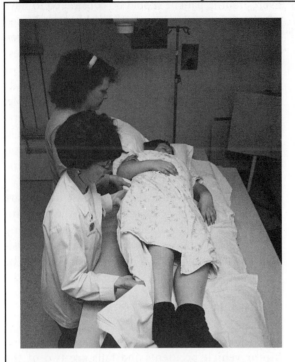

A Pull table pad toward you and lift edge, keeping spine in one plane.

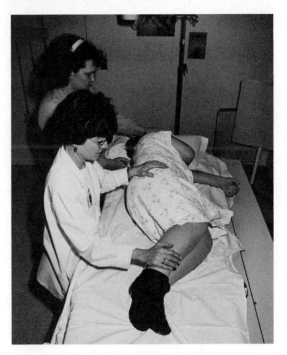

B As patient approaches lateral position, stabilize with hand on hip. Flexing knees helps to maintain position.

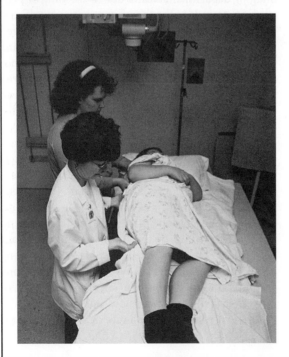

C The sheet alone may serve as support for returning patient to supine position.

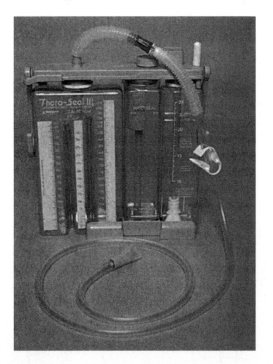

FIG. 8-11 Disposable commercial chest drainage system.

unit, not to put tension on the tube or allow it to become kinked, and to always keep the unit below the level of the patient's chest. When taking a radiograph, assess the situation carefully before moving the patient. If the patient becomes short of breath, cyanotic, or complains of chest pressure, notify the nursing staff immediately. Further discussion of treatment situations involving chest tubes and drainage units is found in Chapter 11.

Multiple rib fractures may result in a flail chest, in which the structural integrity of the chest wall is lost, and the lung collapses. When working with patients injured this severely, observe closely for signs of shock or **hemorrhage** (excessive bleeding). After their condition has been stabilized, these patients may be positioned supine or recumbent on the injured side. This allows the uninjured lung maximum expansion and aids in adequate respiration. These patients must not be positioned for radiographic examination without the assistance of the trauma team or ICU staff.

A blunt blow to the chest may cause bruising of the heart and hemorrhage into the pericardium. This serious condition is called **cardiac tamponade.** As the pericardial sac fills with fluid, it prevents the heart from expanding and soon results in a critical situation. Since little exterior trauma may be apparent, this cause for serious concern should be considered whenever the driver in a motor vehicle accident has hit the steering wheel.

Extremity Fractures

Trauma involving the long bones of the body may be classified in two categories: (1) compound fractures, in which the splintered ends of bone are forced through the skin, and (2) closed fractures. Compound fractures are usually partially reduced and a dressing applied before radiographic examination. Fractures may also be classified according to the nature of the injury. Some common fracture types are illustrated in Fig. 8-12.

There are many ways of temporarily immobilizing extremity fractures. The two legs may be fastened together for stability during transportation (self-splinting), or a stiff object, such as a board or rolled-up magazine, may serve as a splint. Ambulances often carry pneumatic splints, which are air-filled sleeves that protect and immobilize the extremity (Fig. 8-13). Splinting devices should not be removed except under the physician's direct supervision.

When you must position a fractured extremity that is not supported by a splint, maintain gentle traction while supporting and moving the arm or leg. Two people may be required to support and position patients with a potential long bone fracture, since the extremity must be supported at sites both proximal and distal to the injury. It is important to minimize motion of the fracture fragments. This helps avoid unnecessary pain and, more importantly, the initiation of a muscle spasm that could interfere with the physician's attempt to reduce and immobilize the fracture more permanently. Movement of fracture fragments may tear surrounding soft tissues, nerves, and blood vessels, seriously complicating the patient's condition.

Special care is required when positioning extremities following application of a plaster cast. Undue pressure against a fresh (wet) cast may cause it to

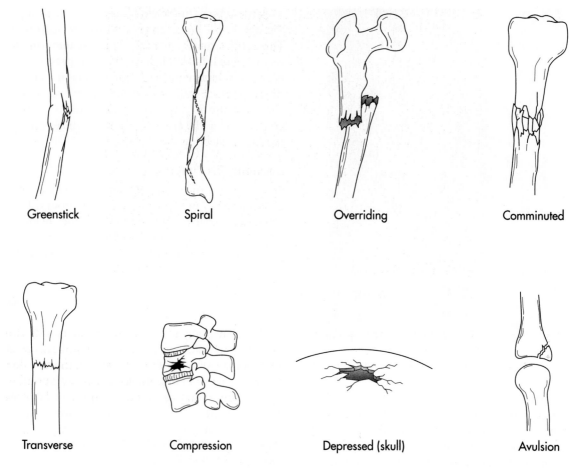

Greenstick   Spiral   Overriding   Comminuted

Transverse   Compression   Depressed (skull)   Avulsion

FIG. 8-12 Fracture types.

change shape. Lift the cast by placing your open hands underneath it; never grasp it from above. Observe the patient's fingers or toes for evidence of impaired circulation. They should be warm, pink, and sensitive to touch and pressure. Coldness, numbness, or lack of normal coloration should be reported to the physician immediately. Swelling within the cast and subsequent pressure can cause permanent nerve and tissue damage if not relieved promptly.

Wounds

Patients with open wounds have usually been treated before you see them in the radiology suite. Bleeding has been controlled, and dressings have been applied.

The radiographer's primary responsibility regarding open wounds is to maintain the dressings and to report promptly any significant amount of fresh bleeding. This is usually considered to be the amount of bright red blood sufficient to soak through a fresh dressing. If a laceration or incision opens, causing severe hemorrhaging, apply direct pressure to the site of bleeding while summoning immediate assistance.

Burns

While burns themselves do not require radiographic evaluation, burn patients may also have traumatic injuries such as fractures. Burns are frequently associated with respiratory complications. Inhalation of

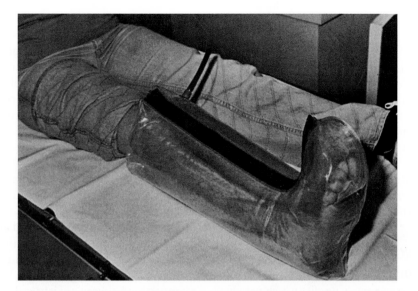

FIG. 8-13 Pneumatic splint for lower leg.

hot gases may result in **pleural effusion** (fluid in the pleural space) or the development of **pneumonia** (inflammation of the lungs), which must be monitored radiographically.

Burns may be categorized by cause of injury, percentage of body surface involved, and depth of tissue destruction. The depth of burns is classified as first-, second- or third-degree. A first-degree burn involves the epidermis only. The skin is red, warm, tender, and painful. There may be swelling, but without blistering. A second-degree burn involves the dermal layer, but not sufficiently to prevent the growth of new epidermis during healing. Pain, swelling, and blisters may be extensive and require medical attention. Full-thickness or third-degree burns destroy nerve endings. The skin appears charred, or white and lifeless, such as those burns caused by scalds or exposure to steam. Dermis and epidermis are involved, and skin transplants may be needed.

When a burn patient needs a radiograph, coordinate your examination with the nursing staff to ensure that the patient has had pain medication about 30 minutes before the procedure. If burns are extensive, the patient may be under protective precautions to avoid infection. You may wish to review this technique in Chapter 5.

Burn patients may have grafts or healing skin that is extremely tender. Such tissue is easily damaged during transfers or positioning, so you should allow these patients to move themselves as much as possible. Use a transfer sheet to avoid abrasion and ask for help if necessary.

Postsurgical Complications: Wound Dehiscence

Patients who have had major surgery may require radiographic examination. Wound **dehiscence** occurs when a suture line parts and the underlying tissues or organs protrude through the opening. While this is rare, it may happen, particularly in obese patients who have had extensive abdominal surgery. It is possible for **evisceration** (loss of organs from a body cavity) to result when extensive suture lines spread apart or split. This may occur when infection has weakened the tissues or when an obese patient experiences a sudden strain such as a fall or a severe attack of coughing or vomiting. If postsurgical patients are ambulatory or assist themselves onto the table, stand nearby to steady them and prevent a fall. When dehiscence occurs, the patient may tell you that something has given way and may complain of pain, or a rush of liquid may saturate the dressings. If this occurs, ease the patient to a sitting position and summon a physician immediately.

An abdominal binder that consists of a wide elastic belt with Velcro closure may be applied to help support abdominal tissues postoperatively. Unless specific orders exist to the contrary, leave abdominal binders in place during the examination, since these supports help prevent wound dehiscence. If you must remove the binder, wait until the patient is comfortably situated on the radiographic table. Replace the binder before the patient is transferred back to the stretcher or wheelchair.

MEDICAL EMERGENCIES
Reactions to Contrast Media

It is not possible to accurately predict which patients may have an allergic response to a contrast medium. An appropriate history is helpful, but a patient who had no adverse reaction to an iodine contrast agent at one time might experience a reaction on a subsequent occasion. For this reason, once the intravascular line has been established, the initial injection of a very small amount of contrast medium is followed by a pause to allow symptoms of an impending allergic reaction to appear. The length of time before the remainder of the injection will vary with radiologists and with the patient's allergy history.

The cause of reactions to iodinated contrast agents has been studied at length but is still unknown. These reactions have been shown *not* to result from antibody formation, which is the usual cause of allergic response. Reactions occur most frequently following intravascular administration of the large doses of ionic iodinated contrast medium used during such examinations as intravenous urography, angiography, and enhanced computed tomography studies. More reactions are associated with intravenous administration than with arterial injections. Patients allergic to food and airborne particles are twice as likely to be affected, and those suffering from asthma are three times as likely to suffer an adverse response. Severe reactions are not common, occurring in only 1 out of approximately 14,000 cases. Fatal reactions to contrast media are quite rare, with an incidence of approximately 1 in 40,000 cases.

Intravascular agents require special precautions, because adverse reactions can occur with devastating speed. Radiographers must be alert for the onset of these reactions and be prepared if they occur. Patients suspected of being sensitive are often premedicated with diphenhydramine (Benadryl), which is sometimes supplemented with cimetidine (Tagamet) and/or cortisone (Solu-Medrol). Although most reactions occur almost immediately, delayed responses may be seen and should be anticipated for at least 30 minutes after the injection. In rare instances, reactions have occurred as long as several hours after the injection. Interestingly, patients do not experience allergic reactions under general anesthesia. One investigator, A. F. Lalli, has demonstrated a connection between anxiety and adverse reactions. He speculated that the deterrent effect of antihistamine drugs may be caused as much by the soporific (causing sleep) effect of the antihistamine as by its specific action. To alleviate anxiety as a factor in potential adverse reactions, you must tell the patient what to expect without causing alarm.

Most patients experience a feeling of warmth during the injection of an ionic iodinated contrast medium and may feel flushed for 1 to 3 minutes afterward. A metallic taste in the mouth is another short-term sensation that can occur. If other minor symptoms such as nausea, vomiting, or coughing occur, provide an emesis basin, alert the radiologist, and continue to observe the patient carefully. These mild reactions pass quickly and may not produce vomiting if the patient is relaxed. No treatment is usually necessary.

An intermediate reaction is characterized by **erythema** (reddening of the skin), **urticaria** (hives), and/or bronchospasm. The physician should be notified while you remain with the patient. The usual treatment is to administer an antihistamine medication such as diphenhydramine orally, intravenously, or intramuscularly, depending on the reaction's severity. If hives are severe, cimetidine may also be given. Bronchospasm, especially when seen as an isolated sign, may be treated with 2 or 3 deep inhalations of Alupent or Proventil. Some physicians prefer to give epinephrine at this point, especially if hypotension is present.

A severe allergic reaction is called anaphylactic shock. This life-threatening condition may result in respiratory or cardiac arrest and less often, in seizures. The early symptoms of anaphylaxis include a sense of warmth, tingling, itching of palms and soles, dysphagia (difficulty swallowing), constriction in the throat, a feeling of doom, an expiratory wheeze, and then progression into laryngeal and bronchial edema. The drug of choice for treatment of anaphylaxis is epinephrine. Solu-Cortef, Aramine, Benadryl, Tagament, and aminophylline are drugs that may also be ordered, in addition to the infusion of IV fluids. The treatments for shock, respiratory arrest, and cardiac arrest may also be appropriate and are outlined elsewhere in this chapter. At the onset of anaphylaxis the radiographer should maintain the patient's airway, alert the radiologist, and call a code.

A vasovagal reaction to a contrast medium can be triggered by cardiovascular changes with a resulting increase in vasodilation of arterioles. This can cause diaphoresis, hypotension, and sinus bradycardia. A steady drop in blood pressure can cause unconsciousness and may be life-threatening. Place the patient in the Trendelenburg position, and notify the physician. Intravenous fluids and atropine may be administered if bradycardia is present.

Chapter 10 provides more information about contrast media and the typical responses to various types of contrast agents.

Drug Reactions

A drug reaction can range in severity from a sudden bout of nausea and vomiting to a cardiac arrest, and the seriousness of the reaction may be found at any point along this continuum. The nature of the symptoms will determine the appropriate treatment. Treatments for the various conditions seen in response to drug administration are found throughout this chapter.

Not all drug reactions result from parenteral administration or even from prescribed medications. Individuals who have been sensitized to an over-the-counter medication may be just as prone to an allergic reaction as those who are receiving an intravenous medication, although the effects of the IV will appear faster.

Diabetic Emergencies

Patients who have diabetes are seen for the same variety of problems that bring other patients to the imaging department. Since diabetes is sometimes associated with circulatory problems, these patients may be candidates for arteriograms as well as for more routine procedures. The diabetic patient can often be identified by means of the Medic-Alert bracelet (Fig. 8-14). These bracelets are also worn by individuals with other medical conditions that could require emergency treatment. The nature of the problem is stated on the bracelet and can indicate an appropriate emergency response.

There are two distinct types of diabetes, diabetes insipidus (DI) and diabetes mellitus (DM). Diabetes insipidus is a disease induced by problems with the kidneys or the pituitary gland that causes glucose to be excreted in the urine while blood glucose levels remain normal. DI is characterized by polyuria and thirst. If untreated, the subsequent water depletion may result in fever, vomiting, and convulsions. Emergency responses to both vomiting and convulsions are discussed in other sections of this chapter. Fluid replacement is essential.

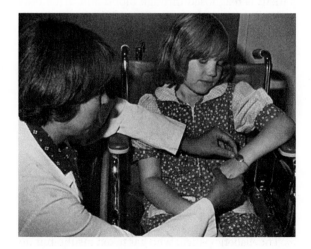

FIG. 8-14 Medic-Alert bracelet identifies diabetic patient.

There are two major classifications of diabetes mellitus. Type I, or insulin-dependent diabetes, is frequently characterized by a lean individual under age 25 who produces little or no insulin and may develop circulatory impairment of vision, kidneys, or extremities. Family history appears to be of minor importance. Blood glucose levels must be closely monitored, and insulin is administered parenterally. Type II, on the other hand, occurs most commonly in the obese individual over age 40 with a marked family tendency. This type of diabetes usually responds to oral hypoglycemic medications and changes in diet and lifestyle.

Diabetes mellitus is characterized by an inability to metabolize blood glucose. Insulin is an enzyme normally produced in the pancreas in response to food intake. Insufficient insulin prevents the use of glucose by the muscles. When the muscles cannot use glucose, the liver forms ketone bodies to supply the energy for muscular contraction. When excess ketone bodies appear in the blood, ketoacidosis develops. The body attempts to compensate for the acidosis by hyperventilation (air hunger) and the loss of minerals and water in the urine. When the blood glucose level is very high, sugar also "spills over" into the urine. The individual who is terribly thirsty, urinates copious amounts frequently, and has fruity smelling breath may be approaching diabetic coma. This condition is characterized by a relatively slow onset. The patient is diagnosed through blood and urine tests and treated with diet, exercise, and medication such as insulin or oral hypoglycemic agents. Diabetic coma is more likely to occur with Type I DM.

Nonketotic hyperglycemic hyperosmolar coma (NKHHC) is a severe condition that can occur when patients with neglected Type II DM become dehydrated and hyperglycemic. This may be induced by sepsis, by fluid loss from either dehydration or diuresis, or by hyperglycemia, tube feeding, or IV glucose overload. The level of consciousness may vary from initial confusion to coma or seizures. Treatment includes fluid administration to rapidly expand intravascular volume to increase circulation and urine output.

The diabetic patient who has taken insulin but no food may develop hypoglycemia, or low blood sugar.

Unlike the slow onset of diabetic coma, hypoglycemia is characterized by a sudden onset of weakness, sweating, **tremor** (quivering), hunger, and finally, loss of consciousness. While the patient is still alert and cooperative, hypoglycemia can be quickly treated by giving the patient a small amount of candy or sweet fruit juice. Squeeze tubes containing a measured amount of glucose may be stored with the emergency medications. These prepackaged tubes are useful because the gel-like material can be placed inside the patient's cheek. This decreases the chance that a semiconscious or confused patient will aspirate it, as might be the case with candy or juice. A parenteral injection of 0.5 to 1.0 mg of glucagon may be ordered if hypoglycemia is severe, especially if the patient is unconscious. Intravenous infusion of dextrose solution may be ordered as well.

Report the occurrence of hypoglycemia to the physician. You must help these patients to sit or lie down until the sugar takes effect. Occasionally individuals with the same symptoms may be adamant that they do not have diabetes. They may have hypoglycemia without diabetes; the treatment is the same. Table 8-3 summarizes the physical findings associated with high blood sugar, indicative of approaching diabetic coma, and low blood sugar, which may signify an impending insulin reaction.

Cerebrovascular Accident

A cerebrovascular accident (CVA), also called a stroke, occurs most frequently in the elderly but can occur at any age. Rupture of a cerebral artery can cause a hemorrhage into the brain tissue, or an artery may become occluded, causing an interruption in the blood supply to the area beyond the occlusion. The symptoms may occur very suddenly or may develop over a period of hours. Warning signs may include:

- Slurred or difficult speech
- Extreme dizziness
- Severe headache
- Muscle weakness on one or both sides
- Difficulty in vision or deviation in one eye
- Temporary loss of consciousness

These symptoms may be only temporary, but they should be reported immediately to a physician.

TABLE 8-3

DIABETIC CRISES

CRISIS	CAUSE	SYMPTOM	TREATMENT
Diabetic coma	Food consumption over dietary allowance Fever, infection, stress Insufficient insulin	Increased thirst Increased urinary output Decreased appetite Nausea, vomiting Weakness, confusion Coma	Inform physician Administer sugar-free liquids if conscious Insulin may be administered
Insulin reaction	Insufficient food Excessive exercise	Headache Hunger Diaphoresis Tremors Tachycardia Impaired vision Personality change Loss of consciousness	Administer food or liquid with high sugar content Inform physician immediately Glucagon may be administered

The patient should be helped to a recumbent position with the head elevated. Do not leave the patient, but summon assistance and have the emergency cart and oxygen at hand. Monitor vital signs every 5 minutes or as ordered by the physician. Transient ischemic attacks (TIAs) present similar symptoms but usually last only minutes, a few hours at most. These temporary attacks should not be ignored, because they are frequently precursors to more permanent damage.

Seizure Disorder

Seizures occur as a result of a focal or generalized brain function disturbance and are accompanied by a change in the level of consciousness. Patients with seizure disorders may come to the imaging department for any reason but are often seen for examinations such as a skull series, cerebral arteriogram, or CT scan. A major motor (tonic-clonic or grand mal) seizure may be preceded by an aura or premonitory sign. The patient may say, "I'm going to have a spell," and should be assisted to a supine position as rapidly as possible. Frequently the seizure is signaled by a hoarse cry when air is forced past the vocal cords by a sudden contraction of all the abdominal and chest muscles. When a seizure occurs, your first duty is to keep the patient as safe as possible. Notify a physician immediately, request assistance, and do not leave the patient. If the patient is on an imaging table, your first concern is to prevent a fall. Remove any objects that might be hazardous, and place padding under the patient's head. Do not attempt to restrain the patient, and do not try to force objects into the patient's mouth. If a padded tongue blade is available and can be easily inserted, it may help avoid a laceration of the tongue. Loss of consciousness and a rigid arching of the back are followed by alternate relaxation and rigidity of the muscles until the seizure passes and the patient slowly regains consciousness. Have diazepam ready for administration in the event of prolonged or repeated seizures (*status epilepticus*). While the patient is unconscious, involuntary voiding and defecation may occur. As the seizure passes, turn the patient to a lateral recumbent position to prevent aspiration of secretions, and remain with the patient to provide reassurance and assistance. In the immediate period following the seizure (postictal period), the patient may be somewhat irritable or confused and may wish only to sleep.

Less intense partial (focal) seizures may cause severe, uncontrollable tremors. This condition often causes extreme anxiety and hyperventilation in a conscious patient. These seizures are exhausting to the patient and may persist for over an hour without treatment. Instruct the patient to breathe slowly, and place a paper bag over the patient's nose and mouth if hyperventilation is otherwise uncontrollable.

Another type of seizure is characterized by a brief loss of consciousness (absence) during which the patient stares or may lose balance and fall. Many patients are unaware that they undergo this loss of consciousness.

Patients taking anticonvulsant medications may not have seizures for long periods. Most of these medications have a relatively slow excretion rate, which allows the patient to miss a dose or two without precipitating an attack. On the other hand, fatigue, apprehension, and the demands of a rigorous preparation for examination may initiate a seizure in a previously stable patient.

Realize that the seizure will run its course. It is most important for you to protect the patient from harm and to be an accurate observer. Note when the seizure began and how long it lasted. Did it involve both sides of the body equally, and did the contractions start in one area and progress from one extremity to another? These observations can help the physician reach an accurate diagnosis.

Remember that not all seizure-prone individuals have the same diagnosis. Seizures may be a response to drug sensitivity, infection, epilepsy, tumor, or fever. Myths and superstitions about seizure disorders have only recently begun to be dispelled. No direct, consistent correlation exists between seizures and mental acuity, emotional instability, or heredity.

Alcoholics hospitalized for medical treatment do not always reveal the extent of their alcohol addiction to their physicians. After 48 hours they may have withdrawal symptoms, including visual and auditory hallucinations and tremors. Some may also experience major motor seizures. Barbiturate or benzodiazepine withdrawal can also contribute to seizure activity.

Vertigo and Postural Hypotension

A "light-headed" or dizzy sensation is common after prolonged bed rest; postural hypotension is the usual cause. This results from the same basic mechanism that causes syncope, or fainting, which is discussed later in this chapter. Blood pools in the extremities when the torso is elevated and causes a transient cerebral **anoxia** (lack of oxygen). This condition can usually be avoided by having the patient sit up gradually. This sensation frequently affects elderly patients, so remain close to them and provide support when a sudden change in position is necessary.

Vertigo has a different cause. The patient does not feel light-headed but describes the room as moving or whirling. These patients frequently cling to the table and will fall if not assisted to lie down. They may experience violent nausea. This sensation is usually attributed to either an inner ear disturbance or to a lesion in the brain or spinal cord. A sudden onset in a patient who does not have a history of vertigo should be reported immediately to the physician, because this may be associated with a TIA or CVA. Alcohol or certain drugs may affect individuals in a similar manner and should also be called to the physician's attention.

Epistaxis

A nosebleed, or **epistaxis,** can be rather frightening to the patient but is usually not serious. Remove eyeglasses when necessary, and provide an ample supply of tissues. Instruct the patient to breathe through the mouth and to squeeze firmly against the nasal septum for 10 minutes. The patient should not lie down, blow the nose, or talk. Provide an emesis basin, instructing the patient to spit out blood that runs down the nasopharynx rather than swallow it. If bleeding lasts more than a few minutes, inform the physician, who may want to apply more direct treatment.

Nausea and Vomiting

Nausea and vomiting are frequently encountered, and a well-prepared radiographer learns to cope easily with this situation. Occasionally patients may feel nauseated for a specific reason, such as after swallowing a barium preparation. Vomiting can often be prevented by the radiographer's reassuring presence and by offering breathing suggestions. "Breathe through your mouth, taking short, rapid, panting breaths," or "Take some long, slow, deep breaths through your nose," are both effective instructions, and each has strong adherents. These suggestions are helpful because they encourage a focus on breathing that distracts the patient from the nausea until it passes. On the other hand, if a patient expresses a need for an emesis basin, offer it immediately. Bring the patient a clean emesis basin before removing the soiled one. Provide tissues and water to rinse the mouth. It is especially important to support the patient in a sitting or lateral recumbent position to avoid aspiration of vomitus. If the patient loses consciousness, be sure to turn the head to the side and clear the airway.

SHOCK

Shock is a general term used to describe a failure of circulation in which blood pressure is inadequate to support oxygen perfusion of vital tissues and is unable to remove the by-products of metabolism.

Shock is a dangerous, potentially fatal condition. Early signs of shock are pallor, increased heart rate and respirations, and restlessness or confusion. There are five main types of shock: hypovolemic shock, septic shock, neurogenic shock, cardiogenic shock, and allergic (anaphylactic) shock.

Hypovolemic Shock

Hypovolemic shock occurs when such a large amount of blood or plasma has been lost that an insufficient amount of fluid is available to fill the circulatory system. This may result from external hemorrhage, lacerations, or plasma loss from burns. Internal bleeding, such as that into the peritoneum from trauma or a perforated gastric ulcer, can also cause shock. Severe dehydration from vomiting, diarrhea, or extreme diuresis can also contribute to hypovolemic shock. Low-volume shock is treated with fluid replacement, oxygen administration, and medications to promote vasoconstriction.

Septic Shock

Septic shock occurs when a massive infection, such as one caused by gram-negative bacteria, produces toxins that increase capillary permeability and vasodilation, causing the blood pressure to drop

sharply. Although radiographers are least likely to encounter this type of shock, you may see cases in the intensive care unit or ED. In addition to antibiotic therapy, emergency treatment for the shock itself must be initiated immediately (see below).

Neurogenic Shock

Neurogenic shock, the failure of arterial resistance, causes a pooling of blood in peripheral vessels. It occurs in reaction to an injury to the nervous system and is an acute situation that demands immediate, drastic intervention. Patients with head or spinal trauma must be monitored closely for a decrease in blood pressure.

Cardiogenic Shock

Cardiogenic shock results from cardiac failure or interference with heart function. A pulmonary embolus or a reaction to anesthesia may initiate such an event. In trauma patients, cardiac tamponade may be the precipitating factor. As stated earlier in this chapter, this occurs when a blow to the chest causes hemorrhage into the pericardium. The resulting pressure interferes with the heart's pumping ability.

Allergic Shock or Anaphylaxis

Allergic shock, often called anaphylaxis or anaphylactic shock, occurs when individuals are exposed to foreign substances to which they are sensitized. An allergic reaction develops that directly affects blood vessels and other tissues. Blood pressure falls rapidly, severe dyspnea caused by respiratory obstruction from edema may develop, and death can result if this is not recognized and treated rapidly. Bee stings and injections of certain medications, including iodinated contrast media, are the most common causes of anaphylactic reaction. In the imaging department, this is most likely to occur during or immediately after the injection of a contrast medium.

Recognizing and Treating Shock

The following symptoms indicate some degree of shock in any or all combinations:
- Restlessness and a sense of apprehension
- Increased pulse rate

- Pallor accompanied by weakness or a change in thinking ability
- Cool, clammy skin (except in patients with septic or neurogenic shock)
- A fall in blood pressure of 30 mm below the baseline systolic pressure

You are responsible for recognizing symptoms of impending shock, knowing the location of emergency medical supplies, and being thoroughly familiar with the code routine of your institution. The physician may call on your knowledge of medications and your medication administration skills during treatment. The radiographer's role in suspected shock is as follows:

- Stop the procedure.
- Assist the patient to a dorsal recumbent position to avoid a fall.
- Obtain help. Notify the radiologist. If in doubt, call a code. It is much better to be mistaken than to have a patient die because of inadequate treatment.
- Check blood pressure.
- Assist the dyspneic patient with oxygen.
- Be ready to perform CPR.
- Assist the code team or physician as necessary.
- Chart the occurrence, the treatment administered, and the patient's response on an incident report form and/or in the chart.

Syncope

Fainting, or syncope, is a very mild form of neurogenic shock that sometimes occurs when fright, pain, or unpleasant events are beyond the coping ability of the patient's nervous system. Blood pressure falls as the diameter of the blood vessels increases and the heart rate slows. When the blood pressure is too low to supply the brain with oxygen, the patient faints. Placing the patient in a dorsal recumbent position with the feet elevated usually relieves this type of shock. Patients who have been allowed nothing by mouth (NPO) for 12 hours and are feeling anxious and stressed may undergo syncope. Patients who feel faint should be assisted into a sitting or recumbent position. If a chair is not within reach, ease the patient to the floor. If the patient does not rouse immediately, spirits of ammonia held under the nose

usually cause a rapid return to consciousness. Small, crushable vials of ammonia are usually kept in imaging departments for this purpose. A physician's order is not usually required for their use. Anyone who has more than a momentary loss of consciousness should be evaluated by a physician before the examination is resumed.

CONCLUSION

Since one of the functions of a modern hospital is to provide care in acute situations, radiographers must expect to use the knowledge contained in this chapter on a daily basis. You should be prepared to recognize and respond appropriately to any acute condition or sudden change in a patient's status, from a simple nosebleed or wave of nausea to a major motor seizure or cardiac arrest. Remember that you are part of a team. Hospital emergency procedures require the expert assistance of physicians, nurses, and code teams, so that you don't have to cope with a crisis alone.

REVIEW QUESTIONS

1. While you are positioning Margaret Dunne for an upright chest radiograph, she collapses against you and slowly slips to the floor. The **first** thing you should do is:
   A. call a code
   B. "shake and shout"
   C. get the emergency drug box
   D. provide oxygen
   E. start CPR
2. John Gaffney is sitting in the waiting room waiting for his wife to get dressed following an upper gastrointestinal (GI) series. Mr. Gaffney looked well when he arrived at the department, but when you go to tell him that his wife will be out in a moment, you notice that he is pale, diaphoretic, and seems distracted. When you ask if he is all right, he says, "Gee, I don't know. I can't seem to get my breath." Which of the following actions is **not** appropriate?
   A. help him to lie down
   B. call for help

C. "shake and shout"

D. check for a diabetic identification bracelet

E. check vital signs

3. A patient who reports that he feels as if the room is spinning is experiencing:

A. a heart attack

B. hypoglycemia

C. postural hypotension

D. vertigo

E. none of the above

4. Epistaxis is another name for:

A. a seizure

B. diabetic coma

C. nosebleed

D. syncope

E. angina

5. While taking radiographs on a trauma patient, you should be especially alert for signs of:

A. absence

B. syncope

C. hypoglycemia

D. shock

E. vertigo

CRITICAL THINKING EXERCISES

1. A motor vehicle accident has brought three victims through the emergency department, and all three need radiographs:

• Dave Black has abrasions and pain in his right leg.

• Paul White has displacement of his left shoulder and has become increasingly cross and drowsy.

• The driver of the car, Mary Green, has no visible injuries but complains of a painful sternum.

Which patients would cause you the most concern? What would you do?

2. What signs might alert you that a patient was experiencing airway obstruction? Would you give CPR?

3. What a week in the imaging department! Three patients went into shock:

• Mrs. Doble was having an excretory urogram.

• John Dix was having an x-ray examination for minor injuries suffered in a motor vehicle accident (MVA) in which his daughter was killed.

• Joseph Marsan had nearly amputated his own leg when he dropped a circular saw.

What type of shock was most likely in each case? How would the treatment differ for these three patients?

4. Suppose it was necessary to "call a code" and the patient has been successfully resuscitated. What tasks remain to be completed before and after the patient leaves the department?

Preparation and Examination of the Gastrointestinal Tract

At the conclusion of this chapter, the student will be able to:

- Explain the purpose of contrast media use in gastrointestinal (GI) studies.
- List three types of patients who should be examined as early in the day as possible.
- Discuss the purpose of bowel preparation for various studies and select a method appropriate for the patient's age and condition.
- List two steps that may be taken to make barium more palatable for oral administration.
- List the temperature, amount of fluid, and height at which the bag should be hung when preparing for administration of cleansing enemas and barium enemas.

- Position a patient correctly for enema administration.
- Give two reasons for discontinuing the examination or preparation of a patient having lower gastrointestinal studies.
- Discuss complications that could arise during an examination for Hirschsprung's disease.
- Compare and contrast procedures for routine upper GI series, double-contrast upper GI series, and hypotonic duodenography.

catheter
commode
congenital megacolon
hemorrhoids
hiatal hernia
Hirschsprung's disease
hygroscopic
hypervolemia
irrigation

mucosa
normal saline
peristalsis
pylorospasm
spasm
suppository
Valsalva maneuver
viscosity

THIS CHAPTER FOCUSES on the use of barium sulfate, or "barium," as a contrast medium in examination of the gastrointestinal (GI) tract. It also discusses the preparation and follow-up care for contrast studies of the GI tract and for the other abdominal soft tissue examinations discussed in Chapter 10.

Radiographic examination of the gastrointestinal tract requires visualization and differentiation of soft tissue structures. Because soft tissues are more difficult than bony structures to demonstrate, substances are introduced into the body that absorb radiation to a different degree than the tissues themselves. These substances are called contrast media (singular, contrast medium) and may generally be classified into four groups:

1. Barium sulfate products
2. Water-soluble iodine compounds
3. Oily iodine compounds
4. Gases

Many soft tissue examinations using contrast media require some type of advance preparation to ensure that the procedure will not cause untoward side effects such as nausea, but the principal reason for preparation is to cleanse the GI tract so that gas and fecal material will not obscure the structures to be demonstrated radiographically. Some preparations require several steps to ensure optimum visualization.

SCHEDULING AND SEQUENCING

One of the more challenging problems shared by nursing services and imaging departments involves the scheduling of multiple diagnostic procedures that may all be ordered at one time by the referring physician. With outpatients, this can be just as difficult, since communication involves both the imaging department and the nurse or receptionist in the physician's office. Consultation is often needed to decide how many procedures can be done in one day and to sequence them in such a way that they will not interfere with each other. For example, an upper GI series usually results in barium scattered throughout the intestinal tract for several days. Even tiny amounts of residual barium cause complications in radiographic examinations of the urinary tract and biliary system, where tiny opacifications are diagnostically significant. Residual barium in the digestive tract also causes unacceptable artifacts on abdominal computed tomography (CT) scans. For this reason, barium studies are scheduled last in any series of procedures.

Some departments may schedule a series of several examinations in one day for patients who are able to tolerate this approach. In some ways, this may be less stressful, resulting in a single bowel preparation, a single period of fasting, or perhaps a shortened hospital stay. However, a debilitated patient can only tolerate so much. After one study the patient may need to rest. Also, radiologists prefer various scheduling practices. For some, it may be common procedure to schedule gallbladder and upper and lower GI studies on the same day. Others may insist on 2 or 3 days for the completion of the same examinations. Whatever the practice in your institution, it should be stated in the procedure manual and the standing orders and be easily available to those involved in scheduling, ordering, and planning preparation.

When fiberoptic studies, such as gastroscopy or sigmoidoscopy, are ordered in conjunction with radiographic examinations requiring barium as a contrast medium, fiberoptic studies are usually done first. This avoids the possibility of the barium interfering with visual assessment during the fiberoptic examination. Patients undergoing gastroscopy should have nothing by mouth (NPO) for 12 hours preceding the examination. They usually receive sedation and a muscle relaxant before the physician inserts the gastroscope. When an upper GI series is to follow, it will be delayed to allow sufficient time for the patient to become responsive and alert before administering the oral barium. Oral administration of barium to a sedated patient increases the risk that barium will be aspirated.

When sequencing diagnostic procedures, thyroid assessment tests must be performed before any iodinated contrast medium is administered because contrast media containing iodine can cause inaccurate results in thyroid tests for at least 3 weeks. Box 9-1 provides a guide to sequencing multiple diagnostic studies for patients undergoing a comprehensive workup.

An additional consideration in patient scheduling involves deciding which patients should be scheduled first in the morning and which should be scheduled later in the day. Imaging departments always begin the daily routine with patients who must fast in preparation for examination so that they will not have to go without food for too long. If several fasting patients are scheduled, decisions are required to determine which should be examined first. After emergency patients have been scheduled, the next priority should be pediatric and geriatric patients, since they have the most difficulty being NPO for long periods and extended fasting may actually interfere with their recovery.

Diabetic patients who must postpone their insulin until their morning meal may also receive priority in scheduling. Diabetic outpatients should be reminded to postpone their morning insulin until the examination is complete, even if they have been scheduled for an early appointment. If an emergency should cause a delay, the patient who has had insulin may suffer a reaction (see Chapter 8).

ENSURING COMPLIANCE WITH PREPARATION ORDERS

For inpatients, the nursing service is primarily responsible for performing patient preparation. The radiographer, however, has the duty to ensure that standing orders for preparations are current and to check with both the patient and the chart to ensure that the orders have been carried out before the examination.

Scout films may also be taken to evaluate patient preparation. Caution at this point may avoid the needless repetition of an examination because of inadequate preparation. Unnecessary repeat studies waste time, money, and energy in the radiology department and result in additional radiation exposure and inconvenience to the patient. If the patient is to maintain confidence in the care received, such repetitions must be avoided.

Although the radiologist establishes the procedures, the radiography supervisor usually ensures that orders are distributed and properly followed. A representative of the imaging department should meet regularly with the nursing staff to clarify any questions regarding preparations and to provide rationale. Radiographers tend to assume that "nurses know all about these things," when preparation for radiography is not a significant part of their education. The rationale for the examination, as well as the particulars of preparation, must frequently be learned on the job. Person-to-person follow-up is

---

BOX 9-1

GUIDE TO SEQUENCING ORDER FOR DIAGNOSTIC STUDIES

- All radiographic examinations not requiring contrast media and any laboratory studies for iodine uptake
- Radiographic examinations of the urinary tract
- Radiographic examinations of the biliary system
- Lower gastrointestinal (GI) series (barium enema)
- Upper GI series

Note:

- Computed tomography (CT) studies requiring intravenous contrast may be done any time after blood has been drawn for iodine uptake studies. CT studies of the abdomen or pelvis should precede examinations involving barium.
- When scheduling multiple studies involving administration of iodine contrast, care must be taken that the total maximum dosages of iodine compounds are not exceeded (see Chapter 10).

especially important whenever a standard procedure has been changed by the radiologist or when the two departments have recurring problems concerning preparations.

When instructing an outpatient regarding preparation for an examination, it is most helpful to have printed instructions prepared in advance. If more than one alternative is printed on any given paper, be certain to indicate, both orally and in writing, which instructions are to be followed. Review the sheet with the patient slowly, explaining any words or procedures that may not be familiar. Have the patient explain back to you what is to be done. If the patient is too young, too ill, confused, or incapable of understanding and following the instructions, give the instructions (oral and written) to the person who will be responsible for assisting the patient. Be sure to include the telephone number of the radiology department so that the patient or the patient's family may call if any questions arise after leaving the department.

When scheduling and giving instructions over the telephone it is especially important to have patients repeat the instructions back to you in their own words, since you have fewer clues to determine whether you have been understood. Patients may sometimes say, "Yes, yes," in an effort to sound cooperative. An agreeable response does not necessarily imply comprehension.

PREPARATION FOR EXAMINATION

Specific preparations vary among institutions and radiologists, and the radiographer is again referred to the procedures at the institution. The most common radiographic preparation is for cleansing purposes. Certain examinations almost invariably require cleansing preparation, the primary one being the barium enema or lower GI study. For this examination the inner lining of the large intestine must be clean and free of all fecal matter. It is a complex undertaking to cleanse all the irregular surfaces of the bowel and usually requires several steps. These may include diet, cathartics, suppositories, or enemas, and the process often consists of several or all of these methods. Once mastered, these techniques

may be applied to preparations for other examinations as well. Cleansing preparation is also routine for studies of the urinary tract (see chapter 10).

Diet

An examination scheduled well in advance offers the opportunity to employ diet as an effective preparation. Patients may be placed on a low-residue diet for several days preceding the examination. At the same time, liquid intake, particularly water, is encouraged or forced, resulting in rapid transit of waste through the digestive tract and less residue in the bowel. For the 24 hours immediately before the examination, the patient's diet may be restricted to clear liquids. These are foods that are entirely absorbed through the intestinal wall, leaving no residue. A clear liquid diet may consist of consommé or bouillon, apple juice, gelatin, and tea. Some soft drinks may also be taken. A good rule to follow is to avoid any food or drink that is not transparent. Milk products are definitely to be avoided, because they curdle during digestion, producing high-residue solids.

Fasting is another dietary regimen that may be used in patient preparation for radiographic examinations. The NPO order is usually instituted for a limited period, approximately 8 to 12 hours, before the procedure. This ensures that the stomach will be empty at the time of examination, which is important for two reasons:

1. If the stomach is to be examined, it must be empty and "clean" so that it will produce an accurate radiographic image of its inner surfaces.
2. If the examination might cause nausea, as intravenous (IV) contrast agents occasionally do, the patient is less likely to vomit. Fasting decreases the possibility that vomitus may be aspirated.

Cathartics

Cathartics, or laxative preparations, are often prescribed to aid in cleansing the bowel. Research has demonstrated that increased fluid intake enhances the effectiveness of cathartics and aids in minimizing patient discomfort. For this reason, standing orders for cathartics are accompanied by a fluid intake schedule that suggests at least 8 ounces of water or clear liquid every 2 hours between noon and midnight on the day preceding the examination.

Cathartic preparations, such as bisacodyl (Dulcolax), a laxative preparation in tablet form, and citrate of magnesia, a carbonated beverage, are commonly used. One or both of these drugs may be specified in the standing orders. Commercial bowel preparation kits are available and may be used in your institution. They often contain one or more types of cathartics, a suppository, a low-volume enema, and illustrated instructions in several languages.

Heavy doses of cathartics may have such strong, thorough action that patients experience painful **spasms** (involuntary muscle contractions) of the bowel and irritation of the intestinal lining after administration. Persistent diarrhea may last through the night, preventing sleep. Although patients may find this preparation uncomfortable and inconvenient, its effectiveness in cleansing the bowel usually outweighs these considerations.

A usual dosage of a specific cathartic should be stated in the procedural manual and in the standing orders, but a degree of flexibility in this regard is essential. Caution must be exercised in implementing an aggressive preparation for elderly or frail patients who are likely to be adversely affected. In addition to providing a gentler alternative for the debilitated patient, those with chronic or acute diarrhea may require a lower dosage or less active preparation than is usually given. When decreasing the routine strength or amount of cathartics, use of a low-residue diet and increased fluid intake become critically important to the success of the preparation. The cleansing dietary regimen previously described may sometimes be substituted for cathartics when strong cathartics are contraindicated.

On the other hand, a more active drug or a higher dose may be required for those patients who have chronic constipation or are habituated to the use of laxatives. A brief history of the patient's bowel habits helps in assessing whether the usual preparation is appropriate. Patients should always be advised of the nature of the action expected from the cathartic when it is given.

Suppositories

A rectal **suppository** is a semisolid nugget of medication that is inserted into the rectum to stimulate peristaltic action in the colon to cause evacuation of the distal portion of the lower bowel. To insert a suppository, wear disposable gloves and insert the suppository gently into the anus with one hand while holding the buttocks apart with the other hand. Using one finger, gently push the suppository past the internal sphincter and approximately 2 to 3 inches into the rectum in a superior-posterior direction. Be certain that the suppository rests in contact with the rectal **mucosa** (lining membrane), since it will not be effective if lodged in a fecal mass. Almost immediately the patient will have an urge to defecate. If this urge is acted on too quickly, the result will be evacuation of the suppository only. The patient should be encouraged to retain the suppository for at least 30 minutes before evacuation.

Cleansing Enemas

Enemas are another method of bowel cleansing that may be used in preparation for radiographic examination. This procedure consists of filling the colon with liquid to aid in dislodging and flushing out any fecal contents remaining in the lower intestinal tract. Orders for enemas are usually carried out by the nursing service in the patient's room for an inpatient, or by the patient at home in the case of an outpatient. Occasionally this duty is assigned to the radiographer, however, and the procedure is included here for that reason. The radiographer must also be familiar with this procedure to be able to instruct those patients who need advice on taking enemas at home. An understanding of this procedure provides a basis for learning the technique of administering the barium enema, which is routine for every radiographer.

The liquid used for a cleansing enema may be tap water or soapsuds in water. Normal saline solution, glycerin in water, and olive oil are also used occasionally. The equipment needed consists of an enema bag or pail with attached plastic or rubber tubing, a disposable rectal catheter and apparatus from which to suspend the enema bag. An IV pole is especially useful for suspending the bag because of its mobility and its height adjustability. If tap water is to be used, fill the container with 1000 ml of tepid (105° F) water from the tap. If soapsuds are to be used, add 30 ml of liquid Castile soap and mix well. Castile soap is a very pure product and is ideal for this purpose; other soap products are likely to contain additives that may be irritating or toxic to the bowel and should not be used. Attach the rectal catheter to the tubing and, holding them over the sink, open the clamp. When the tubing and catheter have filled completely with the liquid, close the clamp. Filling the tubing and catheter before administration avoids instillation of air into the colon. You also need a water-soluble gel to lubricate the catheter tip. If the patient is unable to walk to the bathroom, obtain a bedpan, toilet tissue, and cleansing towelette and keep them at hand.

When you are ready, explain the procedure to the patient and give instructions for assuming the Sims' position (left anterior oblique, Fig. 9-1). Cover the patient with a bath blanket for warmth and modesty. Avoid exposing the patient more than is necessary. Hang the enema container approximately 18 inches above the level of the table or bed. The proper height is very important, since the position of the enema bag regulates the liquid flow pressure. When the bag is too high, the increased pressure may produce a flow that is too rapid, causing abdominal cramping. Excessive pressures could also cause serious harm to patients with conditions that weaken or inflame the bowel, such as diverticulitis or ulcerative colitis.

To insert the catheter, wear disposable gloves, spread the buttocks with your fingers, and gently push the lubricated tip through the anus, directing it superiorly and anteriorly into the rectum 2 to 4 inches. At first, point the tip in the general direction of the umbilicus. If resistance is encountered, redirect the tip posteriorly to accommodate the posterior flexure of the rectum (Fig. 9-2). When inserting a rectal catheter in a female patient, take

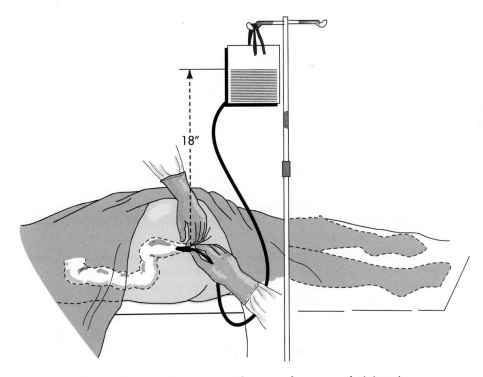

FIG. 9-1 Patient and equipment placement for enema administration.

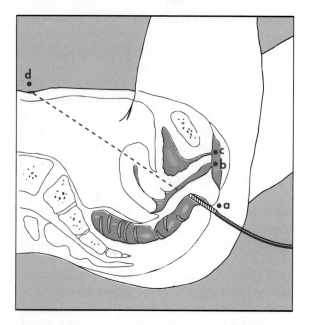

FIG. 9-2 Rectal anatomy in relation to other anatomic structures (female patient). *a,* Anus; *b,* vaginal orifice; *c,* urethral orifice; *d,* umbilicus.

care to ensure that the catheter enters the anus and not the vagina. If you encounter any resistance to the insertion of the catheter, do not exert more force. Sometimes feces in the rectum may prevent proper insertion. In this case the patient may be requested to defecate before continuing with the enema. If extensive **hemorrhoids** (enlarged rectal veins) or other pathologic conditions interfere with catheter insertion, seek the assistance of a nurse or physician.

When the catheter is properly situated, open the clamp, allowing the liquid to flow. If the patient complains of abdominal cramping, stop the flow temporarily and encourage the patient to relax by breathing through the mouth and panting lightly. Spasms of the bowel may occur during enema administration and often produce discomfort as well as an urge to defecate. The patient may feel "full" and believe that no further liquid can be tolerated. A spasm often occurs after the administration of about 200 ml of liquid, which is the approximate amount required to fill the sigmoid colon. When viewing the fluoroscopic image during a barium

enema examination, you will have an opportunity to observe this occurrence. If the patient has received less than 400 ml of the enema, you can be certain this feeling is caused by spasm rather than actual filling of the colon. A brief pause, perhaps with a change of position, should relieve the spasm and allow the procedure to continue. When the bag is empty, or if the patient complains of fullness after the administration of at least 750 ml, stop the flow and remove the catheter. Encourage the patient to hold the enema for 10 minutes, if possible, before going to the bathroom.

Assist the patient to the bathroom or onto the bedpan, and allow as much privacy as is consistent with patient safety. When patients require help onto the **commode** (toilet), use the same face-to-face assist learned in Chapter 4 for helping patients into wheelchairs. Make certain the back of the gown is clear of the seat. As soon as safety is ensured, leave the patient alone, calling attention to the emergency call button if one is available. Check with the patient at frequent intervals. If the patient or gown has become soiled, provide a clean gown, warm wet washcloth, towel, and assistance with cleansing, as needed. A pleasant, helpful attitude reassures patients who may feel very embarrassed about having soiled themselves.

Permit ample time for the patient to expel the enema. This is very important, since spasm of the colon may deceive the patient into thinking that evacuation is complete. If the patient has expelled only a part of the enema and is unable to expel the remainder, encourage some physical activity. The process of standing up and walking around the room for a few minutes usually results in relaxation of the spasm, allowing the patient to complete the evacuation.

One large enema that fills the entire colon is much more effective than several small ones that fill only the sigmoid colon and are discontinued at the first sign of discomfort. If the order calls for "enemas until clear," the procedure is repeated until no solid material can be detected in the stool. If you are checking for this result, instruct the patient not to flush the commode.

When inspecting the stool, evidence of bleeding may be noted. A black, tarry substance is indicative of blood from the upper GI tract. Fresh, red blood may result from hemorrhoids or pathologic conditions in the colon. Report these findings immediately, and when there is more than a trace of blood in the stool, continue with additional enemas only on the direct order of a physician. Since visualization of the causative lesion may be the reason for the examination, the physician may want the preparation to be continued, or perhaps modified to fit the patient's condition.

The sodium phosphate (Fleet) enema is a complete, disposable enema unit containing a salt solution that is highly efficient as an evacuant. It is very effective for the distal portion of the large bowel but does not contain enough fluid to cleanse the entire colon. This enema is sometimes used as a final step in a more comprehensive regimen and is often the method of choice for impromptu use in the radiology department when the patient's prior preparation has not been adequate. Complete instructions come with the product and are easily followed by radiographers and most outpatients.

When excessive gas and feces are present, cleansing preparation may be desirable for examinations of the sacrum and coccyx. This application is not usually found among standing preparation orders. With increasing stress on the limitation of radiation, especially to the pelvic area, perhaps bowel cleansing before sacrum and coccyx radiography deserves to be reconsidered. A Fleet enema for this purpose is inexpensive, easy to give, and relatively tolerable for the patient. It may decrease the number of repeat exposures while increasing diagnostic accuracy.

CONTRAST MEDIA AND OTHER DIAGNOSTIC AIDS FOR GASTROINTESTINAL EXAMINATIONS

Barium Sulfate

Barium sulfate is an inert inorganic salt of the chemical element barium. In the jargon of radiology, barium sulfate is typically referred to simply as "barium." It is used exclusively for radiography of the GI tract and is administered either orally or rectally. Barium is packaged in many forms, ranging from 100-pound drums of plain barium sulfate to premeasured packets containing a finely pulverized form of the medium combined with artificial flavoring and coloring. The dry powder is mixed with water just before use, forming a suspension that may be thick or thin, depending on the proportions of barium and water. Barium is also supplied in concentrated liquid suspensions, and this is the type of product most commonly used. These suspensions may be ready to use or may require dilution. Instructions for specific applications are provided with the products. Barium is also supplied in tubes in the form of an oral paste that is used for studies of the pharynx and the esophagus.

The barium itself has no flavor, but many patients find it difficult to swallow because of its chalky consistency. For oral administration, it is most palatable when cold and offered with a drinking straw, which helps prevent it from coating the mouth.

For rectal administration (barium enema), disposable enema kits are available that include a plastic bag, enema tubing, and a rectal catheter. A liquid barium suspension may be poured into a disposable enema bag and diluted, if required, with cold water. Although a warm solution would seem more comfortable for the patient, a cold liquid is less likely to cause bowel spasms with the discomfort of cramping. Some kits contain powdered barium, to which the radiographer must simply add water and shake vigorously. The bags are usually printed with graduated markings to aid in measuring the water as it is added. A bead may be situated at the junction of the bag and the tubing to prevent premature emptying of the bag. After the barium is mixed in the bag, a squeeze at the junction will dislodge the bead, allowing the tubing to fill. If the unit has a clamp rather than a bead to prevent flow through the tubing, close the clamp while filling the bag and open it briefly to allow the tubing to fill.

The proper **viscosity** (thickness) of the barium suspension is important in GI examinations. Studies of the esophagus require a thick mixture, whereas single-contrast barium enemas demand a thin one. Radiologists' preferences vary regarding the proportions to be used in regulating viscosity. This can usually be controlled with sufficient accuracy by following established standard measurements for the amounts of barium and water to be combined for each study.

Since barium sulfate is an inert compound, it does not react chemically with the body to any appreciable extent. Allergies are almost never a problem, and few side effects occur. If oral barium preparations contain coloring or flavoring additives, it may be standard practice to check with patients about possible allergies to these substances. The principal problem complicating the use of barium is its **hygroscopic** nature (i.e., its tendency to absorb water). When mixed with water, it slowly absorbs the liquid and tends to solidify in the same manner as plaster of Paris, although to a lesser degree. This problem is increased by the normal function of the colon, which is to absorb water from the bowel contents. Care must be taken so that patients with restricted bowel action do not develop a bowel obstruction as a result of barium impaction. Geriatric patients who are inactive are most prone to this problem. To decrease the risk of these complications, patients should increase intake of fluids and bulk in their diet. A laxative or cathartic preparation may also be prescribed following barium studies of either the upper or lower GI tract.

Reports of allergic reactions to latex (rubber) products, including a few severe anaphylactic responses to latex enema tips, have been reported. Products have now been introduced that do not contain latex, and these have largely replaced latex enema tips. If latex tips are used in your facility, it may be necessary to take a patient's allergy history before barium enema studies (see Chapter 10).

Iodinated Media

Special water-soluble iodine compounds, such as Gastrografin and Hypaque Sodium Oral, are available for contrast examination of the GI tract. These media are used only in special cases when the administration of barium sulfate may be hazardous to the patient. They are especially useful when a rupture of the GI tract is suspected, such as perforated ulcer or ruptured appendix, because these compounds can be absorbed into the bloodstream from within the peritoneal cavity. For this reason they are advantageous when the risk of perforation

during the procedure is a concern, and they are also indicated when abdominal surgery is likely in the immediate future. Barium sulfate extravasation (leakage) into the peritoneal cavity cannot be absorbed and therefore presents a much more serious complication. The iodinated media are also used when there is high risk of barium impaction, and they are also occasionally selected for neonatal studies.

Compared with barium, iodinated media are more expensive and generally produce less radiographic contrast. Iodinated media are not without risk either. They sometimes cause serious dehydration and are hazardous if aspirated. These media are therefore contraindicated for examinations of the esophagus or when a fistula connecting the esophagus and the trachea is suspected. The radiologist chooses which medium to use.

Air Contrast

Barium and iodine compounds provide positive contrast; that is, they absorb more radiation than surrounding tissues and make a white or light shadow on the radiograph. Air and gases, on the other hand, absorb less radiation and produce negative contrast, or dark shadows on the film. When used in combination for double-contrast GI examinations, the barium coats the mucosal lining of the alimentary canal while the air fills the lumen. The result is a high degree of contrast, which tends to enhance the visualization of the GI mucosa.

Glucagon

Glucagon was introduced in Chapter 8 as one of the drugs used to treat hypoglycemia. In addition to increasing the level of blood glucose, it causes relaxation of the smooth muscle of the gastrointestinal tract. This effect is useful as a diagnostic aid in examinations of the GI tract because it slows **peristalsis** (contractions that propel food through the digestive tract) and prevents cramping. Anticholinergic drugs such as atropine have a similar effect, but glucagon is most commonly used for this purpose due to a lower incidence of side effects.

Glucagon is a polypeptide hormone identical to human glucagon. It is supplied in lyophilized (freeze-dried) form as part of a kit that includes a diluent

TABLE 9-1

RECOMMENDATIONS FOR GLUCAGON ADMINISTRATION

DOSE	ROUTE OF ADMINISTRATION	TIME OF ONSET OF ACTION	APPROXIMATE DURATION OF EFFECT
0.25-0.5 mg (0.25-0.5 units)	IV	1 minute	9-17 minutes
1 mg (1 unit)	IM	8-10 minutes	12-27 minutes
2 mg* (2 units)	IV	1 minute	22-25 minutes
2 mg* (2 units)	IM	4-7 minutes	21-32 minutes

From *2001 Mosby's GenRx*, ed 11, p. III-1164, Table 1, St Louis, 2001, Harcourt Health Sciences.
*Administration of 2 mg (2 units) produces a higher incidence of nausea and vomiting than do lower doses.
IV, Intravenous; *IM,* intramuscular.

and specific instructions. The drug is mixed with the diluting solution immediately prior to use. When using glucagon, the following general instructions must be followed*:

- The diluent is provided for use only in the preparation of glucagon for parenteral injection and for no other use.
- Glucagon should not be used at concentrations greater than 1 mg/ml (1 unit/ml).
- Reconstituted glucagon should be used immediately. *Discard any unused portion.*
- Reconstituted glucagon solutions should be used only if they are clear and of a water-like consistency.
- Parenteral drug products should be inspected visually for particulate matter and discoloration before administration.

Table 9-1 lists recommended dosages, routes of administration, and anticipated timing of effects. Since the stomach is less sensitive to the effect of glucagon, 0.5 mg (0.5 units) IV or 2 mg (2 units) intramuscularly (IM) are recommended for examinations of the stomach, duodenum, and/or small bowel. For colon examinations, the recommended dose is 2 mg (2 units) IM approximately 10 minutes prior to the procedure. The most common side effect of glucagon administration is nausea and vomiting, which is most likely to occur with doses of 2 mg (2 units).

---

*From *2001 Mosby's GenRx*, ed 11, St Louis, 2001, Harcourt Health Sciences.

EXAMINATIONS OF LOWER GASTROINTESTINAL TRACT
Routine Barium Enema

A preliminary radiograph of the abdomen may be taken before the instillation of barium (Fig. 9-3). This "scout film" has diagnostic value from the radiologist's viewpoint and also provides technical assistance to the radiographer. In addition, it provides a further opportunity to assess the efficacy of the preparation. If fecal material is seen in the colon on this radiograph, further preparation may be required for an optimum study. If glucagon is routinely used, it is usually administered intramuscularly following evaluation of the preliminary radiograph. Colon relaxation and reduction of patient discomfort may allow the radiologist to perform a more satisfactory examination.

The administration of the barium enema is very similar to the procedure for the cleansing enema, with several significant exceptions:

- A larger amount of liquid is prepared for a barium enema than for a cleansing enema, usually 1200 to 1500 ml.
- The enema bag is suspended a greater distance above the table, usually 24 to 30 inches. This is necessary because the greater viscosity of the barium suspension requires greater hydrostatic pressure to maintain an adequate flow rate.
- A larger rectal catheter is used. This may be a disposable plastic enema tip or a disposable retention catheter with an inflatable cuff (Fig. 9-4).

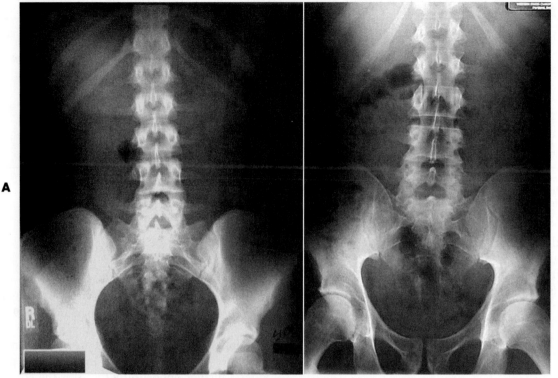

FIG. 9-3 Preliminary radiographs for barium enema examination. **A,** Good preparation results in very little gas or fecal matter within the abdomen. **B,** Extensive gas and fecal material demonstrate lack of adequate preparation.

The retention catheter helps the patient retain the barium for the duration of the study. Some radiology departments use retention catheters for all patients. In other facilities, the radiographer must decide when a retention catheter is required. Patients who are alert, competent, and cooperative may be more comfortable with a plain enema tip. Others may feel more secure with a retention cuff in place. The patient's expectation regarding enema retention may help the radiographer in deciding which tip to use. The cuff of the retention catheter is inflated with an air pump. Most disposable retention catheter kits include a disposable pump in the form of a plastic bag that is squeezed to inflate the cuff. Follow the directions provided with the unit. Overinflation of the catheter cuff may injure or rupture the rectum, which could be very hazardous to the patient.

This risk is minimized when the radiologist inflates the cuff under fluoroscopic control at the beginning of the procedure.

Place the patient in the lateral recumbent or Sims' position for insertion of the enema tip. Don protective gloves, and insert the lubricated tip as instructed for the cleansing enema. If a retention catheter is used, inflate the cuff unless it is the radiologist's practice to do so. After the tip is in place, the patient is placed in the supine position in readiness for the fluoroscopic study. The radiologist will indicate when to start and stop the barium flow. After fluoroscopy, routine radiographs are taken (Fig. 9-5).

When the study is complete, the tube may be removed and the patient escorted to the bathroom. If a retention catheter is used, be certain to deflate the cuff before attempting to remove the catheter.

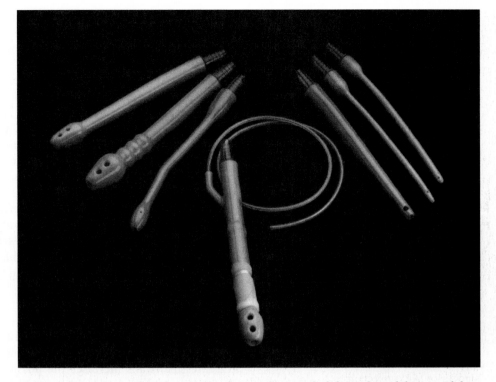

FIG. 9-4 An assortment of tips for enema catheters. Those on the left are plain adult tips, and those on the right are pediatric tips. At the center is an adult tip with an inflatable retention cuff.

In some cases it may be beneficial to place the bag below the level of the table and allow part of the barium to drain back into the bag before removing the catheter.

Most barium enema examinations include one or more postevacuation radiographs (Fig. 9-6). The best result is obtained when the patient has evacuated the barium as completely as possible. As with the cleansing enema, allow ample time for evacuation and encourage physical activity if appropriate.

Barium Enema Considerations and Precautions

Patients with colon enlargement

Patients with unusual conditions may require special care by the radiographer when undergoing a barium enema examination. Barium enema studies are important in diagnosis and evaluation of these conditions, but they may also prove hazardous.

One example is the patient with enlargement of the colon, often caused by chronic constipation. An extreme example of colon enlargement is the infant or child who has **congenital megacolon** (colon enlargement present at birth), also called **Hirschsprung's disease.** This condition involves a segment of distal colon in which no peristalsis occurs because of a neurological deficiency. This causes chronic constipation and resulting enlargement of the colon to an extreme degree (Fig. 9-7).

Whenever the colon is enlarged, the increased area of the mucosal lining provides greater opportunity for rapid, excessive absorption of water from the barium suspension. This predisposes these patients to barium impactions. An aqueous iodine contrast

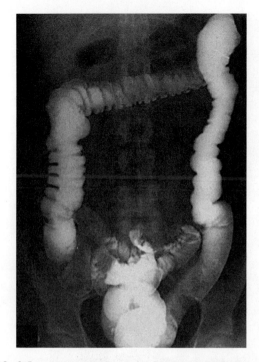

FIG. 9-5 Barium enema study demonstrates lumen of colon (anteroposterior [AP] projection).

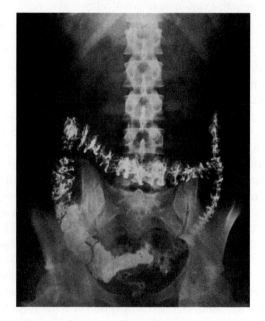

FIG. 9-6 Postevacuation radiograph demonstrates mucosal pattern of colon (posteroanterior [PA] projection).

may be used; if not, follow-up care to avoid impaction is essential. This may involve diet, forced fluids, cathartics, and/or cleansing enemas, similar to the preparation for the examination.

Colon enlargement may also cause excessive fluid absorption during a barium enema. On rare occasions this may result in a massive change in the fluid concentration in the blood, known as fluid overload or **hypervolemia.** While this is not common, you should be alert to the possibility with patients who have congestive heart failure. In such cases extreme fluid overload could lead to total physical collapse.

The hazards of excessive water absorption are minimized by mixing the barium with normal saline solution instead of tap water. **Normal saline** is a solution of 0.85% sodium chloride (table salt) in water and can be prepared by dissolving two level teaspoons of salt in 1 liter of tepid water.

Potential colon perforation

As previously mentioned, any condition that causes weakening, inflammation, or degradation of the intestinal walls increases the possibility that perforation of the colon could occur during enema administration. In the case of a barium enema, extravasation of barium into the peritoneal cavity causes a very serious complication known as barium peritonitis. Patients particularly at risk include the elderly, patients receiving long-term steroid medication, and those with diverticulitis or ulcerative colitis. Precautions involve lowering the enema bag to maintain a relatively low flow pressure and/or using aqueous iodinated media instead of barium, when indicated. A rigorous bowel preparation may not be appropriate for patients at risk of bowel perforation. In these cases, several days of clear liquid diet may be substituted for the usual preparation.

Ostomies

Another situation requiring special knowledge and skill in the performance of a barium enema involves patients with ostomies, that is, colostomies or ileostomies. These patients have undergone surgical resections of the colon for the treatment of disease, trauma, obstruction, or birth defect. As explained in Chapter 6, the distal end of the remaining functioning

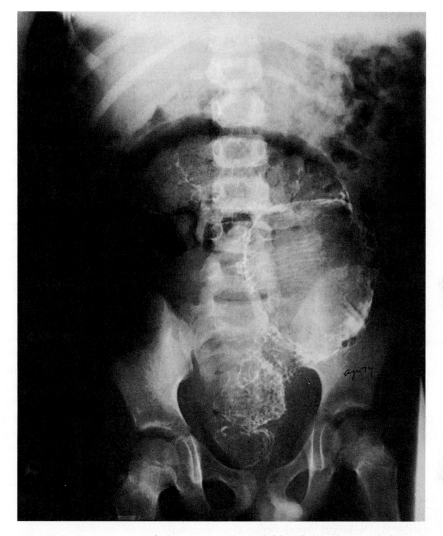

FIG. 9-7 Barium enema study (post evacuation): child with Hirschsprung's disease.

bowel (proximal colon or, if the entire colon has been removed, the distal ileum) terminates in an artificial opening in the abdominal wall called a stoma. The stoma appears as a small hole surrounded by a rosette of mucosal tissue similar in appearance to the lining of the mouth (Fig. 9-8). Since the patient has no voluntary control over the stoma, fecal matter is expelled through this opening automatically. In the case of a "double barrel" colostomy, there are two stomas, the distal end of the proximal

segment and the proximal end of the distal segment. Fecal matter is expelled from the proximal segment and mucus from the distal portion.

The location of the stoma is determined by the nature of the surgery and the size of the bowel portion that has been removed. Figure 9-9 illustrates the common types of colostomy and ileostomy and lists the characteristics of each that may be of concern to radiographers. To determine a patient's ostomy type, check the history section of the chart.

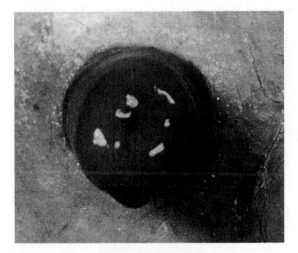

FIG. 9-8 Typical colostomy stoma.

For the sake of simplicity in the material that follows, we will refer to all of these artificial openings into the gastrointestinal tract as colostomies.

Colostomies may be temporary or permanent. Sometimes a temporary colostomy is done to allow the distal portion of the bowel to rest and heal. The remaining bowel portions may later be surgically reconnected (anastomosis). If the distal portion of the bowel must be removed, the colostomy is permanent.

Patients with colostomies must wear a colostomy bag, a receptacle that fits over the stoma and is sealed to the skin surrounding it. Appliances for this purpose are designed to receive fecal matter, minimize odor, and protect the skin surrounding the stoma. Fecal matter expelled from a colostomy may be highly odorous and irritating to the skin. The more proximal the colostomy, the more severe these problems tend to be. Patients with colostomies may be quite sensitive about this condition, and it is important to avoid any display of disgust or revulsion while caring for them. Until the procedure is sufficiently familiar to instill confidence, the student should work with an experienced radiographer.

Patients who have had a colostomy for any length of time are accustomed to performing their own colostomy care and are often most comfortable when they are allowed to empty their colostomy bag

and cleanse the area themselves. Many colostomy patients irrigate their stoma daily to initiate a bowel movement at a convenient time. This allows them to wear a smaller bag or simply a protective cover. If a cleansing enema is necessary, the competent colostomy patient may do a much more effective job than the radiographer. If you must perform an **irrigation** (cleansing enema) on a colostomy patient, the procedure is essentially the same as that for the barium enema (described in the following paragraphs), except that water is used instead of barium.

A special catheter is needed for the barium enema. A urinary retention (Foley) catheter may be used, since it is smaller than a rectal catheter and has a small inflatable cuff to hold it securely in place. Wearing disposable gloves, remove the colostomy bag and cleanse the area. Place the patient in the supine position, and lubricate the catheter tip. The catheter tip is inserted into the stoma approximately 4 to 6 inches and is held in position by inflating the cuff with a syringe. Catheter insertion and cuff inflation are usually performed by the radiologist. If it is your duty, insert the catheter gently and do not force it if you encounter any resistance. When the catheter is properly situated, use a syringe to inflate the catheter cuff to hold it snugly in place. Take care not to overinflate the cuff; 5 to 10 ml of air is usually sufficient. Special enema kits for colostomies are commercially available and may be used instead of the Foley catheter. The manufacturer's directions for such a kit, including illustrations, are shown in Fig. 9-10.

From 500 to 700 ml of barium is usually adequate for a colostomy enema. It is instilled under fluoroscopic control as the radiologist directs.

When the examination is complete, drain as much barium as possible back into the enema bag, deflate the catheter cuff, and remove the catheter. Provide the patient with an emesis basin or disposable colostomy bag in which to empty the barium. A suitable bag is a part of most disposable barium enema colostomy kits. If you are using this type of product, the bag will be in place during the examination.

The patient then requires the necessary supplies to cleanse the area and apply a fresh colostomy bag.

TYPES OF OSTOMIES

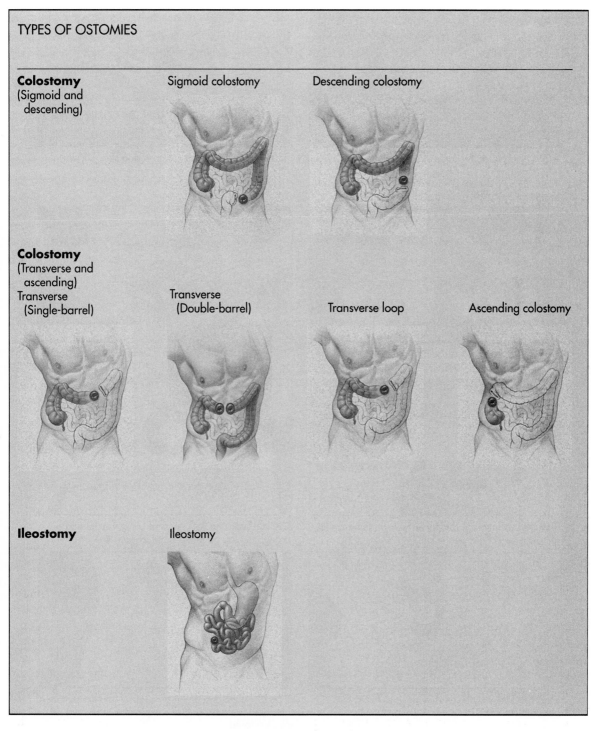

Colostomy (Sigmoid and descending)

Sigmoid colostomy

Descending colostomy

Colostomy (Transverse and ascending)

Transverse (Single-barrel)

Transverse (Double-barrel)

Transverse loop

Ascending colostomy

Ileostomy

Ileostomy

FIG. 9-9 Types of ostomies.

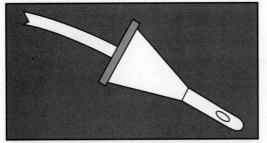

STEP 1 - Lubricate the catheter tip with the water soluble jelly (provided) and slide the catheter through the cone shield. Be sure the small end of the cone shield taper is pointing toward the blunt end of the catheter.

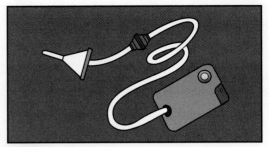

STEP 2 - Attach the catheter to a standard barium solution bag by using the 5-1 connector which is attached to the catheter.

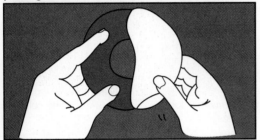

STEP 3 - Remove the release paper from the adhesive ring on the irrigation sleeve.

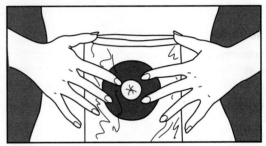

STEP 4 - Attach the irrigation sleeve to the skin around the stoma.

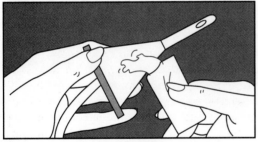

STEP 5 - Lubricate the soft cone shield with the water soluble jelly included in the kit.

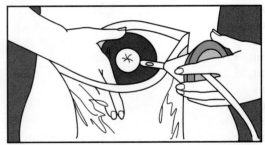

STEP 6 - Insert the catheter and cone into the stoma through the top opening of the irrigation sleeve.

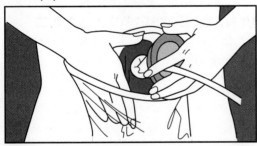

STEP 7 - Cone may be held in place to retain the barium.

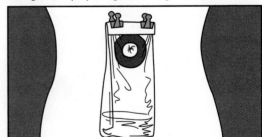

STEP 8 - At the end of the procedure, fold the bottom of the sleeve to its top and clip in place with the two (2) clips enclosed.

FIG. 9-10 Instructions for use of commercial barium enema colostomy kit.

Instructions should be given in advance to outpatients so that the necessary supplies can be brought from home to replace the colostomy bag after the examination. Instructions for assisting the patient to apply a fresh colostomy bag are given in Chapter 6.

Occasionally the distal portion of the remaining colon may be studied. For this part of the examination the procedure is the same as for any routine barium enema except that much less barium is needed. Following this study it may be necessary to irrigate the distal colon to remove the barium, since this part of the colon is no longer active in the elimination process.

Double-Contrast Barium Enema

Some radiologists prefer the enhanced visualization of the mucosal lining provided by double-contrast studies for some or all of the colon examinations they perform (Fig. 9-11). A special barium mixture may be purchased for this purpose, or a preparation is thoroughly mixed to provide a suspension that is very smooth and somewhat thicker than for single-contrast studies. After the colon is filled, examined, and partially evacuated, air is instilled via the enema tip using a special insufflation device or an air pump such as the bulb used with a sphygmomanometer. Air must be instilled slowly to avoid cramping and patient discomfort. After the study the patient returns to the bathroom to evacuate the air and any residual barium.

Disposable double-contrast enema kits are available commercially. After routine instillation of barium, these kits allow barium to be siphoned back into the bag by lowering the bag below the height of the table. Thus evacuation is accomplished without removing the patient from the fluoroscopic table. Air retained in the bag may then be instilled into the colon by turning the bag upside down and squeezing it gently. Some kits are supplied with a special enema tip that has a double lumen, allowing separate passages for air and barium and providing better control of air instillation.

Defecography

Defecography is a procedure for the evaluation of patients with defecational dysfunction. It is also

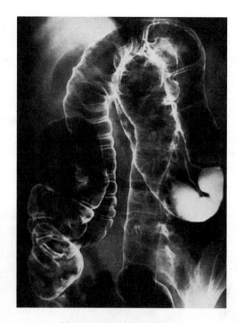

FIG. 9-11 Double-contrast barium enema enhances visualization of mucosal pattern (oblique projection).

known as evacuation proctography or dynamic rectal examination.

Kits for this procedure include a high-density barium sulfate paste with a special injector to instill the barium. No patient preparation is needed. After the barium is instilled into the rectum, the patient is seated on a special radiolucent commode in front of the fluoroscopic unit. Video recording or serial spot films of the defecation process produce images in the lateral projection.

UPPER GASTROINTESTINAL STUDIES
Routine Upper Gastrointestinal Series

An upper GI series is a fluoroscopic and radiographic examination of the esophagus, stomach, and duodenum. Barium is usually the contrast medium for this study and is administered orally. Patient preparation is usually quite simple, consisting of an NPO order for approximately 8 hours before the examination. Some radiologists prefer that patients not smoke on the day of the examination, since smoking may increase gastric secretions, resulting in liquid dilution of the contrast medium in the stomach. Chewing gum is avoided for the same reason. Fig. 9-12 demonstrates the importance of adequate preparation for an upper GI study.

The examination usually begins with the fluoroscopic table in the upright position and the patient standing on the footboard. While that patient drinks the barium, the radiologist observes the fluoroscopic image of the esophagus. The table is then placed in the horizontal position and the recumbent patient is turned into various positions to coat the lining of the stomach and to demonstrate all aspects of the mucosal lining of the stomach and proximal duodenum. The table may also be placed in the Trendelenburg position and the patient asked to stop breathing and bear down as if having a bowel movement. This is called the **Valsalva maneuver** and is sometimes useful in the diagnosis of **hiatal hernia** (protrusion of a portion of the stomach through the diaphragm into the thoracic cavity).

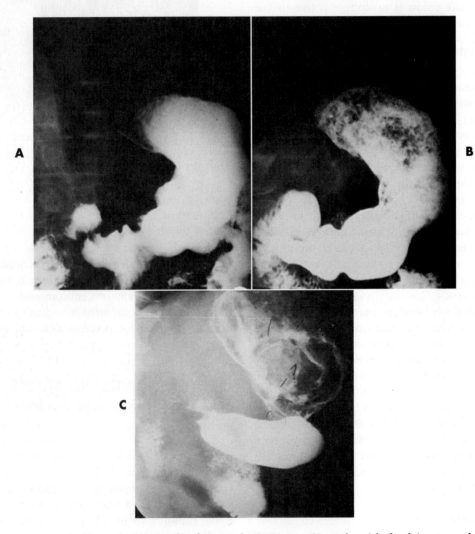

FIG. 9-12 **A,** Normal radiograph of stomach. **B,** Upper GI study with food in stomach. **C,** Cancer of stomach. Note similarity of appearance of **B** and **C**.

The patient care role of the radiographer in this examination consists of preliminary explanations and instructions, handing the patient the cup of barium, receiving the cup when the patient has finished it, and assisting the patient to assume various positions as directed by the radiologist during fluoroscopy. Occasionally the examination is delayed when the barium in the stomach does not empty into the duodenum because of **pylorospasm** (constriction of the sphincter muscle between the stomach and the duodenum). In this event it is helpful to place the patient in the right anterior oblique position, which allows gravity to assist the normal flow of gastric contents. Following the fluoroscopic examination, routine radiographs are taken.

Double-contrast upper gastrointestinal study

Double-contrast examination is a more frequently used method to evaluate the upper GI tract. It enhances visualization of the mucosal surface (Fig. 9-13) and involves several variations in procedure. At the beginning of the examination, the patient is given a gas-producing substance in the form of a tablet, powder, or carbonated beverage. This is followed by a small amount of a high-density barium mixture. The patient may feel the need to belch but should not do so, since the gas must be retained in the stomach to provide radiographic contrast.

Glucagon may be injected IM or IV before examination to induce relaxation of the stomach and duodenum to improve visualization. The technical aspects of this fluoroscopic and radiographic procedure are essentially the same as for the routine upper GI series.

Hypotonic Duodenography

This examination is useful for the detection of lesions in the duodenum distal to the duodenal bulb and for the diagnosis of pancreatic disease. It involves passing a tube through the mouth or nose and into the duodenum after the administration of glucagon to relax the GI tract and halt peristalsis. Barium and air are injected through the tube via syringe to provide radiographic contrast. The procedure is similar to

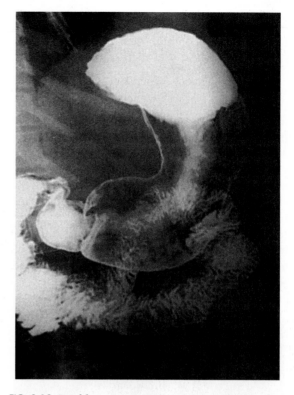

FIG. 9-13 Double-contrast upper gastrointestinal study.

the enteroclysis examination of the small bowel discussed in the following section, the differences being the placement of the tube and the extent of bowel to be evaluated. The use of this study is declining and is being replaced by ultrasound studies and double-contrast upper GI examinations for duodenal visualization and by CT studies, needle biopsy, or endoscopic retrograde cholangiopancreatography (ERCP) for pancreatic evaluation. These imaging methods are discussed in Chapters 10 and 12.

SMALL BOWEL STUDIES

There are three methods of introducing contrast into the small bowel for radiographic evaluation: oral, complete reflux filling, and enteroclysis, or small intestine enema, in which an intestinal tube is used to instill the contrast.

Oral Method

By far the most common method of studying the small bowel is the oral method. For this study, the patient drinks the barium suspension and a series of timed radiographs follows its progress through the small bowel. The first radiograph is usually taken 15 minutes after the ingestion of the barium, and subsequent films are taken at 15- to 30-minute intervals until the entire small bowel is visualized (Fig. 9-14). Fluoroscopy with spot films may be utilized at any time during the procedure to study portions of the intestine as they become opacified with the contrast medium. Ice water, coffee, tea, or a food stimulant may be used to increase intestinal motility and speed the filling of the small bowel. Often this procedure follows an upper GI series, utilizing a single dose of barium for both studies. A limited study of the small bowel may be a routine part of the upper GI series, consisting of a single radiograph of the abdomen taken 30 to 60 minutes after barium ingestion.

Complete Reflux Method

A complete reflux examination of the small bowel is accomplished by retrograde flow using essentially the same method as for the barium enema (Fig. 9-15). A large volume (4500 ml) of thin barium is needed to fill the colon and the small intestine. Glucagon may be given to relax the intestine in preparation for this procedure. Diazepam is also sometimes prescribed to help the patient relax and cope with the discomfort associated with the filling of the bowel. The barium is instilled under fluoroscopic control. The enema bag is lowered to drain the colon, and radiographs are then taken.

Enteroclysis

Enteroclysis is the injection of nutrient or medicinal liquid into the small bowel. For the radiographic

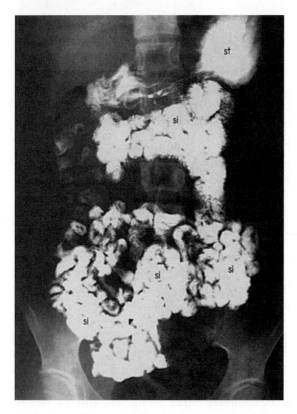

FIG. 9-14 Small intestine demonstrated 30 minutes after oral ingestion of barium.

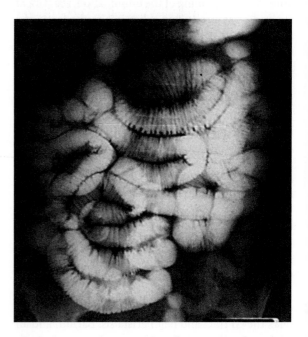

FIG. 9-15 Normal retrograde reflux examination of the small intestine.

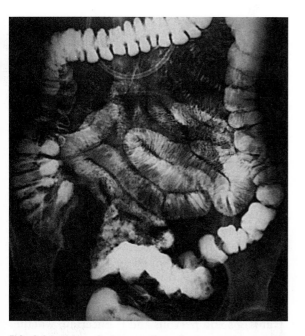

FIG. 9-16 Enteroclysis procedure demonstrates contrast filling of both small bowel and colon.

procedure, a special catheter with a stiff wire guide (Bilbao or Sellink tube) is advanced to the distal portion of the duodenum, and barium is injected through the tube under fluoroscopic control. The flow rate should be approximately 100 ml per minute. Fluoroscopy and spot film radiography are followed by routine radiographs (Fig. 9-16). Once the contrast has reached the cecum, air or methylcellulose may be injected through the tube to provide double contrast.

Thorough cleansing of both the large and small bowel is essential to the success of the enteroclysis study and must be accomplished without the use of enemas, because enema fluid may be retained in the small bowel and degrade the quality of the visualization. The routine preparation is usually a combination of diet and cathartics.

FOLLOW-UP CARE

As mentioned earlier, bowel care is very important after all barium studies because of the tendency of barium to clump and harden in the bowel. This may cause constipation and, in severe cases, barium impaction with resulting bowel obstruction. To prevent these complications, patients should be instructed to increase their intake of fluids and high-bulk foods following barium examinations. It is also a common practice to administer a cathartic preparation following the examination. This may be a liquid, such as milk of magnesia or citrate of magnesia, or a tablet, such as bisacodyl. For inpatients, this is often given by the nursing service when the patient returns to the unit. For outpatients, the radiographer may administer the cathartic when the examination is completed, or the patient may simply be instructed to take a laxative on returning home.

If the departmental policy is merely to prescribe a laxative and leave its procurement and administration to the patient, the radiographer must be very specific when explaining the rationale for this instruction. Otherwise, the patient who has just undergone a major catharsis in preparation for the examination may not feel inclined to follow the advice and may not follow through as directed. In some hospitals it has been found that the most effective method of ensuring compliance is for the radiographer to administer the cathartic to every outpatient on completion of the examination. If this is your duty, use the method for oral administration of medication described in Chapter 7.

CONCLUSION

Radiographic and fluoroscopic examinations of the gastrointestinal tract frequently require preparation by diet, cathartics, suppositories, and/or enemas. Radiographers prepare barium sulfate suspensions that are then administered orally or rectally to enhance soft tissue contrast for adequate visualization. The radiographer may be responsible for scheduling examinations and for providing instructions for preparation and follow-up care that will best serve the diagnostic requirements and the patient's physical needs. Precautions are needed to reduce the risk of adverse effects from both the preparations and the procedures.

REVIEW QUESTIONS

1. Preparation for an upper GI series usually involves:
   A. cathartics
   B. suppositories
   C. enemas
   D. nothing by mouth for 8 hours
   E. all of the above
2. A medication used to slow peristalsis and prevent cramping for GI studies is:
   A. glucose
   B. glucagon
   C. Glucophage
   D. Gastrografin
   E. barium sulfate
3. A position that assists the gravity flow of barium from the stomach is:
   A. supine
   B. prone
   C. right anterior oblique
   D. left anterior oblique
   E. left posterior oblique
4. Oral administration, reflux filling, and enteroclysis are three methods of administering the contrast medium for examination of the:
   A. esophagus
   B. stomach
   C. small bowel
   D. colon
   E. rectum
5. Follow-up care after an upper GI series or other barium study usually involves:
   A. a clear liquid diet
   B. cleansing enemas
   C. a cathartic such as citrate of magnesia
   D. a suppository
   E. glucagon

CRITICAL THINKING EXERCISES

1. Leah McKelvey calls from Dr. Rahaman's office to schedule a series of examinations for Martha Logan. Ms. Logan needs to have a chest x-ray, an intravenous urogram, and an upper GI series. She also needs to stop by the clinical laboratory to have fasting blood samples drawn for multiple blood chemistry tests. Leah wants to know whether this can all be done on the same day. Is this possible? Explain to Leah the advantages and disadvantages of scheduling these exams on one day, compared to two or more separate appointments. In what order should these examinations be done?
2. Eleanor Buss, age 70, is an outpatient and has just arrived for her barium enema appointment with her daughter, who will be waiting to drive her home after the procedure. She seems to be very anxious and nervous and is uncertain whether she wants to have the examination. List possible causes of Mrs. Buss's anxiety. What would you say to her?
3. Richard Meyerson, age 42, stops by the radiology department to arrange an appointment for a barium enema examination. The history on his requisition form states that Mr. Meyerson had colon surgery 6 months ago and has a sigmoid colostomy. Explain to Mr. Meyerson what will be involved, how he should prepare, and what he should bring with him to the examination.
4. Nathan Purdy, age 55, is scheduled for a barium enema. Upon reviewing the scout film, the radiologist notes that there is excessive fecal material in the colon and instructs you to reschedule the examination. Tell Mr. Purdy why the examination must be rescheduled, and explain what he must do to ensure a good result.

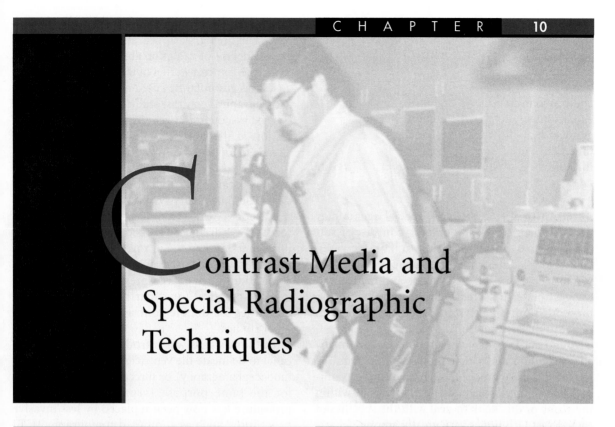

Contrast Media and Special Radiographic Techniques

At the conclusion of this chapter, the student will be able to:

- Name four types of contrast media and give two examples and two applications for each.
- List four types of adverse responses to contrast medium injection.
- Demonstrate how to take an appropriate history prior to injection of an iodine contrast medium.
- Describe the radiographer's role in performing an intravenous urogram.
- List steps to be taken in preparation for an oral cholecystogram.

- Name the blood chemistry tests that may be significant in patients having cholecystography and those scheduled for urography.
- Describe three methods used to introduce contrast media into the biliary system.
- Describe the procedure for the injection of contrast media for myelography.

aqueous	ionic
arthrography	manometer
bolus	myelography
cholecystectomy	nephrogram
cholecystitis	nonionic
cystogram	osmolality
diuretic	stent
intrathecal	

AS CHAPTER 9 HAS SHOWN, special agents may be used to enhance radiographic contrast of soft tissues. Among these are barium sulfate, air, gases, and various iodine compounds. Chapter 9 discusses primarily barium sulfate products and their use in the gastrointestinal tract. This chapter focuses on procedures using contrast media other than barium outside the gastrointestinal system. Special knowledge and skill in patient preparation, contrast media administration, and patient monitoring are required to perform these procedures. Some of these examinations are very sophisticated, and it is not within the scope of this book to deal with the specifics of each. Exact techniques vary greatly among departments and radiologists, and procedures are subject to frequent change. Some of these studies, however, are so integral to the radiographer's work that they are performed routinely. A more thorough understanding of them will help you form the judgments required for professional performance in these situations.

CONTRAST MEDIA
Air and Gases

As discussed in Chapter 1, the mass density or atomic weight of a substance determines the degree to which it will attenuate radiation. Air and gases are very light and therefore absorb x-rays to a significantly lesser degree than do soft tissues; as a result, structures containing gases appear black or very dark on a radiograph. This appearance is referred to as negative contrast, and air and gases are called negative contrast agents. Cavities filled with air demonstrate a clear outline of the surrounding soft tissues, which have a lighter gray appearance because of their greater degree of radiation absorption. In addition to double-contrast studies of the colon and stomach, air or gas is sometimes used as a contrast agent in **arthrography** (contrast studies of joints). Gas may be used as a contrast agent in **myelography** (visualization of the spinal canal) for patients who are allergic to iodinated contrast media. Gas is also used to fill the peritoneal cavity for fiberoptic studies of various organs, including the female reproductive system and the biliary system.

Carbon dioxide (CO_2) has clear advantages over room air as a diagnostic gas because the body absorbs it much faster than the nitrogen in air. CO_2 is commercially available in small cartridges for individual applications or in a large, pressurized cylinder that is more practical for departments that use large quantities for double-contrast enemas as well as other studies.

In the past, gas was introduced into the spinal canal to delineate the ventricles of the brain (pneumoencephalography) or directly into the ventricles for the same purpose (ventriculography). This procedure has now been replaced by less invasive procedures, such as computed tomography (CT) and magnetic resonance examinations.

Iodinated Media

Most organs and blood vessels have x-ray absorption characteristics very similar to those of the surrounding soft tissues. This causes their radiographic images to be only faintly distinguishable, if visible at all. With an atomic number of 53 and a mass number of 127, iodine is a heavy element compared to the composition of the body. Iodine compounds therefore absorb radiation to a greater degree than blood or soft tissues, causing any organ or blood vessel that contains the contrast agent to stand out by appearing white or much lighter than the surrounding tissues. This is referred to as positive contrast, the opposite of the dark or negative contrast seen with air or gas. Using iodine compounds, many different structures can be delineated more clearly than with plain film radiography.

Most iodinated contrast agents are **aqueous;** that is, water is the principal solvent for the iodine compound. These agents mix readily with blood and other body fluids.

Table 10-1 lists procedures that use contrast agents. Appendix I provides an extensive list of contrast agents used for diagnostic imaging. Specific information on content, strength, contraindications, and precautions for all of these products can be found in the drug package inserts.

Ethiodized Oils

Oily iodine compounds called ethiodized oils are specialized contrast agents that were developed for studies in which absorption of contrast into the surrounding tissues, or mixing of contrast with body fluids, is not desired. At one time oil-based iodine media were commonly used in bronchography and myelography as well as other studies, but other imaging methods and the newer aqueous iodine agents have replaced oily media for most applications. The principal use of ethiodized oil today is for lymphography. It is injected into the lymphatic vessels to visualize these vessels and the lymph nodes. This procedure is primarily used to evaluate the clinical extent of lymphomas, and the most commonly used product is Ethiodol. Other imaging modalities such as CT are more commonly used today for the diagnosing and staging of lymphomas.

Because oil-based iodine media tend to decompose when exposed to light, heat, or air, they must be properly stored and checked for any sign of decomposition before they are used. The following precautions should be observed with any oil-based iodine media:

- Store in a cool, dark place.
- Check the expiration date prior to use.
- Check the color. When fresh, these agents are clear with a pale amber or yellow color. Darkening of the normal coloration indicates decomposition; media that have changed color should not be used.
- Use glass syringes for injection of oil-based contrast agents, since the media can dissolve toxic substances from the plastic composition of disposable syringes.

Since oil-based media are not miscible with body fluids, they are not readily absorbed and excreted and tend to persist in the body for long periods, which is not usually a problem. Although you should be prepared for an allergic reaction when any medication or contrast agent is given, allergic reactions to iodized oils are extremely rare. Inflammation in the area of injection may occur, especially if there is extravasation during lymphography or the injection of small ducts, but adverse reactions are infrequent and rarely of serious consequence.

Water-Soluble Iodine Compounds

Water-soluble (aqueous) iodine compounds are by far the most frequently used contrast agents other than barium. These media are stocked in the radiology department in a wide variety of types, volumes, and strengths. Although some of these products are approved for one specific purpose, many have broader application. These multipurpose agents may be administered intravenously for urography, intra-arterially for angiography (visualization of vessels), or injected directly into the structures to be visualized, such as the common bile duct for cholangiography or the joint capsule for arthrography.

A **bolus** of contrast refers to a substantial intravenous (IV) dose delivered at once. A bolus may be injected directly using a syringe with an IV catheter or butterfly set, or an infusion of the medium may be administered in a diluted form through an IV drip. Either method, or both, may be employed for contrast enhancement when doing CT scans.

All water-soluble iodine contrast media are carbon-based organic chemicals composed of molecules containing iodine atoms and various combinations of other atoms. These molecules vary in size, and some contain more iodine atoms than others. Appendix J provides illustrations of the chemical structure of typical molecules. These products differ with respect to certain characteristics of their strength and chemical nature that affect their clinical performance. These characteristics include iodine concentration, osmolality, viscosity, and toxicity.

Iodine concentration determines the degree to which the medium will attenuate x-rays, with

TABLE 10-1

IMAGING STUDIES USING CONTRAST MEDIA

EXAMINATION	ROUTE OF ADMINISTRATION	STRUCTURES VISUALIZED	EXAMPLES OF CONTRAST MEDIA USED
Angiography			
Aortography	Arterial catheter	Abdominal or thoracic aorta	Omnipaque 350, Optiray 350
Angiocardiography	Arterial catheter	Heart and surrounding great vessels	Imagopaque 350, Iomeron 350, Visipaque 320
Digital subtraction angiography (DSA)	Arterial catheter	Cerebral vasculature, aorta and branches	Iomeron 300, Imagopaque 350, Omnipaque 140
Digital subtraction angiography (DSA)	Intravenous	Cerebral vasculature, aorta and branches	Iomeron 350, Conray-43
Peripheral arteriography	Arterial catheter	Arteries of the extremities	Visipaque, Hexabrix, Isovue-300, MD-76
Peripheral venography	Intravenous	Veins of the extremities	Conray-43, Imagopaque 200 or 250, Visipaque 270
Cerebral angiography	Arterial catheter	Cerebral vasculature	Optiray 240, Visipaque 270
Selective visceral arteriography	Arterial catheter	Renal, celiac, splenic, or coronary arteries, for example	Hexabrix, Imagopaque 300, MD-76, Optiray 320
Biliary System			
Cholangiography, operative and postoperative	Direct injection via T tube	Common bile duct	Conray, Reno-60, Hypaque Meglumine 60%, Hypaque 76
Cholecystography	Oral	Gallbladder	Telepaque, Oragrafin Capsules, Oragrafin Granules
Endoscopic retrograde cholangiopan-creatography (ERCP)	Catheter via endoscope	Common bile duct and pancreatic duct	Conray, Reno-60, Hypaque Meglumine 60%, Hypaque 76
Percutaneous transhepatic cholangiography (PTC)	Direct injection	Common bile duct	Conray, Reno-60, Hypaque Meglumine 60%, Hypaque 76
Spinal Studies			
Myelography	Intrathecal injection via lumbar puncture	Spinal canal (subarachnoid space)	Omnipaque 180, Isovue 200, Isovue 300
Discography	Direct injection	Intervertebral disk	Conray, Reno-60, Hypaque Meglumine 60%, Hypaque 76
Urinary Tract Studies			
Excretory urography	Intravenous	Kidneys, ureters, and bladder	Iomeron 350, MD-76, Optiray 240, Reno-60, Reno-Dip (infusion), Conray-43, Hypaque 60%

TABLE 10-1

IMAGING STUDIES USING CONTRAST MEDIA—cont'd

EXAMINATION	ROUTE OF ADMINISTRATION	STRUCTURES VISUALIZED	EXAMPLES OF CONTRAST MEDIA USED
Retrograde urography	Ureteral catheter via cystoscope	Kidney pelves, calyces, and ureters	Hypaque-Cysto 30%, Iomeron 200, Cysto-Conray II, Cystografin, Reno-30
Cystourethrography	Direct injection via Foley catheter	Urinary bladder, urethra	Hypaque-Cysto 30%, Iomeron 200, Cysto-Conray II, Cystografin, Reno-30
Gastrointestinal Studies			
Esophagram	Oral administration	Esophagus	Barium sulfate products
Upper GI series	Oral administration	Esophagus, stomach, and duodenum	Barium sulfate products, Gastrografin, Hypaque Sodium Oral Powder, MD-Gastroview
Lower GI series	Rectal administration	Colon	Barium sulfate products, Hypaque Sodium, Gastrografin, MD-Gastroview
Small bowel series	Oral administration or enteroclysis	Small intestines	Barium sulfate products, Gastrografin, Hypaque Sodium Oral Powder, MD-Gastroview
Miscellaneous Studies			
Arthrography	Direct injection	Joints (e.g., knee, shoulder, ankle)	Conray, Visipaque 320, Hypaque Meglumine 60%, Hypaque 76
Computed tomography (CT)	Intravenous	Contrast enhancement of anatomy examined	Imagopaque 300, Conray-30
Computed tomography (CT)	Oral administration	Contrast enhancement of gastrointestinal tract	Gastrografin, Hypaque Sodium Oral Powder, MD-Gastroview
Hysterosalpingography	Direct injection via cervical cannula	Uterus and fallopian tubes	Iomeron 300, Sinografin
Lymphography	Direct injection into lymphatic vessels in feet	Lymph vessels and lymph nodes	Ethiodol
Magnetic resonance imaging (MRI)	Intravenous	Brain, spinal cord, vascular structures	Magnevist, ProHance (These paramagnetic agents are not iodinated.)

higher concentrations producing a greater degree of positive radiographic contrast. Many different concentrations of contrast agents are available, and the concentration required for a given application depends largely upon the degree to which it will be diluted by body fluids. For example, a high concentration is needed to study the aorta, where dilution by a large volume of blood is a factor, whereas a lower concentration is adequate for the visualization of veins and smaller arteries. Greater concentrations have a greater viscosity and greater osmolality and tend to be more toxic.

Osmolality refers to the number of particles in solution per kilogram of water. The osmolality of human blood is about 300 milliosmoles per kilogram (mOsm/kg), whereas the osmolality of water-soluble contrast media ranges from 600 mOsm/kg to more than 1000 mOsm/kg. Compounds that contain more iodine atoms per molecule can provide the desired contrast with fewer molecules and therefore will have a lower osmolality. Since osmolality is largely responsible for the adverse effects of contrast media, risk is reduced when osmolality is lowered.

Some contrast media molecules dissociate into two charged particles when placed in solution, resulting in higher osmolality. This process is called ionization, and media whose molecules dissociate in this way are termed **ionic.** Media whose molecules remain whole in solution are termed **nonionic.**

To compare the relative osmolality of both ionic and nonionic contrast agents, it is helpful to use a ratio of the number of iodine atoms to the number of particles. For instance, a compound with a ratio of 3:2 would contain three iodine atoms and would dissociate into two particles in solution. When the ratio is divided, the numerical value is 1.5. Compare this with a medium that has six atoms of iodine in each molecule and is nonionic; it would have a 6:1 ratio, or a numerical value 6. The higher the numerical value of the ratio, the lower the osmolality for a given iodine concentration.

Viscosity is a measure of the resistance of fluid to flow. Liquids with a high viscosity are sometimes described as "thick" or "syrupy," while those with low viscosity may be thought of as "thin" or "watery." Viscosity is determined by the number of particles in solution, the size of the particles, and the attractions among the particles. Agents with high iodine concentrations tend to be more viscous. Viscosity is also affected by the specific nature of the molecule. This characteristic is an important consideration in determining flow rate, injection time, and needle size. Solutions with high viscosity require greater injection pressures for administration. Viscosity may be reduced somewhat by warming the medium to body temperature before injection.

The toxicity of a contrast medium on body tissues and organs is related to the chemical configuration of the molecules, the iodine concentration, the osmolality, ionization characteristics, the rate of injection, and the dosage administered. Contrast media that are nonionic, have low osmolality with low iodine concentration, and are injected slowly tend to be less toxic and are less likely to result in adverse reactions or side effects. Intra-arterial injections tend to produce fewer toxic effects than do intravenous injections.

Two common, versatile water-soluble iodine compounds are diatrizoate meglumine and diatrizoate sodium. Each chemical has advantageous properties. The sodium salts are made up of relatively small molecules and contain more iodine per molecule, so that in equal concentrations they are more radiopaque than their meglumine counterparts. Meglumine (methylglucamine) salts are somewhat less toxic and are more soluble in water. They are also more viscous. Some contrast agents, such as Renografin-60 and Hypaque 76, contain both chemicals. These agents, which have been in use for decades, are ionic compounds and are now referred to as high-osmolar contrast agents (HOCAs) because of their relatively high osmolality compared with the newer generation of water-soluble iodine contrast media.

In the 1980s low-osmolar contrast agents (LOCAs) were introduced to the radiology market. Although these products were ionic, they delivered a relatively high concentration of iodine with fewer particles in solution than conventional contrast media. The first of these agents was metrizamide (Amipaque), and its primary application was for **intrathecal** (within the spinal canal) injection for myelography. Metrizamide was followed by LOCAs for multipurpose use, such as meglumine ioxaglate (Hexabrix). Many newer LOCAs are also nonionic. Examples include iopamidol (Isovue, Niopam) and iohexol (Omnipaque). These agents are less toxic than conventional contrast media and are less likely to stimulate an anaphylactic response. They are also more comfortable for the patient, producing less heat and discomfort when injected. They are particularly desirable for angiographic cardiac catheterization studies (special procedures where a contrast medium is injected via catheter to demonstrate the coronary arteries of the heart) because they are less likely to cause irregularities in cardiac function.

Risk factors that may influence the choice or dosage of media include any history of compromised renal, cardiac, or respiratory function and a history of allergies. The weight given to various risk factors varies with the institution and physicians involved. Nonionic contrast agents and other LOCA products were very expensive when they were first introduced. Today, however, these agents are comparable in cost to HOCA products. For this reason, most radiology departments are now using LOCAs for most procedures and for all patients whose allergy history or physical condition places them at greater risk.

Pharmacodynamics and adverse responses

When water-soluble media are injected intravascularly, they circulate in the blood and are excreted by the kidneys. When injected into other structures, they are absorbed gradually into the bloodstream before being excreted. The adverse reactions that occur in response to contrast media injections may range from mild and transient to severe and life threatening. The pharmacodynamics of contrast media responses involve the effects of osmolality, ionization, and molecular toxicity.

Osmolality affects the body as a result of tissue response to osmotic pressure. Since water passes through cell membranes in the direction of highest particle concentration (osmosis), media with higher osmolality tend to cause dehydration of blood cells and of the cells of the blood vessels and surrounding tissues. Subsequent circulation causes a reversal of this process, producing changes in hemodynamics, in the red blood cells, and in the capillary lining. This may cause adverse changes in pulmonary artery pressure, blood volume, and cardiac output.

Ionization also affects toxicity and is a factor to be considered when ionic media are used. The central nervous system is sensitive to increased levels of ions in the blood, which may interfere with the normal electrical activity of the body. The resulting risk includes the possibility of seizures and cardiac dysfunction. Generalized effects frequently seen in response to ionic media include a sensation of warmth spreading throughout the body, lightheadedness, nausea, and vomiting.

The release of histamine, causing allergic or anaphylactoid responses, is not the result of antigens in the blood and does not occur in anesthetized patients. This suggests a central nervous system response. Since ionic media have a much more powerful effect on the central nervous system than nonionic media, ionization may also account for the higher incidence of allergic responses to ionic media.

Toxicity may occur as a result of excessive dose or failure of the renal system to excrete the media. It may also result when a contrast medium is combined with an incompatible medication. When iodine media are mixed directly with incompatible medications, the contrast agent may undergo a chemical change, resulting in solid particles that precipitate with potential for very serious consequences. Research has not established the results of all possible combinations of contrast agents and medications, but precipitate formation has been noted with some combinations of contrast media and the following common medications: diphenhydramine, papaverine HCl, cimetidine, and protamine. To avoid the possibility of this complication, flush the intravenous or arterial catheter with saline before and after the injection of the contrast medium.

Precautions

Since procedures involving intravenous, intra-arterial, or intrathecal administration of iodine contrast clearly involve risk, an informed consent is usually required, and a careful history is essential. Patients may have allergic reactions to contrast agents because of sensitivity to iodine or some other component of the contrast medium. Toxic responses, mild or severe, may occur in patients with poor heart or kidney function, or may result from an overdose of the contrast agent.

Renal failure or compromised renal function impairs the patient's ability to eliminate the contrast and may result in a toxic response. As stated in Chapter 6, urea and creatinine are products of cellular metabolism that are excreted by the kidneys, and high blood levels of these substances indicate impaired renal function. Therefore radiographers must check the blood chemistry section of inpatient charts to ensure that the blood urea nitrogen (BUN) and creatinine levels are within normal limits. The usual normal ranges for adults are considered to be approximately, 7 to 18 mg/dl for BUN, and 0.6 to 1.5 mg/dl for creatinine. Creatinine levels of 2.0 mg/dl or greater constitute a contraindication for administration of iodine contrast agents. Report abnormal test levels to the radiologist before the administration of iodinated contrast. With outpatients, screen for history of kidney failure, kidney disease, or diabetes, and report positive responses. The policies of many institutions state that elderly patients and those with histories of kidney problems or diabetes must have BUN and creatinine tests prior to contrast administration.

Patients with diabetes must be identified because this disease predisposes the patient to renal complications. It is especially important to be alert for the possibility that diabetic patients may be taking medications containing metformin hydrochloride, such as Glucophage, Glucovance, Metaglip, or Avandamet, which are agents prescribed to manage hyperglycemia. Metformin products must be withheld on the day the contrast medium is administered and for at least 48 hours afterward. At that point, metformin therapy is only resumed if the attending physician has determined through testing that the patient's renal function is normal. Diabetic patients may suffer acute renal failure as a result of the contrast medium. With inadequate kidney function, metformin could build to dangerous levels in the blood, causing lactic acidosis, a change in blood pH that is potentially fatal.

Contrast agents cause vasodilation, which may produce dangerous changes in blood pressure and cardiac output. Radiographers must identify patients with heart disease before contrast administration because these patients are at greater risk of adverse response.

Since excessive doses of contrast media may have a toxic affect, it is a radiographer's duty to ensure that maximum dosages of contrast agents are not exceeded. While overdose of a contrast agent is unlikely when routine procedures are followed for a single examination, overdose may become an issue when injections must be repeated due to errors or problems in angiographic studies, or when there are multiple examinations. Since several different departments may use iodine contrast (e.g., radiography, cardiovascular laboratory, CT), patients may be scheduled for more than one contrast examination in a limited period. For instance, a patient brought to the emergency department with flank pain may be suspected of having a kidney stone and sent to the imaging department for an excretory urogram. If this study is negative, the patient may be admitted and transferred to the care of another physician, who orders a CT scan of the abdomen. The contrast dose for multiple procedures may exceed the 24-hour maximum dose. Ideally, records are kept, transferred with the patient, and read by those who order additional tests, but it is essential for the radiographer to check the patient's chart and to double-check by asking the patient whether any other tests have been done recently. Recent contrast examinations should be brought to the attention of the radiologist, who will determine whether the proposed study would result in an overdose.

As discussed in Chapter 6, the history you take must document allergies. Of particular concern are previous allergic responses to medication, especially to contrast agents, and a history of asthma. Patients who have experienced asthmatic attacks in the past are three times more likely than others to respond to contrast with an anaphylactoid reaction.

Another common history question involves any routine medications the patient may be taking. Radiologists sometimes want to know whether the patient is taking beta-blockers or antihypertensive drugs. A statement of routine medications may provide clues to various conditions of interest for which the patient is being treated.

While some radiologists prefer to take the history themselves, some institutions use a written form for this purpose. A summary of essential elements for a precontrast history is provided in Box 10-1. If the patient's history suggests a high risk of allergic response, a nonionic contrast medium may be indicated and/or the procedure may be preceded by the administration of an antihistamine or corticosteroid drug to reduce the risk of reaction.

If the patient has a history of allergy to iodine and has not been premedicated, the procedure will be cancelled and perhaps another imaging modality will be substituted.

Since most allergic responses occur within a very short time after injection, a minute amount of the contrast medium may be injected intravenously, followed by a pause during which the patient is observed carefully. If no symptoms are noted, the injection is then continued. The radiographer must be prepared to respond to a reaction from the test dose, since serious allergic responses have been reported in sensitive individuals with only 1 ml of the medium injected.

Severe reactions to contrast media are not common, but they do occur. Although the physician should be within the immediate area, the radiographer often notes the first signs of a reaction. Your ability to cope with such emergencies depends on your recognition of symptoms and your knowledge of the actions and treatment to follow. Chapter 8 includes descriptions of symptoms and appropriate responses to the varying degrees and types of contrast media reactions. A brief summary is printed in Box 10-2. Emergency supplies and equipment must be readily available whenever iodine media are injected.

BOX 10-1

CHECKLIST FOR A PRECONTRAST HISTORY

1. History of kidney disease or kidney failure. Check inpatient charts for BUN and creatinine levels.
2. History of diabetes. If yes, check for Glucophage medication.
3. History of heart disease or high blood pressure. Check current blood pressure.
4. Iodine contrast studies within the past 48 hours? If yes, check to determine when, which agent, concentration, and dose.
5. Any history of allergy.
6. Any history of asthma.
7. Previous allergic reaction to contrast medium. If yes, what agent and what reaction.
8. Current medications. Note particularly any beta-blockers, antihypertensive medications, or metformin products.

BOX 10-2

SIGNS OF ALLERGIC REACTIONS TO IODINATED CONTRAST MEDIA

- Restlessness and a sense of apprehension
- Increased pulse rate
- Pallor accompanied by weakness or a change in thinking ability
- Cool, clammy skin or itching skin
- A red rash, urticaria (hives)
- Throat constriction
- Dyspnea
- A fall in blood pressure of 30 mm below the baseline systolic pressure

Note: A brief period of nausea, with or without vomiting, is a fairly common reaction to ionic contrast media, but it is NOT an indication of an allergic response.

State laws or regulations may govern whether radiographers are allowed to start IV lines and/or perform IV injections. Institutional requirements or prohibitions may exist as well. In most situations when radiographers are permitted to administer IV contrast, some sort of certification and/or skill verification is required. Be familiar with the standards that prevail in your hospital, and keep your qualifications current. See Chapter 7 for IV injection procedures.

CONTRAST EXAMINATIONS OF THE URINARY SYSTEM
Excretory Urography

Excretory urograms are sometimes called intravenous urograms (IVUs) or intravenous pyelograms (IVPs). *Pyelogram* is terminology derived from roots signifying visualization of the kidney pelvis and was once the common name for this study. Since the scope of the examination includes the entire urinary tract, *urogram* is a more accurate term and is now the most commonly used.

The excretory urogram is a functional study of the urinary system accomplished by the injection of a water-soluble iodine contrast medium, such as Hypaque Meglumine 60%, Renografin 60, or Isovue 300. The contrast agent mixes and circulates with the blood until it reaches the kidneys, which extract it. As a component of urine, the contrast medium opacifies first the outer portion of the kidney as it fills the tiny vessels and glomeruli in the cortex and the collecting tubules in the medulla. This imparts a hazy opacification to the entire kidney structure, which quickly disappears with normal function. Films taken within the first 3 minutes after injection to visualize this phase are referred to as **nephrograms** and are used in the evaluation of hypertensive patients.

As the contrast medium is collected, it is channeled into the calyces and pelves of the kidneys, clearly outlining these structures. As the pelves fill, the opaque urine begins to flow through the ureters and into the bladder (Fig. 10-1). This process occurs within 15 to 20 minutes with normal kidney function. Thus each portion of the urinary tract may be

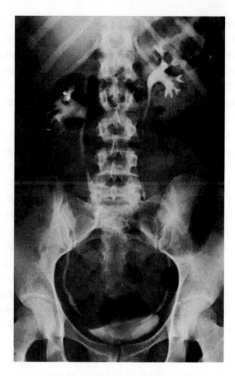

FIG. 10-1 Excretory urogram.

visualized in turn by the timing of the radiographic sequence. Compromised renal function may require delays in the timing of the study to visualize the internal structures of a diseased kidney.

Preparation for urography usually includes cleansing of the bowel to avoid gas and fecal shadows that could obscure structures of interest. Nothing by mouth (NPO) orders are given to avoid nausea and to create a moderate degree of dehydration, resulting in a greater concentration of the contrast medium in the kidneys. Be familiar with departmental policy regarding medications to be withheld before the examination. For instance, drugs that have a **diuretic** effect (promoting increased urination) may be withheld, since they tend to dilute the contrast agent with body fluids during excretion. As mentioned earlier, diabetic patients taking antihyperglycemic agents containing metformin must also have this medication withheld.

In preparation for the injection, the radiographer checks the emergency supplies and equipment and sets up the IV medication tray (see Chapter 7), including the vial of contrast medium, syringe, and an appropriately sized IV catheter or butterfly needle. For drip infusion administration, you need instead a drip bottle of dilute contrast medium and an IV infusion set. Dosage varies depending on the medium used, the radiologist's preference, and the patient's weight and age.

After explaining the procedure and injecting the contrast medium, the radiographer proceeds with the technical aspects of the examination. If a radiologist injects the contrast medium, the radiographer performs introductions and assists with the injection as needed. The patient must be closely monitored for signs of adverse reaction to the contrast medium.

Cystography

Several other studies of the urinary tract deserve mention. The **cystogram** provides contrast imaging of the internal contours of the urinary bladder. The bladder is filled by retrograde injection of a water-soluble iodine medium through a urinary catheter (Fig. 10-2) and examined using fluoroscopy and/or radiographs.

Voiding cystourethrograms (VCUGs) examine the urinary bladder and the urethra. The bladder is filled with contrast as for a cystogram, the catheter is removed, and fluoroscopy with spot films records

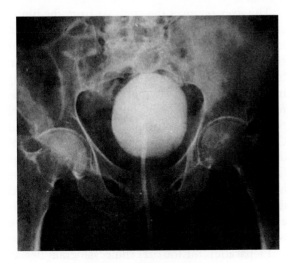

FIG. 10-2 Cystogram.

the contours of the urethra and the action of the bladder as the patient voids. This procedure is useful in the identification of urethral strictures in males and for diagnosis of vesicoureteral reflux (backflow of urine from the bladder into the ureters) in both males and females. This study is more commonly performed on children than on adults. Some institutions have specialized equipment for measuring urinary force and flow rate, and these measurements may be taken in conjunction with the VCUG study.

When a cystogram is ordered, the patient is usually sent to the radiology department with a retention catheter in place. If an outpatient study is being done, or if the catheter must be replaced, the hospital will have a specific standing order indicating who will insert the catheter. A nurse or orderly may be requested to come to the imaging department for this duty, or the radiologist or urologist may catheterize the patient. In some hospitals, this procedure is performed by radiographers who have been trained in catheterization technique (see Appendix K). The audiovisual or nursing education department of your college, or the in-service department of your hospital, will have videotapes or DVDs and anatomical models, which are invaluable in learning catheterization theory and technique.

The chief concern in performing a cystogram is the possibility of introducing bacteria into the urinary tract, thus causing an infection in a patient with an already compromised urinary system. A cystogram is a minor sterile procedure that does not require sterile gowning. When the catheter is in place, the contrast medium (Cystografin or Hypaque-Cysto) is poured into a 50- to 100-ml catheter-tip syringe and allowed to flow by gravity through the catheter and into the bladder. Depending on the specific protocol of your institution, this procedure may be repeated several times until the desired quantity has been instilled. Some radiologists use relatively small quantities of the contrast agent. Others prefer that the bladder be completely filled and distended.

The radiographer's role includes explaining the procedure to the patient, assembling the necessary equipment and supplies, assisting the physician with injection, and completing the technical aspects of the procedure. In some departments, cystography may be performed solely by radiographers. Box 10-3 provides suggested procedures for performing both routine cystography and VCUG studies. Cystography may be performed in conjunction with a cystoscopic procedure (fiberoptic study of the bladder). Under these circumstances the patient is sedated, and a surgical nurse assists the physician. The radiographer's role is almost exclusively technical. These procedures are usually performed in a cystourology room that is part of the surgical suite.

Retrograde Urography

Another urographic examination, often performed in conjunction with cystoscopy, is the retrograde urogram (formerly called retrograde pyelogram). Under cystoscopic visualization, long, slender catheters are inserted into the ureters, and a water-soluble iodine compound such as Reno-30 is injected into the kidney pelves via the catheters. This study provides radiographic visualization of the anatomical form of the pelves, calyces, and ureters (Fig. 10-3). Since this procedure carries a much lower risk of contrast medium reaction than procedures involving intravenous injection, it is sometimes ordered in lieu of an excretory urogram for patients at risk of an allergic response or those with high BUN or creatinine levels. Most hospitals have a cystourology room in the surgical suite with special equipment for performing these studies. The surgical staff provides patient care, and the radiographer's role is almost exclusively technical.

CONTRAST EXAMINATIONS OF THE BILIARY SYSTEM

Before the 1990s, biliary problems such as stones in the gallbladder or common bile duct or acute **cholecystitis** (inflammation of the gallbladder) were treated only with open surgery. Recently developed treatment methods have created much safer and less invasive therapy for many biliary problems. Fiberoptic devices such as the laparoscope and the endoscope are now used in both diagnosis and treatment of biliary disease, so patients who are not good candidates for surgery can now be successfully treated. With

better treatment options available, the diagnostic information required to make treatment decisions becomes more complex. Physicians may need to know the size, number, location, and composition of gallstones, whether the cystic duct is patent, and whether there are anomalies in the structure of the biliary ducts. A number of possibilities exist for obtaining this information. Contrast radiography, ultrasound examination, cholescintigraphy (a nuclear medicine procedure), computed tomography studies (especially spiral CT intravenous cholangiograms), and magnetic resonance imaging (MRI) examinations of the biliary system all play a role in this complex process.

Traditionally diagnosis of right upper quadrant pain began with an oral cholecystogram. Today the initial procedure is usually an ultrasound examination, followed by further studies when necessary, as determined by the initial findings.

Oral Cholecystography

While sonography is the preferred method for demonstrating gallstones, oral cholecystography is still occasionally used because of its ability to demonstrate both stones and gallbladder function. The gallbladder may be examined using an orally administered contrast medium in the form of tablets (Telepaque, Bilopaque, Oragrafin) or Oragrafin granules.

The liver removes the contrast from the blood and uses it to produce opaque bile, which is stored in the gallbladder. Liver disease, such as hepatitis or cirrhosis, may prevent removal of contrast medium from the blood and inhibit bile production, resulting in nonvisualization of the gallbladder. For this reason, patients must have bilirubin levels checked prior to contrast administration. You will recall from Chapter 6 that the bilirubin level is an indicator of liver function. Normal total bilirubin values range from 0.2 to 1.0 mg/dl. When the total bilirubin value is greater than 1.5, or when the direct bilirubin level is above 0.5, the patient must receive medical management to lower the bilirubin before proceeding with the examination.

Preparation for the oral cholecystogram begins early on the day preceding the examination.

BOX 10-3

PROCEDURES FOR CYSTOGRAPHY AND VOIDING CYSTOURETHROGRAPHY

Cystography
1. Obtain all needed equipment, and position it conveniently.
2. Place the patient on the table in the supine position, and cover him or her with a sheet, allowing access to the catheter.
3. Explain the procedure.
4. Fill the syringe with contrast medium.
5. Perform hand hygiene. Don gloves.
6. Cleanse the catheter drainage tube junction with antiseptic if the catheter is to be left in place after the procedure.
7. Separate the catheter from the drainage tubing, taking care not to contaminate either end. Protect the end of the tubing with dry, sterile gauze or a sterile plastic cover.
8. Place the tubing so it will not be contaminated. Hold the catheter in your nondominant hand.
9. Place the syringe tip into the end of the catheter. Hold the catheter and syringe in the vertical position to prevent air from being injected into the bladder, and allow the contrast medium to flow into the bladder by gravity. It is not necessary to push the plunger of the syringe.
10. The contrast will be instilled under fluoroscopic control. When the bladder is full, clamp the catheter.
11. Remove gloves. Repeat hand hygiene.
12. Complete the fluoroscopic and radiographic imaging of the full bladder.
13. When the study is complete, perform hand hygiene, don gloves, and unclamp the catheter. Allow the contrast/urine to drain into a disposable container.
14. Cleanse the end of the catheter with antiseptic. Reconnect to the drainage tubing, taking care not to contaminate the ends.
15. Remove equipment. Remove gloves, and perform hand hygiene.
16. Assist the patient from the radiographic table.
17. Charting should include the amount of urine discarded if the patient is under orders to have intake and output (I&O) recorded.

Voiding Cystourethrography (VCUG)
Follow Steps 1 through 12 above.
13. When the full bladder imaging is complete, position the patient in preparation for imaging while voiding. Female patients will be positioned supine; male patients will be in the posterior oblique position. Take care that the penis does not superimpose the femur.
14. Repeat hand hygiene, and don clean gloves.
15. Deflate the catheter's retention balloon. This may be accomplished by using a scissors to snip off the balloon valve and allowing the water to drain into a basin or by using a 10-ml syringe and needle to withdraw the water through the valve. Do not unclamp the catheter itself.
16. Remove the catheter by pulling gently. Discard the catheter and clamp.
17. Proceed with the established procedure for imaging the voiding process. Usually the urine is collected in a towel that has been placed to absorb it without interfering with the image of the urethra.
18. When the study is complete, cleanse the genital area with a towel and see to the patient's comfort.
19. Remove gloves, and repeat hand hygiene.

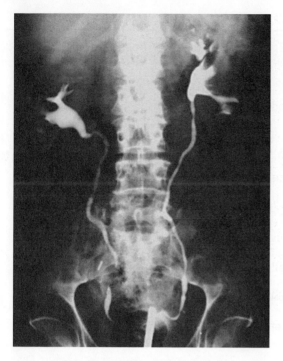

FIG. 10-3 Retrograde urogram.

For breakfast or lunch on this day, the patient's diet must include some fat. Two strips of crisp bacon or two pats of butter adequately fill this requirement. This is especially important for patients who have been on a low-fat diet by preference or by prescription. The presence of dietary fat causes the gallbladder to contract and release bile into the duodenum to aid in the digestion of fats. If no stimulation occurs to cause contraction, the gallbladder tends to remain full and does not receive or concentrate new bile. In fact, the liver is not stimulated to produce bile if the gallbladder is full, and the gallbladder will not be seen radiographically.

On the evening preceding the examination, the patient eats a fat-free supper, and takes 6 to 12 contrast tablets, depending on body weight. They are swallowed one at a time, 5 minutes apart, with minimal water. After ingestion of the tablets, the patient is NPO except for sips of water until the examination is completed.

A preliminary radiograph is taken and evaluated before proceeding with the remainder of the study.

The examination is discontinued if the gallbladder is not opacified.

When the gallbladder has been successfully demonstrated, a radiograph may be taken 20 to 30 minutes after a fatty meal (Fig. 10-4). Films taken following a fatty meal are useful in demonstrating gallbladder function as well as in visualizing the cystic and common bile ducts.

Common Bile Duct Examinations

At one time the intravenous cholangiogram (IVC) was the preferred method of examining the common bile duct, but a relatively high degree of risk was associated with the contrast used. The examination consisted of an IV injection of Cholografin, followed by repeated radiographs of the right upper quadrant over a period of 2 to 6 hours until adequate visualization was obtained. Today, IV cholangiograms using spiral CT with nonionic contrast media provide safer, quicker, and more comprehensive visualization. Percutaneous transhepatic cholangiography (PTC), T-tube cholangiography, endoscopic retrograde cholangiopancreatography (ERCP), and ultrasound studies also provide information about the common bile duct.

Percutaneous transhepatic cholangiography

PTC, sometimes called thin-needle cholangiography, involves placing the tip of a long, thin needle through the patient's right side, through the liver, and directly into the common bile duct. From 20 to 40 ml of a multipurpose contrast medium of 50% to 60% strength is injected under fluoroscopic control for fluoroscopic and radiographic visualization of the biliary system.

The radiographer's role is to assist the radiologist with the skin preparation and sterile techniques required for the injection and to complete the procedure's technical aspects.

PTC presents risk to the patient and is usually attempted only when immediate information is needed and more conservative approaches are not practical or have been unsuccessful. Possible complications include leakage of bile into the peritoneal cavity, hemorrhage, pneumothorax, and sepsis (infection).

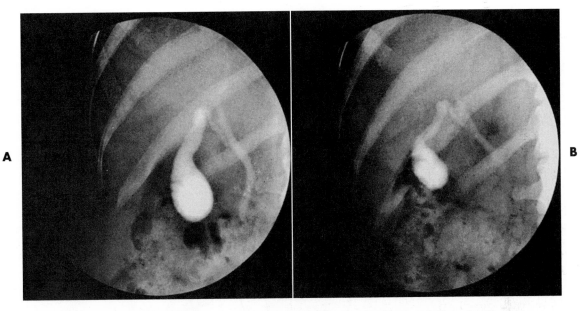

FIG. 10-4 Oral cholecystograms. **A,** Opacified gallbladder. **B,** After fatty meal. Note visualization of biliary ducts.

T tube and surgical cholangiography

After surgical **cholecystectomy** (removal of the gallbladder), a tube is sometimes left temporarily in the patient. This flexible rubber tube is about the size of a drinking straw in the shape of a T. The crossbars of the T extend into the hepatic and common bile ducts. The base of the T extends through the stump of the cystic duct or a tiny surgical opening in the common bile duct and exits through a small opening left in the original incision (Fig. 10-5).

The T tube serves primarily as a drain for bile until the postsurgical edema in the common bile duct subsides and bile can pass normally into the duodenum. It also serves as an avenue for the administration of a contrast agent if it is necessary to examine the biliary system postoperatively. This study may be performed to detect residual calculi in the hepatic or common bile duct, but it is most frequently used to determine the patency of the ducts before removing the drain.

A surgical T-tube cholangiogram may be performed in conjunction with cholecystectomy to ensure that any calculi remaining in the ducts are detected and removed before closing the incision (Fig. 10-6). Following an operative study, the T tube may or may not be left in place when the incision is closed. During surgery the radiographer's duties are strictly technical. Patient care is accomplished by the anesthesiologist, and contrast injection is performed by the surgeon with assistance from the surgical staff (see Chapter 11).

A postoperative study done in the radiology department requires that the radiographer assume a more prominent role. The procedure is summarized in Box 10-4. You should review the availability and contents of the emergency supply kit before any procedure involving contrast, but reactions to this study are extremely rare compared with those involving IV injections.

Endoscopic retrograde cholangiopancreatography

ERCP is a fiberoptic examination of the common bile duct that uses an endoscope. The tubular

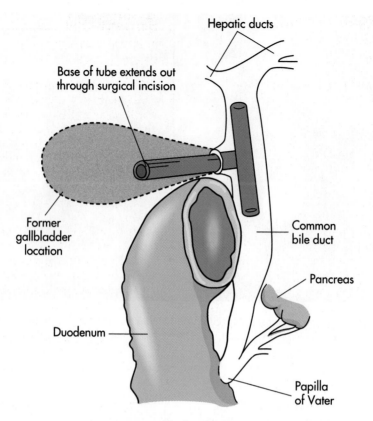

Hepatic ducts

Base of tube extends out
through surgical incision

Common
bile duct

Pancreas

Former
gallbladder
location

Duodenum

Papilla
of Vater

FIG. 10-5 **T** tube placement.

portion of the endoscope is passed through the patient's mouth (Fig. 10-7), down the throat, and through the stomach into the duodenum under fluoroscopic control. A small catheter is then passed through the endoscope into the distal end of the common bile duct through the papilla of Vater. Contrast is injected through the catheter, and spot films are taken to record the cholangiogram radiographically.

Attachments for the gastroscope include a "stone basket" for removal of biliary calculi and a tiny rotary blade for excising scar tissue or other obstructions. Sometimes a small plastic tube called a **stent** is left in the papilla to facilitate bile drainage.

This procedure may be performed in the radiology department or in a minor surgical setting using the C-arm fluoroscope. Some departments have a dedicated suite with fluoroscopic and endoscopic equipment for performing this procedure.

OTHER CONTRAST EXAMINATIONS
Myelography

The myelogram is an examination that uses contrast media to visualize the internal surfaces of the spinal canal. This study helps in diagnosis of conditions characterized by deformity or crowding of the spinal canal, such as spinal cord tumors and intervertebral disk herniations.

The injection procedure is called a spinal tap or lumbar puncture and involves the insertion of a needle into the subarachnoid space. A small amount of spinal fluid is usually removed and sent to the clinical laboratory for analysis. The contrast medium is then injected through the needle.

The usual medium is a water-soluble, nonionic contrast agent such as Isovue-M. The aqueous medium is miscible in spinal fluid and outlines the

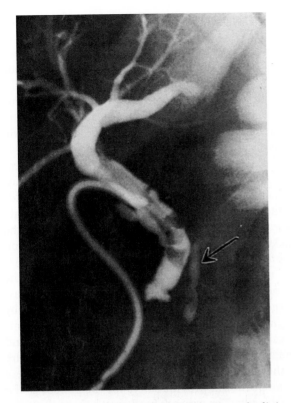

FIG. 10-6 T-tube cholangiogram showing calculi in common bile duct and visualization of pancreatic duct (*arrow*).

nerve roots as the fluoroscopic table is tilted into various positions. Fluoroscopic spot films record regions of interest. A CT study may be performed after the myelogram to obtain axial images of the spinal canal while the contrast is present.

The water-soluble contrast is readily absorbed from the spinal fluid and excreted via the urinary tract. This characteristic is a disadvantage in a prolonged procedure because the contrast medium may begin to disappear before the study is complete. For this reason, it is important to avoid delays between the time of injection and the examination.

The radiographer's role during a lumbar puncture is to assist the physician. In preparation the radiographer assembles the following items:

- Sterile myelogram tray or lumbar puncture tray
- Antiseptic for skin preparation (e.g., Betadine)
- Ample supply of the contrast medium
- Sterile gloves for the physician (two pairs)
- Sterile spinal manometer and specimen tubes (if needed and not included on the tray)

Additional spinal needles may also be added to the tray to meet the physician's preferences.

When these items are ready, the patient is positioned according to the physician's preference, either prone with a bolster under the abdomen or laterally recumbent with the hips flexed and knees drawn up toward the chin. In either position the objective is to provide convenient access to the puncture site for the physician while providing maximum lumbar flexion to separate the spinous processes at the level of the injection (Fig. 10-8). The site may be any intervertebral interspace from the twelfth thoracic–first lumbar (T12-L1) through the fifth lumbar–first sacral (L5-S1). The L2-L3 and L3-L4 interspaces are frequently used. The physician or the radiographer may prepare the skin. The physician then drapes the area and proceeds with the puncture.

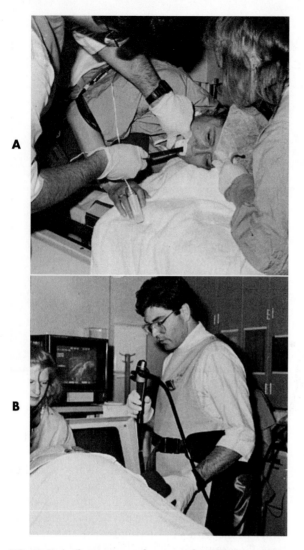

FIG. 10-7 **A,** Gastroscope placement for ERCP examination. **B,** Radiologist manipulates catheter through gastroscope under fluoroscopic control.

When a sample of spinal fluid is removed, it is placed in sterile specimen tubes. The radiographer is responsible for ensuring that the specimens and requisition form are delivered promptly to the laboratory. Often the radiographer delegates this duty to another member of the staff and continues to assist the radiologist. The person who delivers the specimens must be instructed to notify the medical technologist that a spinal fluid specimen has been delivered. This is very important because a delay in processing the specimen may invalidate the results.

The lumbar puncture procedure may also include the measurement of spinal pressure using a special device called a **manometer.** When this is done, the physician states the pressure readings aloud, and the radiographer records them for later inclusion in the chart and the radiologist's report.

When the physician is ready to make the injection, the radiographer prepares the vial of contrast medium, shows the physician the label, and holds the container steady at a slight angle to facilitate withdrawal into the syringe. After the injection, the needle is withdrawn and the fluoroscopic examination proceeds.

During the fluoroscopic portion of the study, the radiologist will tilt the table, causing the contrast agent, which is heavier than spinal fluid, to move by gravity in the spinal canal and fill the areas of clinical interest. Don't forget to check the footboard and shoulder guard on the fluoroscopic table to ensure they are secure before the table is tilted. These supports will provide safety for the patient as the table tilts. The patient's head must be kept above the level of the spine, and the head of the radiographic table should not be lowered more than 15 degrees. The patient is usually in the prone position during the examination. When the cervical region is to be studied, the patient's neck is extended with the chin supported on a radiolucent sponge. This position prevents the contrast agent from flowing into the cerebral region, causing adverse effects.

During the examination, observe the patient for any change in appearance that might indicate a change in status. Listen for any complaint, and provide reassurance. Occasionally a patient may faint during the lumbar puncture or subsequent myelogram. Seizures and allergic reactions are rare but may occur at any time from the moment of injection to as long as 8 hours afterward.

Loss of spinal fluid with resulting lowered spinal fluid pressure tends to cause severe headaches following lumbar punctures. This discomfort can be minimized by controlling activity and encouraging fluid intake for 24 hours after the examination.

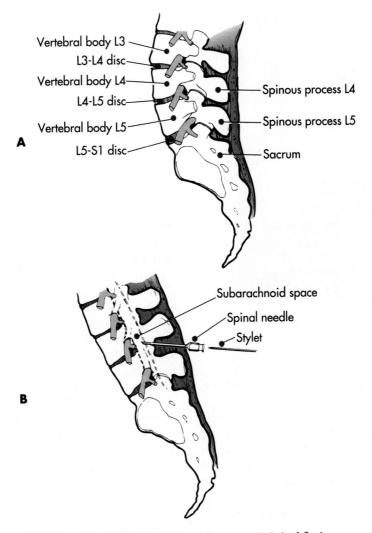

FIG. 10-8 Lateral aspect of lumbar spine. **A,** Normal posture. **B,** Spinal flexion separates spinous processes, allowing needle access to subarachnoid space.

The patient is kept supine with his or her head elevated 20 to 30 degrees for the first 4 to 8 hours, and activity may be restricted for an additional 16 hours. Failure to keep the head elevated allows the contrast medium to flow upward to the hypothalamus, causing severe nausea with vomiting and potential dehydration.

Contrast Arthrography

Arthrography, or contrast radiography of joints, is a special procedure used to detect injury and disease of the joint cartilage as well as abnormalities of the joint capsule (Fig. 10-9). The contrast medium for these studies may be a gas, one of the water-soluble iodine compounds (50% to 60%), or a combination of both (double-contrast arthrography). The shoulder and knee are the most common sites for this study, but methods have also been developed for the examination of the ankle and other joints arthrographically. Contrast arthrography is not as common as it once was due to the increased use of

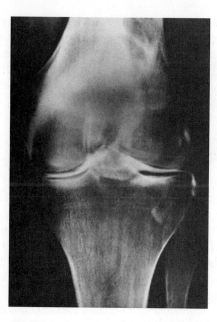

FIG. 10-9 Contrast arthrogram of knee.

MRI studies to evaluate the soft tissue components of joints.

Patient care for these examinations consists mainly of providing explanation and support to the patient and assistance to the radiologist with the injection procedure. The necessary items are available commercially in a sterile disposable tray, to which the radiographer may need to add antiseptic for skin preparation, contrast media, local anesthetic, and gloves for the radiologist.

After injection the radiographer may assist the patient to perform a range of joint motions to distribute the contrast agent. The radiographer may also be called upon to wrap the extremity with an elastic bandage to maintain even pressure on the area for contrast localization and best visualization. The wrap must be firm but not too tight. Periodically check the distal portion of the wrapped extremity for signs of decreased circulation including numbness, discoloration, or swelling that may indicate that the bandage is too tight. Bring any of these signs to the radiologist's attention. Fasten the wrap with adhesive tape rather than the usual metal clip, which

is radiopaque and may obscure an anatomical area of interest.

The radiologist may stress the joint during the arthrographic procedure, using considerable pressure. Sometimes this is required for the contrast to reach damaged areas or to fill splits in the joint cartilage for adequate visualization. This procedure can be quite painful, so stay close to the patient and provide plenty of support and reassurance.

CT arthrography may follow the radiographic procedure.

CONCLUSION

Radiographic examinations employing contrast media are used extensively in the hospital to enhance visualization of many soft tissue structures. Many media and methods are used, depending on the area to be studied and individual and departmental policies.

Contrast radiography provides opportunities for the radiographer to use patient care skills. These include patient assessment, effective communication, providing explanations and reassurance, promoting asepsis, and medication administration.

Since there is a potential danger of serious allergic reactions or toxic responses to contrast media, especially when injected intravenously, the radiographer must be prepared with equipment, supplies, and knowledge to deal with such occurrences and must be constantly alert to recognize their early signs.

REVIEW QUESTIONS

1. When molecules of water-soluble iodine contrast do not dissociate, but remain whole in solution, the medium is described as:
   A. ionic
   B. nonionic
   C. LOCA
   D. HOCA
   E. viscous
2. Blood chemistry values that must be checked prior to iodine contrast administration include:
   A. blood glucose and total cholesterol
   B. HDL cholesterol and BUN

C. BUN and creatinine
D. blood glucose and bilirubin
E. total cholesterol and creatinine
3. Which of the following examinations provides images of the urethra?
A. VCUG
B. IVU
C. BUN
D. PTC
E. ERCP
4. PTCs, ERCPs, and T-tube cholangiograms are examinations that may be performed to demonstrate the:
A. pancreas
B. gallbladder
C. spleen
D. common bile duct
E. ureters
5. A sterile manometer and specimen tubes might be needed when preparing to perform a(n):
A. cystogram
B. myelogram
C. excretory urogram
D. oral cholecystogram
E. arthrogram

CRITICAL THINKING EXERCISES

1. Meg Munsey's allergy history states that she has experienced several mild asthma attacks that were attributed to a pollen allergy. During an excretory urogram, she becomes agitated and short of breath. What should you do?

2. Your supervising technologist has asked you to prepare the supplies and tray for urinary catheterization and cystography. What technique must you follow? Why is this technique important?

3. George LeForte is gowned and ready for his cervical myelogram. What should you do to prepare for the injection procedure? How should Mr. LeForte be positioned for the contrast injection? What should you watch for as you monitor his condition after injection? What is your responsibility with regard to his spinal fluid specimens? What instruction should he receive for follow-up care?

4. The package insert information supplied with Mallinckrodt's Optiray, a multipurpose water-soluble iodine contrast agent, provides the following information regarding pediatric dosage for excretory urography:

Children: OPTIRAY 320 at doses of 0.5 ml/kg to 3 ml/kg of body weight has produced diagnostic opacification of the excretory tract. The usual dose for children is 1 ml/kg to 1.5 ml/kg. Dosage for infants and children should be administered in proportion to age and body weight. The total administered dose should not exceed 3 ml/kg.

The radiologist has requested a dose of 1 ml/kg for an 8-year-old child weighing 60 pounds. What is the volume of contrast to be administered? Is this order consistent with the manufacturer's recommendations? What is the recommended *maximum* dosage for this child?

Note: You may find it helpful to review the information on dosage calculation in Chapter 7.

Bedside Radiography: Special Conditions and Environments

At the conclusion of this chapter, the student will be able to:

- Demonstrate the appropriate procedure for gathering information before performing a bedside radiographic examination.
- List three situations in which bedside radiography may be preferable to examination in the imaging department.
- State the purposes of gastric, nasoenteric, tracheal, and thoracic suction.
- List precautions to be taken when doing a bedside examination of a critical neonate in the intensive care unit (ICU).
- List four important factors to be noted during an initial survey before radiography in the intensive care or coronary care unit.
- List three types of special beds or mattresses that may be seen in special units, and state the

- precautions to be used when doing mobile radiography with each type.
- List three essential precautions to be taken with patients who have a tracheostomy.
- Demonstrate the procedure for discontinuing gastric suction.
- Define the term *sterile corridor,* and explain the significance of this concept to the radiographer.
- List and describe two types of central venous catheters.
- Identify the correct locations for the tips of Swan-Ganz, Groshong, and PICC catheters.
- State the consequences of dislodging a thoracic tube, and explain how to avoid this occurrence.

atelectasis
CCU
decompression
ICU
Isolette
laparoscope

lithotripsy
nasogastric (NG)
nasoenteric (NE)
neonate
orthopedic traction
osseous

MOBILE RADIOGRAPHY

SO FAR WE HAVE primarily discussed patient care in the radiology department. This chapter deals with bedside imaging and with the conditions encountered when radiography or fluoroscopy is needed outside the radiology department. Emphasis is given to patient conditions that are usually seen in special care units but may occasionally be encountered in the radiology department or other areas of the hospital.

Hospital radiology departments are equipped with mobile x-ray generators. These are used primarily for bedside radiography and may also be used in the surgical suite. Studies done with this equipment are frequently called "portable" examinations, but this is not a very accurate term. Portable means "capable of being carried," and few x-ray machines fit this description. When equipment is on wheels or capable of being moved around, *mobile* is the better word. Two types of units are generally used: the mobile radiographic unit and the C-arm mobile image intensifier, a fluoroscopic unit. The C-arm unit is also capable of producing radiographs of a relatively small anatomical area.

Bedside radiography is ordered when a patient's condition makes transfer to the radiology department difficult or hazardous. It is often more advantageous to do bedside radiography for patients in special care units, **orthopedic traction** (treatment to correct bone deformity), and isolation (see Chapter 5 for isolation procedures). Since mobile radiography equipment has significant technical limitations compared with the facilities in the diagnostic imaging department, it is seldom possible to do bedside examinations with the same ease and radiographic quality possible in the radiology suite. If the

examination ordered can be done in the radiology department with a better outcome, the radiographer should consult the nurse in charge regarding the advisability of moving the patient. If the attending physician has ordered a mobile study, however, the examination must be done that way, or the physician's consent must be obtained to change the order.

With the exception of chest radiographs, bedside examinations are seldom routine. Standard positioning may not be possible, and situations often demand creative, innovative approaches. The skills gained by observing and assisting experienced radiographers will help you learn to handle these difficult situations competently.

The following list provides general guidelines for any bedside examination:
- Call the nursing station before leaving the imaging department unless responding to a "stat" (immediate) request.
- Check with the nurse in charge to inquire about the patient's condition.
- Confirm the order in the patient's chart.
- Always greet the patient, and inspect and prepare the room before bringing in the x-ray equipment.

These guidelines will be expanded as needed to meet special care unit requirements in the sections that follow.

SPECIAL CARE UNITS

Intensive care, coronary care, neonatal intensive care, postanesthesia care, and emergency trauma units in the emergency department (ED) are considered special care units. Patients in these settings are in critical condition and need continuous monitoring and care by specialized nurses and physicians.

Postanesthesia Care Unit

The postanesthesia care unit (PACU) is sometimes referred to as "postanesthesia recovery" (PAR), or simply the "recovery room." It is located just outside the operating room, allowing for the unimpeded transfer of patients and immediate access to surgeons, anesthesiologists, and operating room nurses. Special dress is generally not required for personnel entry. PACUs may also be located near critical care units for the expeditious transfer of patients requiring continuous monitoring when they leave the PACU.

The PACU is designed and staffed for close observation and care of patients following operative procedures that require an anesthetic agent. Each patient admitted is retained until the effects or possible complications of anesthesia have been eliminated. Because of the effects of the anesthesia and pain medication, patients in this unit are generally not fully responsive. Patients may be on oxygen, with or without a ventilator. They may also have central venous catheters and various drainage tubes. These treatment situations are frequently seen in the intensive care unit and are described in detail in a later section of this chapter. A nurse will be nearby to assess patient condition and to provide intravenous (IV) fluids, medications, and simple comfort measures.

These patients are often monitored radiographically. Chest x-rays are frequently requested to demonstrate line placement or to diagnose a possible pneumothorax. **Osseous** (of bone) x-rays are sometimes ordered to check an artificial joint or the alignment of fractures and placement of screws and plates. The mobile x-ray unit is used to demonstrate these anatomical areas. The nurse will inform you of any patient precautions and will assist you during the examination if necessary.

Patients in the PACU generally complain of being cold. This is due to the effects of anesthesia, premedication, and the cool atmosphere of the operating suite and PACU. Keep patients covered with warming blankets during examination whenever possible. While obtaining films, follow the same precautions described later in this chapter for patients in the intensive care unit (ICU) or the coronary care unit (CCU).

Emergency Trauma Unit

Patients with severe trauma are often x-rayed in the trauma room as part of the total assessment of their injuries. The patient is immobilized on a backboard and placed on top of the trauma bed until radiographs rule out fractures and spinal injury. Mobile x-ray examinations of the cervical spine, chest, and pelvis are commonly ordered. The radiographer must wear a lead apron and must also don protective attire to prevent contact with the patient's blood or body secretions. Assessment and stabilization of the patient create a flurry of activity as nurses, physicians, and laboratory, respiratory therapy, and electrocardiography (ECG) technicians perform their specialized tasks. The radiographer must carefully maneuver the x-ray equipment around these other professionals, place the cassettes, center the x-ray tube, and obtain the radiographs as efficiently as possible. Only minimal movement of the patient can be tolerated. Disturbance of the equipment, tubes, and lines used to monitor and treat the patient must be avoided. Lead aprons must be provided for staff members who cannot leave the patient.

Trauma patients arrive at the ER in a variety of emotional and physical conditions. They may be agitated, intoxicated and belligerent, or in an altered state of consciousness (confused, drowsy, or comatose). They may have large and gaping wounds, fractured and distorted extremities, bone piercing their skin, partially severed body parts, or severe burns. You can never anticipate what you will encounter in an ER trauma unit. As a beginning student, you will always work beside an experienced radiographer until you develop the knowledge, skill, perseverance, and patience required for this unique setting.

Neonatal Intensive Care and Newborn Nursery

Although most newborns arrive in perfect health, some have serious problems and are placed in the neonatal intensive care unit. Premature and low-birth-weight infants, or those with health problems, may require frequent imaging. For example, pediatric respiratory distress syndrome (PRDS) or newborn **atelectasis** (failure of the lungs to expand completely) may require chest radiographs for evaluation. Newborns with skeletal, cardiac, urinary tract, or gastrointestinal congenital anomalies may need chest, abdomen, or osseous studies. Skull

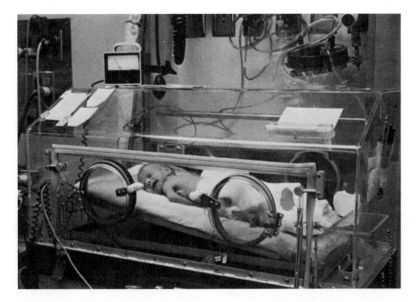

FIG. 11-1 The Isolette provides warmth, moisture, and oxygen while premature infants and those at risk gain maturity and strength.

radiographs may be requested for infants with neurological problems. Even infants in the newborn nursery who are not in critical condition sometimes require a radiograph (e.g., when a clavicle fracture is suspected at birth or a chest radiograph is required to confirm aspiration pneumonia).

The **neonate** (newborn) at risk may be placed in an open incubator under a radiant warmer or in an **Isolette.** The Isolette (Fig. 11-1) is more frequently used because this closed environment provides extra warmth, moisture, and oxygen while reducing exposure to airborne infection.

Procedure

Infants needing radiography may require protective precautions to avoid nosocomial infections. These include disinfecting the x-ray equipment before coming into the unit, hand hygiene, and possibly covering your uniform with a gown. A mask is generally not necessary, and gloves are worn only if you handle the baby. Refer to the infection control guidelines established by your institution. If procedures for protective precautions are not in place,

attention to the general principles of medical asepsis is essential for the infant's safety. There are generally fewer restrictions on handling and positioning babies who are not in critical condition.

The neonate at risk must be radiographed within the Isolette with assistance from a nursing staff member (Fig. 11-2). Some Isolettes are designed with a sliding tray below the unit for cassette placement. If you must open the unit to place the cassette, it is imperative that you work quickly to preserve the warmth of the infant. The cassette is covered and placed under the patient by the nurse, who positions the patient according to the radiographer's instructions. A short length of stockinet may be slipped over the arms and/or legs to aid in immobilizing and positioning (see Chapter 4). If the infant is in an open incubator with a radiant warmer, remember to move these lamps out of the way before centering the x-ray tube. Before making the exposure, provide a gonad shield for the infant, a lead apron for yourself, and one for the nurse, if necessary. Good immobilization techniques should eliminate the need to hold the infant.

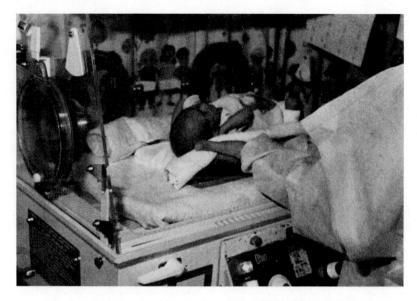

FIG. 11-2 A neonate at risk must be radiographed within the Isolette.

Intensive Care and Coronary Care Units

The intensive care unit (**ICU**) and coronary care unit (**CCU**) are designed for patients in critical condition whose treatment and status require frequent monitoring. Depending on the size of your institution, the intensive care unit may be subdivided into medical, surgical, trauma, neonatal, and pediatric units. The coronary care unit may also be subdivided, with patients recovering from cardiac surgery in one area and those receiving medical and nonsurgical treatment (e.g., balloon angioplasty) in another.

The ICU and CCU are familiar places to radiographers. Many patients in these units require frequent radiographic monitoring with mobile units. Chest radiographs are most often called for, but other examinations and/or imaging procedures may also be requested. For example, you may be asked to bring the C-arm mobile image intensifier to the ICU for bronchoscopy or to the CCU for placement of a central venous catheter or a pacemaker.

The inexperienced radiographer entering these units need not expect great difficulty in coping with the acutely ill patient. Since there is always adequate staff to provide constant patient care, the radiographer's duties are limited almost exclusively to technical considerations. The special problems faced in this environment may be twofold: dealing with your own anxiety about confronting near-death situations and dealing with an assortment of life-sustaining equipment connected to the patient and to other equipment by a network of cords, cables, pumps, tubes, and lines (Fig. 11-3).

Today's ICUs and CCUs are equipped to monitor the heart's electrical activity, cardiac output, cardiovascular function (through the placement of special catheters), blood pressure (through placement of an arterial line), internal body temperature, oxygenation, intracranial pressure, and ventilation. Continuous support equipment, such as cardiac assist devices (e.g., aortic balloon pump) and dialysis machines may also be found connected to patients in ICUs and CCUs.

Radiographers working in major medical centers may be called to the ICU to radiographically check line placement on a patient who is biologically dead. As discussed in Chapter 3, potential organ donors are kept on support systems to maintain the integrity of organs until donation is completed.

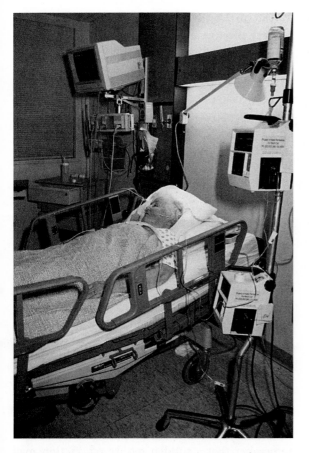

FIG. 11-3 The ICU can be intimidating with its vast array of technical equipment.

Procedure

Before bringing your equipment into the ICU or CCU, confer with the nurse in charge. You will be more successful in obtaining a diagnostic radiograph and minimizing any harm to the patient if you coordinate your efforts with the nursing staff. Explain what you need to do to accomplish the procedure and inquire about any necessary precautions. Next you will need to assess how much the patient can cooperate with the procedure. Speak to patients, even when they are not responsive, providing a brief explanation and calm reassurance as you work. Do not assume that they are unable to hear you, and avoid making any qualitative remarks about any patient's condition during the examination.

Since space is sometimes limited, you may need to move some equipment to make room for the x-ray unit. Check the bed rails and the area under the bed to locate cords, tubes, and drainage receptacles so that you will be aware of their location and not damage them accidentally as you move equipment. Newly designed ICUs and CCUs have an overhead system that provides support for monitors, oxygen, suction, and compressed air for the ventilator. A freely moveable unit containing bottles for chest tube drainage and nasogastric suction may be located at the head of the bed. These innovations allow more room and mobility when it is necessary to move the bed or to care for the patient from the head of the bed. If the bed must be moved, obtain help from the nursing service. Usually two people are needed to move the bed safely without placing undue stress on cables or tubes connected to the patient. When a mobile C-arm and monitor will be used, locate the most convenient electrical outlet and decide where you will place the equipment. The beds in the ICU and CCU are usually "fluoro capable" (radiolucent), permitting operation of the C-arm through the bed.

When the plan is clear and the area is ready, bring in the x-ray equipment and complete the study as efficiently as possible. Since drainage tubes, intravenous lines, and dressings all have a tendency to leak, cover the cassette with a plastic or cloth cover and don gloves before lifting or turning the patient. Check that all lines and tubes are clear as you place the cassette under the patient. Accidentally dislodging lines or tubes during cassette placement is a common and dangerous error. Sliding the cassette between the mattress and the sheet may facilitate placement. Always employ radiation protection measures for yourself and others. Provide lead aprons for the staff, place a gonad shield on the patient, if applicable, and announce, "X-ray!" before making the exposure. Correct procedure requires all nonessential staff to leave the immediate area. When the examination is complete, return everything carefully to its original location.

The monitoring units have auditory and visual signals that are activated by a change in the patient's condition or position, or when there are equipment problems. An alarm could indicate that a patient is breathing too fast, a tube or line has been dislodged, or the ventilator has disconnected from the patient or equipment. When an alarm is activated while positioning the patient, check the patient's condition before summoning the nurse. If the alarm does not terminate within 15 seconds, a nurse will come to check the patient.

Patients with ventilators, heart monitors, and other specialized equipment may be found in different parts of the hospital but are most frequently encountered in the ICU or CCU. Whatever their location, patients being monitored need the same precautions and attention to detail as those in a specialized unit.

TREATMENT SITUATIONS INVOLVING SPECIALTY EQUIPMENT
Special Beds and Mattresses
Many patients in ICU, CCU, and long-term care units are relatively immobile and have circulation problems. Several innovative devices are used to improve circulation in immobilized patients. Alternating pressure mattresses, air mattresses, rocking beds, and various types of wave, flotation, and bead mattresses are among the equipment that enhances the well-being of patients unable to tolerate being moved in the usual manner. The continual changes in position and pressure promote healing and may decrease the frequency of turning patients from side to side.

When bedside radiography is needed for patients on special beds, consult the nursing staff to see exactly what equipment is being used. Beds that have a rocking motion, or waves of alternating pressure, need to be turned off during x-ray exposures to avoid motion blur on the radiograph. Air mattresses need to be fully inflated to firm up and level the bed before placing the cassette under the patient.

Some patients need to lie on an alcohol- or water-filled pad to raise or lower body temperature. Since it is important to place the cassette on top of the pad to obtain the correct exposure, be careful not to snag the pad while positioning the cassette.

The surfaces of Mylar warming blankets or pads are very effective in reflecting body heat back toward the patient's body. Again, you must use care in placing the cassette between the patient and the reflecting surface without damaging the Mylar. The "Bair Hugger" is another version of a warming blanket. It has two layers. The layer in contact with the patient is a flat, non-woven fabric; above this lies a series of connected plastic tubes that are filled with warm air. An attached electrical unit, controlled by a thermostat, supplies the air. Since the blanket does not contain any metal parts, radiographs can be taken without removing it. Use care to avoid damaging the plastic.

Orthopedic Traction
Orthopedic traction is a mechanical method that uses weights to provide a constant pull on part of the body for therapeutic reasons. In the past, fractured long bones, such as the femur, were placed in traction to maintain the alignment of bone fragments as they healed. Today, however, traction is used only until muscle spasm subsides and the bone is surgically immobilized with a pin or plate. This permits a cast to be applied and allows the patient to convalesce at home.

When you encounter a patient in traction, remember that a sudden release of traction may result in serious harm and should never be attempted by the radiographer. Even an accidental bump against the bed or the traction weights may cause severe pain. Since patients are usually aware of which motions are tolerable, let them assist as much as possible with any moving or lifting. Often the traction apparatus includes a trapeze bar that the patient grips to assist in elevating the torso. If you have any doubt about certain movements, ask the nursing service.

Tracheostomies
A tracheotomy is a surgical procedure that creates an opening into the trachea to provide a temporary or permanent artificial airway. This opening, through which a tube may be placed, is called a tracheostomy (Fig. 11-4). A tracheotomy may be necessary due to obstruction in the upper respiratory tract caused by laryngospasm, cancer of the larynx, or burns in

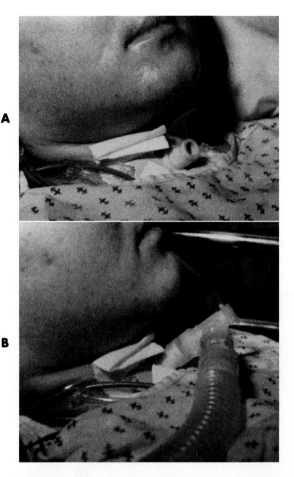

FIG. 11-4 Tracheostomy. **A,** Open. **B,** Attached to respirator.

the mouth and throat. Another reason may be to provide controlled respiration with a ventilator in patients with respiratory collapse due to paralysis, pulmonary edema, trauma, or adult respiratory distress syndrome (ARDS).

Patients with new tracheostomies are monitored in the ICU. Because these patients require frequent suctioning to keep the tube free of secretions, close monitoring and immediate access to suction equipment are required. For these reasons a nurse will accompany them when they are brought to the diagnostic imaging department.

The tapes holding the tracheostomy tube are never untied because a sudden cough can expel the tube,

and the edges of the tracheostomy may close sufficiently to obstruct respiration. Remember to observe the following precautions:
- Monitor tracheostomy patients closely.
- Never untie the tapes holding the tracheostomy tube in place.
- Have suction equipment and supplies immediately available.

Mechanical Ventilation

Patients who need mechanical assistance with respiration are intubated; that is, an endotracheal tube is passed through the mouth and into the trachea. The tube is then connected to a ventilator (mechanical respirator), which assists breathing, either by supplementing the patient's breath or by forcing respiration under pressure. Ventilators may also be connected directly to tracheostomies.

When doing an x-ray examination of the chest or abdomen, do not turn off the ventilator to eliminate respiratory motion. If the ventilator is controlling both the rate and the volume of breathing, you may be able to determine when a brief pause in respiration will occur by paying attention to the breathing rhythm. If the exposure time is short and your sense of rhythm is good, you will be able to take a motion-free exposure.

Position the patient carefully so you don't disconnect the endotracheal or tracheostomy tube or apply tension to the ventilator tubing. If the ventilator alarm is activated during positioning and the patient appears distressed, notify the nurse immediately. Protect yourself when positioning patients on ventilators. Wear gloves and avoid placing your face too close to the patient's head and neck area. These precautions will help prevent contamination by mucus if the tubing disconnects.

Patients may also be ventilated manually by a nurse or respiratory therapist with an Ambu bag, a device that is squeezed regularly by hand to force respirations. This method is used briefly during the time between intubation and setting up the ventilator. Manual ventilation, often referred to as "bagging," may also be used while the patient is being transferred for diagnostic studies.

Nasogastric and Nasoenteric Tubes

Another treatment situation that may be encountered in the ICU and elsewhere involves the insertion of **nasogastric (NG)** or **nasoenteric (NE)** tubes. These tubes are passed through the nose and down into the stomach or small intestine.

Nasogastric tubes are passed into the stomach (Fig. 11-5) and have several purposes:
- Feeding
- Decompression
- Radiographic examination

It may be necessary to feed a patient with an NG tube when trauma, disease, an altered state of consciousness, or a surgical procedure (e.g., tracheostomy) prevents normal swallowing. A commonly used feeding tube is the Dobbhoff nasogastric feeding tube (Fig. 11-6). **Decompression,** the removal of gas and secretions by suction, is prescribed to prevent vomiting in patients who have recently had surgery. The Levin and the Salem-Sump tubes are the most common NG tubes used for this purpose. The Levin is a single-lumen tube with several holes near its tip. The Salem-Sump tube is a radiopaque double-lumen tube. One lumen is used to remove gastric contents, and the other functions as an air vent (Fig. 11-7).

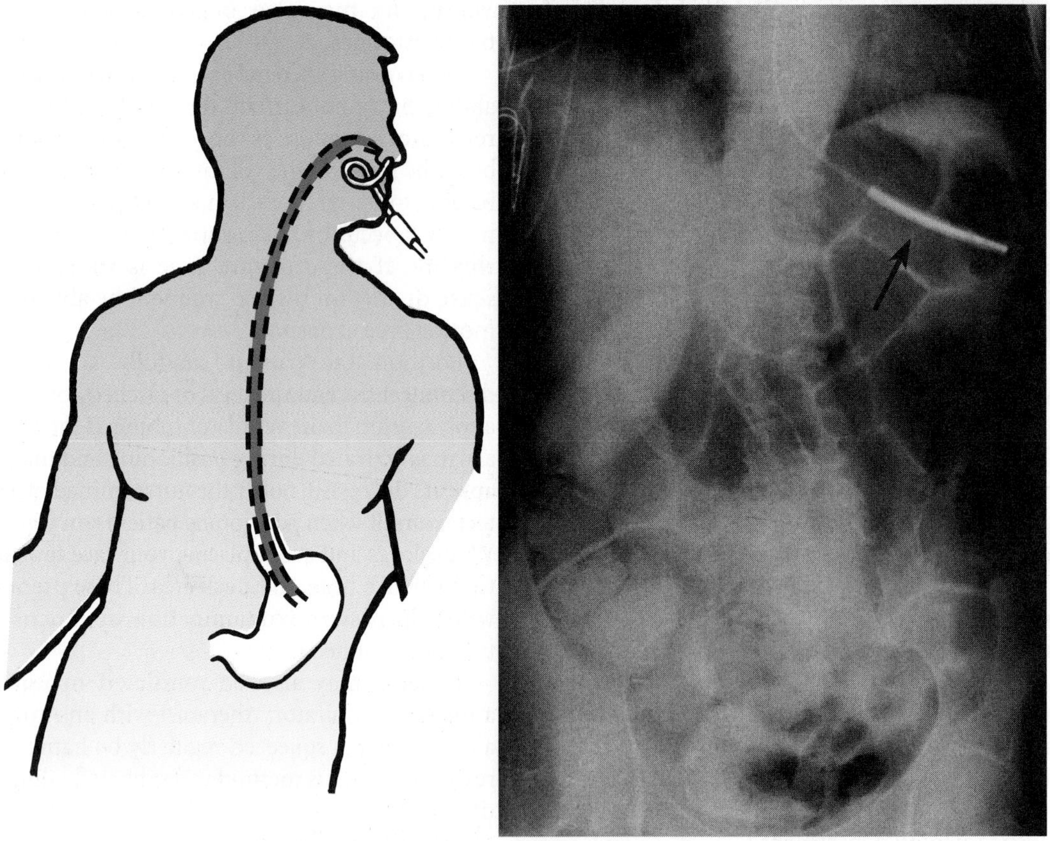

FIG. 11-5 **A,** Nasogastric tube placement. **B,** Abdomen radiograph demonstrates nasogastric feeding tube in stomach *(arrow).*

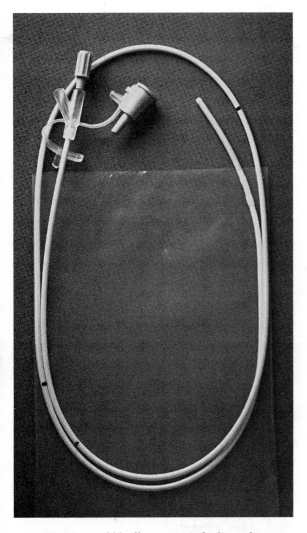

FIG. 11-6 Dobbhoff nasogastric feeding tube.

The nasogastric tube may also be used for radiographic examination of the stomach. The radiographer draws up a thin barium mixture or oral aqueous iodine solution into a large syringe; the syringe is connected to the NG tube, and the radiologist instills the contrast under fluoroscopic control. Oral contrast mixtures for computed tomography (CT) examinations may also be instilled through the NG tube. This is done before the examination by the nursing service.

Nasoenteric tubes (Fig. 11-8) are placed in the stomach, and peristalsis advances them into the small intestine. They generally have two purposes:
- Decompression
- Radiographic examination

Nasoenteric tubes can remove gas and fluid that occurs postoperatively or as a result of a bowel obstruction. Much like the procedure for studying the stomach, nasoenteric tubes may be used to instill contrast media for radiographic examinations of the small intestine (see Chapter 9).

Some typical nasoenteric tubes include Miller-Abbott, Harris, and Cantor tubes. The Cantor and Harris tubes have a single lumen with one opening for drainage. The Miller-Abbott has a double lumen, one for drainage and the other for a balloon. The balloon is weighted to simulate a bolus of food and promotes peristalsis to advance the tube into the small intestine. Nasoenteric tubes are frequently localized radiographically; they may be placed fluoroscopically if advancement beyond the stomach is difficult.

When doing bedside radiography of a patient with an NG or NE tube, there is little cause for concern except to avoid disturbing the tube. It is uncomfortable when tugged on and very messy if the drainage end is dislodged from the bottle or the suction machine.

When the tube is connected to suction for decompression, it may be temporarily disconnected to bring the patient to the diagnostic imaging department. Before discontinuing suction, get approval from the nurse in charge. With permission, turn off the suction, clamp off the tube with a hemostat, and then disconnect the tube. Wipe the tube with a tissue or gauze sponge, then double the end and wrap the bent portion tightly with a rubber band so that it will not leak. Remove the hemostat, and tape or pin the loose end of the tube to the patient's gown to prevent the tube from being pulled out of position by its own weight. Take care not to remove the gown without first remembering to unfasten the tube. It is very unpleasant for the patient to have the tube reinserted.

Closed Chest Drainage

Closed chest drainage is a method used to remove fluid or air that has accumulated in the pleural space.

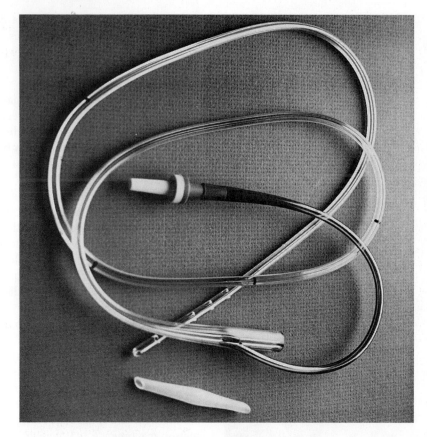

FIG. 11-7   Salem-Sump nasogastric tube.

It consists of a tube placed within the pleural cavity and connected to a suction device through a drainage receptacle. Chest tubes are inserted in different locations depending on the type of treatment desired. Tubes inserted through the anterior superior chest wall remove air, which rises (Fig. 11-9); they are placed through the posterior inferior chest wall to drain fluid, which collects at the base of the pleural space (Fig. 11-10). A typical drainage system is demonstrated in Fig. 11-11. Disturbance of the drainage system at either end may result in a rush of air into the pleural space, reversing the intent of the treatment and possibly causing collapse of a lung. Extra caution is therefore required to see that the suction and drainage apparatus is not disturbed, that the chest tube is not dislodged when positioning the cassette for a chest radiograph, and that the drainage unit remains below the level of the patient's chest.

Specialty Catheters

The radiographer encounters a variety of catheters with specialized functions. They have been developed to help monitor and manage critical patients and patients requiring long-term care. You may see the Swan-Ganz catheter and various central venous catheters such as central venous pressure (CVP), Hickman, peripherally inserted central catheter (PICC), Groshong, Raaf, and Port-A-Cath. In general, all these catheters are tubes that provide access to the circulatory system on a repeated or continuing basis. Since improper use may jeopardize the physical status of patients with specialized catheters, only specially trained personnel are permitted to use or care for them.

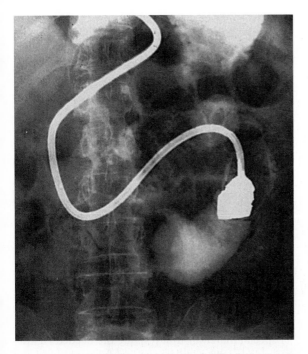

FIG. 11-8 Nasoenteric tube (Miller-Abbott) in small bowel. Note that an aqueous iodine contrast medium has been injected through tube to outline intestine just distal to opaque weight at tube tip.

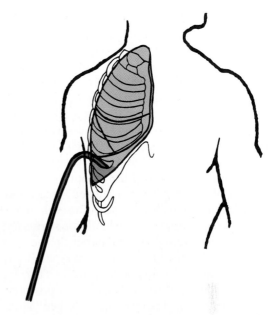

FIG. 11-10 Chest tube placed to drain fluid from pleural space.

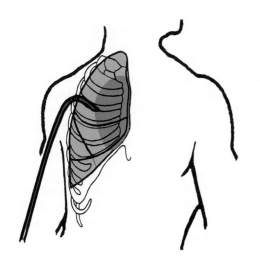

FIG. 11-9 Chest tube placed to relieve pneumothorax.

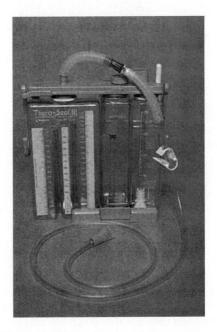

FIG. 11-11 Disposable chest drainage system.

Pulmonary artery flow-directed catheters such as the Swan-Ganz measure cardiac output, right heart pressures, and indirectly, left heart pressures. These catheters (Fig. 11-12) diagnose right and left ventricular failure and monitor the effects of specific medications, stress, and exercise on heart function. If the pulmonary artery catheter has a fiberoptic infrared sensor, it is also capable of measuring mixed venous oxygen saturation, which reflects the balance between oxygen supply and oxygen demand. This simply means it can reveal the amount of oxygen left in the blood after it has circulated through the body. High or extremely low levels of oxygen on the venous side of circulation could indicate significant problems, depending on the patient's age and condition. If the patient is elderly or very weak, any exercise or stimulation may be detrimental. This may help you understand why a nurse might postpone radiography until the patient's oxygen levels improve.

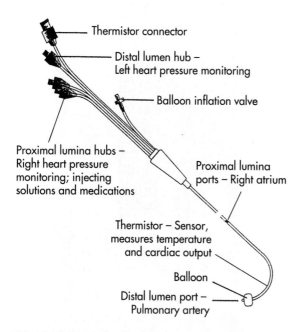

FIG. 11-12 Example of pulmonary artery catheter. This quadruple-lumen catheter measures cardiac output, heart pressures, and core temperature. It has two lumina for administration of fluids and medications.

These catheters are often seen in ICU or CCU patients who have undergone open heart or chest surgery and those who require intensive monitoring. The Swan-Ganz catheter has several lumina and a balloon at its tip. It is inserted through the subclavian, internal or external jugular, or femoral vein and advanced until the tip rests in the right atrium. Inflation of the balloon with air floats the catheter into the pulmonary artery and pulmonary capillary wedge position where pressures can be monitored (Fig. 11-13). This catheter is usually inserted at bedside, and a mobile chest radiograph is requested to verify its placement.

Central venous catheters facilitate the administration of chemotherapy or other long-term drug therapy, total parenteral nutrition, dialysis, or blood transfusions. They may also facilitate the drawing of blood for testing and allow central venous pressure monitoring. Central venous catheters share some common characteristics. Almost all are constructed of special materials that provide the needed rigidity for placement and lower the incidence of blood clot formation. They all possess radiopaque strips or have radiopaque distal ends, allowing x-ray verification of placement. Depending on their purpose, they have either single or multiple lumina. Their distal tips all rest in the vena cava near the right atrium.

Central venous catheters can be classified as follows:

- Short-term, nontunneled external catheters
- Long-term, tunneled external catheters
- Long-term, implanted infusion ports

Short-term, nontunneled external catheters are frequently inserted at the bedside. They are placed through the skin and directly into a vein in the neck, shoulder, groin, or antecubital fossa. To prevent dislodgment, they are secured at the point of insertion with sutures or a dressing. This helps provide protection from infection. The PICC and CVP catheters are examples of this type. The PICC is inserted into a vein in the patient's antecubital fossa and advanced until its tip lies in the superior vena cava (Fig. 11-14). This catheter is used to administer medications and to draw blood. The CVP catheter is inserted into a vein in the

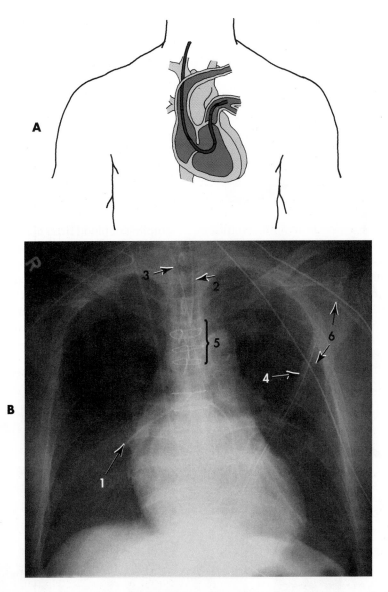

FIG. 11-13 **A,** Swan-Ganz catheter placement. **B,** Anteroposterior (AP) chest radiograph showing *(1)* tip of Swan-Ganz catheter advanced into right pulmonary artery, *(2)* endotracheal tube, *(3)* nasogastric tube, *(4)* chest tube, *(5)* wire sutures in sternum from open heart surgery, *(6)* monitor lines (external).

patient's arm, neck, shoulder, or groin and advanced into the vena cava (Fig. 11-15). It is used to monitor the pressure of the blood as it returns to the right atrium and aids in the evaluation of right heart function.

Long-term, tunneled external catheters are surgically placed beneath the skin and directed to the desired vein (Fig. 11-16). Their access ends are generally located midway between the nipple and the sternum. New tissue formation secures the catheter's

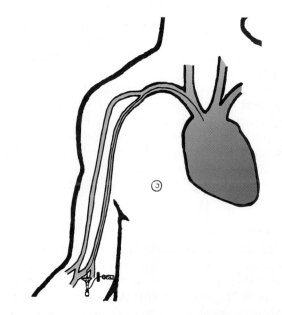

FIG. 11-14 PICC line placed from antecubital insertion point.

Dacron cuff in place, preventing accidental dislodgment while providing a barrier to infection. The Hickman, Groshong, and Raaf are examples of tunneled catheters. They all are advanced into the superior vena cava. The Hickman is used for patients requiring long-term parenteral nutrition. The Groshong is a single- or double-lumen catheter used to administer medications or to draw blood. The Raaf is a large, double-lumen catheter used for dialysis.

Long-term implanted infusion ports, also known as venous access ports (Fig. 11-17), are used for patients who need intermittent infusion of medications or chemotherapy, blood transfusions, or sampling of blood from the superior vena cava. The port, which is encased in plastic or metal (usually titanium), and an attached venous catheter are surgically implanted and sutured under the skin of the upper chest or arm. The port is not externally visible but can be easily felt under the skin. A specially designed needle called the Huber needle is used to

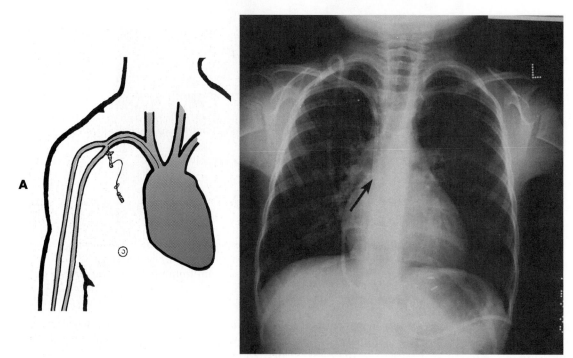

FIG. 11-15 **A,** Nontunneled central venous catheter with tip in superior vena cava placement. **B,** Posteroanterior (PA) chest radiograph demonstrates proper placement of CVP line.

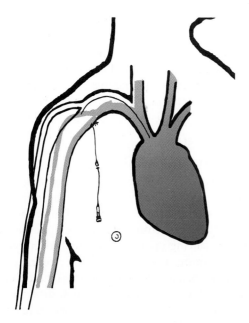

FIG. 11-16 Tunneled placement of catheter for long-term use (e.g., Groshong, Hickman).

access its self-sealing port. An example of a commonly used infusion port is the Port-A-Cath. Other similar products include InfusaPort, Mediport, and Lifeport.

Chest radiographs or mobile C-arm fluoroscopy may be requested to check the position of these specialty catheters or to guide their tips into place. As mentioned previously, observe these lines and use caution as you place the cassette. It may be necessary to move any external wires (fiberoptic sensors) out of the way to avoid artifacts on the radiograph.

Pacemakers

The artificial pacemaker is an electromechanical device that regulates the heart rate by providing low levels of electrical stimulation to the heart muscle. This is very similar to the stimulation normally provided by a nerve impulse. Pacemakers are primarily used to treat conduction defects. If the conduction system of the heart is unable to

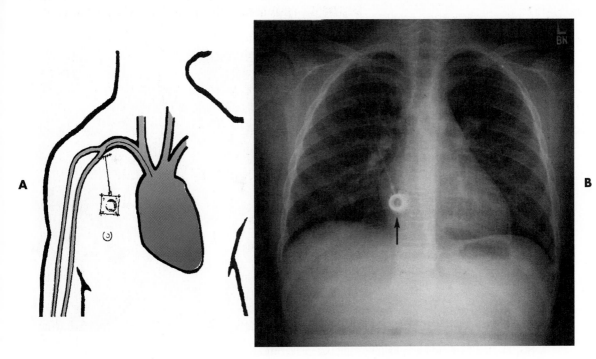

FIG. 11-17 **A,** Placement of subcutaneous venous access port. **B,** Chest radiograph demonstrates venous access port *(arrow).*

maintain an effective rate and rhythm, the pacemaker will electrically stimulate the heart to maintain an adequate rate.

The pacemaker system is composed of a battery-powered energy source and a wire or catheter that delivers electrical stimulation to the heart. Internal pacemakers are surgically implanted within the patient's chest; external pacemakers are usually temporary and the bulk of the instrument remains outside the patient's chest. When the pacemaker is inserted under fluoroscopic control in the imaging department, a radiographer is part of the team and may assist the cardiologist with patient care procedures and with the technical aspects of fluoroscopic imaging. Pacemakers are also inserted in the operating room and in the ICU or CCU. The C-arm fluoroscope is used when the procedure is performed outside the imaging department. If fluoroscopic guidance is not used during the procedure, a chest radiograph is commonly requested afterwards. An overexposed image should reveal the tip of the catheter in the apex of the right ventricle (Fig. 11-18).

The radiographer should carefully position the patient for the chest radiograph and must avoid abducting or elevating the patient's left arm. This restriction is placed on the patient for 24 hours after surgery to prevent dislodging the pacemaker and catheter.

SURGICAL SUITE
Surgical Access and Clothing

The radiographer has a critical role in the operating room. There are many surgical procedures that require imaging before, during, and/or at the completion of the procedure. The radiographer must be skilled at setting up and operating the equipment and obtaining the images with accuracy and efficiency. For this reason the inexperienced radiographer is not sent to the surgical suite alone. An experienced radiographer guide is essential to proper orientation.

To maintain asepsis, all traffic in the surgical suite is limited to personnel and items with a legitimate reason to be there. In addition, special surgical attire

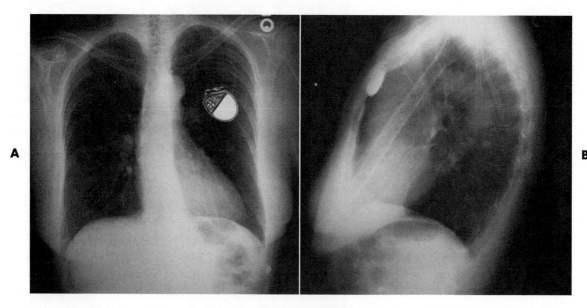

A **B**

FIG. 11-18 Chest radiographs following pacemaker insertion. **A,** PA projection demonstrates pacemaker and catheter placement. **B,** Lateral projection. Note left arm superimposed on thorax; elevation of arm within the first 24 hours risks disturbing catheter or pacemaker placement.

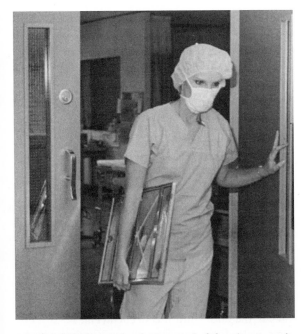

FIG. 11-19 Radiographer leaves surgical dressing room in scrub clothes.

must be worn. Just inside the limited access area is a dressing room where personnel can change into surgical attire (Fig. 11-19), often called "scrub clothes." Beyond this point, access is allowed in clean scrub clothes only. Scrub clothes include nonsterile shirt and pants, a mask to cover your nose and mouth, a hat or hood to cover all hair (including a beard if applicable), and shoe covers, which may be optional. Shoe covers will keep your shoes from becoming soiled and may lower the transfer of microorganisms into the operating room, but there is no evidence that they have any effect on the incidence of wound infections. Shoes with closed heels and toes protect your feet around moving equipment and from heavy objects that may be accidentally dropped. If you must handle anything contaminated with the patient's blood, don gloves.

Before bringing x-ray equipment into the surgical suite, you must wipe it down with a germicidal solution. In some hospitals a mobile x-ray machine is maintained for surgical use only. Some surgical suites also have permanent radiographic installations.

While these measures help reduce contamination, the radiographer is still responsible for equipment cleanliness.

In the past it was considered good practice to wear a "cover gown" over scrub clothes when leaving the surgical suite temporarily or to change to fresh scrub clothes when returning from other hospital areas. Infection control studies reveal that this practice is not required for nonsterile team members, such as radiographers, who do not work in the sterile field. If you must go outside the surgical suite in scrub clothes (e.g., to show a film to the radiologist) follow the established policy at your institution.

Surgical Environment

The average size of a multipurpose operating room (OR) is 400 square feet. Specialty ORs, such as those equipped for trauma or cardiac bypass surgery, may require 600 square feet. Since corridors may have higher microbial counts, the doors to the operating room should always remain closed, and the number of times the door is opened should be minimized. Positive air pressure in each of the rooms minimizes air circulation from outside the room. Filtration systems, air exchanges, and circulation provide fresh air, prevent accumulation of anesthesia gases, and reduce airborne contamination in the operating rooms. Ceiling lights provide general illumination, and the overhead operating light provides high-intensity illumination over the operative site. Some rooms have permanent radiographic and fluoroscopic equipment and x-ray viewboxes on the walls or PACS monitors suspended from the ceiling or mounted on mobile carts.

There are several varieties of surgical tables, depending on the type of procedure. Examples include spinal, cystourology, and orthopedic, to name a few. Most are height-adjustable and tilt for patient positioning. Some contain a tunnel for placing an x-ray cassette beneath the patient. Arranged around the room you will find a wide array of monitoring, surgical, and anesthesia equipment. There will also be strategically placed instrument tables, ring stands with basins, buckets, trash containers, and laundry bags.

The surgical team is subdivided according to function and consists of both sterile and nonsterile members. The sterile members perform a surgical scrub, don sterile attire, and work within the sterile field. This group may include the:

- Surgeon
- Assistant to the surgeon (physician)
- Nonphysician assistant
- Scrub person (RN, LVN, or surgical technologist)

The nonsterile members perform their tasks outside the sterile field. This group may include the following:

- Anesthesiologist or anesthetist
- Circulating nurse or surgical technologist
- Various other technologists (biomedical, orthopedic, and radiologic)

The surgical suite may seem to have a mysterious quality because there is usually a great deal of activity with very little noise. Sudden noises or loud conversations are distracting to the surgical team and may make it difficult for the anesthesiologist to hear heart sounds. Remember that the surgical patient is always at some degree of risk. Prolonged anesthesia increases the risk of surgical complications. This places pressure on the surgical team to work quickly.

The surgical team generally works best in a low-key environment and strives to maintain this type of atmosphere. The tension level may escalate, however, when things are not going well or when errors cause delays. You know how difficult it is to wait patiently when you are tense and anxious. The surgeon and surgical staff may have this state of mind as they wait for you to set up equipment, take radiographs, and process the images. Their work is "on hold," since they cannot proceed without the information your images will provide. When the stress level is high, they may urge you to hurry or may have an impatient attitude or tone of voice. At these times, your ability to proceed confidently and speak calmly will help insulate you from the stress and will allow you to complete your work quickly and accurately.

Surgical Setup

When mobile equipment is used, it is usually kept outside the door until it is needed (Fig. 11-20). For some procedures, however, the equipment may be positioned in advance and the tube head covered with sterile drapes during the setup. You must

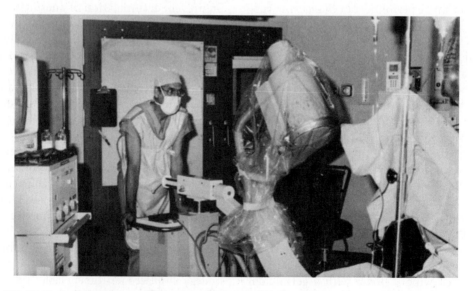

FIG. 11-20 Radiographer carefully moves C-arm mobile fluoroscope into position in operating room. Note wrapping of image intensifier to prevent contamination of sterile field by dust from equipment.

be familiar with the institution's policies and the surgeon's preferences.

When working in the OR, be aware of sterile fields and use caution not to contaminate them with your clothing or the equipment. Do not wear dangling jewelry or other loose items around your neck or wrists. Don't fill your shirt pockets with items that could fall out as you work around the surgical table. Also, watch the cables as you manipulate the equipment.

The area between the patient drape and the instrument table is maintained as a "sterile corridor" (Fig. 11-21) and is the province of the surgeon and the instrument nurse only. Access to this area is permitted only to those wearing sterile gowns and gloves, and the radiographer is excluded from this part of the room. For abdominal surgery and open reduction of the lower extremities, the head end of the table is not a sterile field. This is a safe area from which the radiographer may assess the situation.

Cassettes are sometimes positioned via a tunnel in the operating table that may be reached from the nonsterile area. Otherwise, they are placed in a sterile cover and positioned by the surgeon. The technique of cassette transfer to a sterile cover is the same as that used for protective precautions (see Chapter 5).

Surgical Procedures Requiring Radiography

One study performed by the radiographer in the surgical suite is the surgical cholangiogram, an adjunct to cholecystectomy. The basis for this radiographic examination is explained in Chapter 10 as part of the discussion on T-tube cholangiography. When surgical cholangiograms are anticipated, the radiographer may be notified to come to surgery for a preliminary radiograph before the sterile field is established. This radiograph verifies correct cassette location and exposure factors. If a preliminary radiograph is not taken, the radiographer uses patient height and weight data to estimate exposure

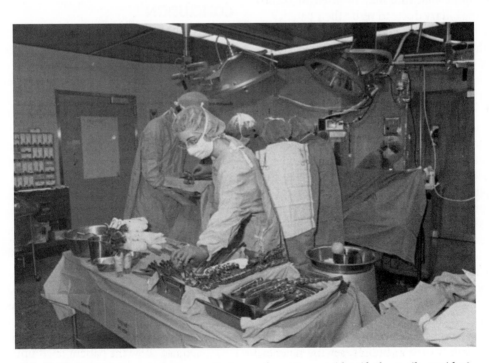

FIG. 11-21 Operating room during surgical procedure. Can you identify the sterile corridor?

factors and relies on the surgical team to indicate the centering point for cassette and x-ray tube placement. In some institutions these methods are considered reliable, and the preliminary image is not a part of the usual routine.

The laparoscopic cholecystectomy is performed more frequently than the operative procedure. Three or four incisions are made in the upper right quadrant between the levels of the xiphoid process and the umbilicus. Long metal tubes (trocars) and a rigid fiberoptic **laparoscope** (device for viewing inside the abdominal cavity) are inserted through these incisions. The peritoneal cavity is insufflated with carbon dioxide through one of the trocars to increase its size. The other trocars are used to pass instruments and equipment into the peritoneal cavity to grasp and remove the gallbladder. The scope is connected to a camera that projects the operative site onto a monitor located at the head of the surgical table. This allows the surgeon to observe and manipulate the instruments during the procedure. Following removal of the gallbladder, the C-arm fluoroscope or radiographic machine may be used to record images of the biliary ducts to verify their patency.

Another common surgical application of radiography is the open reduction of fractures. Plaster or fiberglass casts are used to hold many fractures in position while healing occurs. Some fractures, however, require surgical intervention to align the fragments. Internal fixation by means of rods, nails, plates, or screws maintains the alignment securely. This method is often used to stabilize hip fractures and may also be used for many other types of fractures. Reconstructive orthopedic surgery to correct crippling from developmental defects, previous injuries, or degenerative diseases may also require imaging. A radiographer may be present during these procedures, using the C-arm unit to provide fluoroscopic guidance for aligning bone fragments and placing hardware. A radiographic record is made of the final position of the bones and fixation devices.

Localization is the reason for several types of surgical radiography. Radiographs or fluoroscopic visualization may help determine the exact location of foreign bodies such as bullets, sewing needles, or industrial steel fragments during their surgical

removal. A spinal needle may be positioned in an intervertebral disk space and radiographed to establish the accuracy of the spinal level before proceeding with surgical intervention. A radiograph may be used to locate a surgical sponge or instrument within the abdominal cavity if the surgical count indicates a missing item before final closure of the incision. C-arm fluoroscopy may guide the surgical placement of internal pacemakers or catheters. Ultrasound is used in surgery to precisely localize tumors in the brain, spine, and liver.

Retrograde urograms (see Chapter 10), ureteral stent placements, stone extractions, and **lithotripsy** (stone fragmentation by laser, ultrasound, or some other energy) are urologic procedures requiring radiography in the operating room. Newer cystourology rooms are installed with permanent fluoroscopic and radiographic equipment. Preliminary and/or postcontrast images of the kidneys, ureters, and bladder may be obtained.

CONCLUSION

Radiography outside the imaging department can provide some of the most interesting and challenging opportunities to the radiographer. When working in other departments, the radiographer must respect the rules and wishes of the personnel in charge, communicate clearly, and obtain any information that may be lacking before proceeding. While working in ICU, surgery, or the trauma unit you will be required to deal with patients at great risk. In such acute situations, attention to detail and a high level of performance are essential.

REVIEW QUESTIONS

1. Which precautions must be followed when obtaining a bedside chest x-ray on a patient who has recently had a pacemaker implanted?
   A. Do not abduct his or her left arm.
   B. Do not abduct his or her right arm.
   C. Do not allow the patient to sit upright.
   D. Do not allow the patient to lie flat.

2. Which of the following statements represent(s) the guidelines for performing a bedside radiographic examination?
   A. Check with the nurse in charge to inquire about the patient's condition.
   B. Confirm the order in the patient's chart.
   C. Greet the patient and prepare the room before bringing in the x-ray equipment.
   D. All of the above.
3. Nasogastric tubes are placed in patients for:
   A. feeding
   B. decompression of gas and fluids
   C. imaging purposes
   D. all of the above
4. An example of a nasogastric tube used to feed the patient is called a _____ tube.
   A. Dobbhoff
   B. Miller-Abbott
   C. Harris
   D. Cantor
5. The tip of a PICC or any central venous catheter should be visualized in the:
   A. pulmonary artery
   B. right atrium
   C. right ventricle
   D. superior vena cava

CRITICAL THINKING EXERCISES

1. You have arrived in the ICU to obtain a chest x-ray on Mrs. Squire. In assessing Mrs. Squire, you note that she has a tracheostomy and that a chest tube exiting her left thorax is connected to a suction device below the bed. List the steps you would follow in preparation for taking the radiograph to insure an optimum image while providing proper care to the patient. List the precautions you would take while obtaining her chest x-ray.
2. You are sent to the surgical suite and asked to take an operative cholangiogram film. The surgeon needs to check for possible residual stones in the biliary ducts. List the precautions you would take in preparing and setting up your equipment, placing the cassette, and aligning the tube.
3. Observe an experienced radiographer performing bedside radiography and record the special skills that are required when obtaining radiographs at bedside rather than in the radiology department.

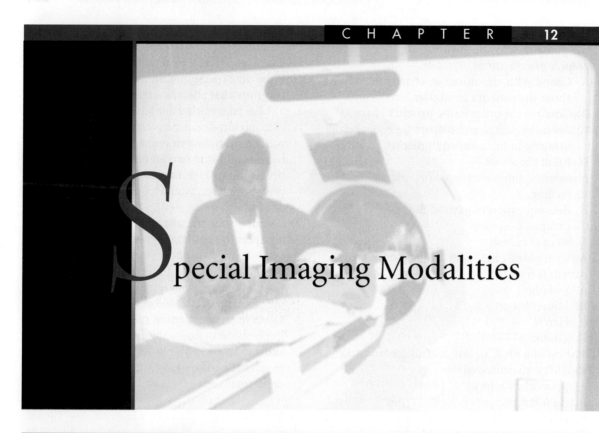

Special Imaging Modalities

At the conclusion of this chapter, the student will be able to:

- List specific angiographic examinations and name the blood vessels that are demonstrated with each.
- Describe Seldinger technique and state its purpose.
- List five specific procedures classed as interventional radiology and state the purpose of each.
- Identify and state the purpose of each of the principal parts of a computed tomography (CT) scanner.
- List advantages of spiral and multislice spiral/helical scanners in comparison to conventional CT scanners.
- Discuss the use of oral and intravenous (IV) contrast media in CT and list precautions for avoiding extravasation of IV contrast agents.
- List common diagnostic applications of magnetic resonance imaging (MRI).
- List safety precautions for personnel working in the area of an MRI scanner.

- Explain the use of contrast agents and medications in MRI and the procedures for monitoring sedated patients during MRI examinations.
- Compare and contrast conventional nuclear medicine procedures, positron emission tomography (PET) and single photon emission computed tomography (SPECT) scans.
- Compare and contrast nuclear medicine procedures with other imaging modalities.
- Describe in simple terms the process of acquiring ultrasound images and list common diagnostic applications for both conventional and Doppler ultrasound.
- Describe the procedure for routine mammography and explain the patient care considerations that are significant with this modality.

THE IMAGING TECHNIQUES in this chapter are not done in every health care institution. They are performed by technologists with advanced training who may also have specialty certification. These topics provide beginning radiographers with an introduction to the nature and purpose of these imaging modalities and highlight the applicable safety procedures and patient care issues. As a student you should know about these procedures and be able to provide preliminary explanations when patients inquire about them while in the radiography department. You should also be prepared to assist with the more routine aspects of patient care if you have scheduled rotations into these specialty areas.

Technological advancements in computers, electronic engineering, and diagnostic pharmaceuticals are producing rapid changes in all of the imaging modalities in this chapter. A scanner that combines positron emission tomography (PET) with computed tomography (CT) provides the speed and flexibility of x-ray CT with data on physiological function from nuclear medicine techniques. Gamma cameras with huge overhead gantries are being replaced with handheld models for some specific applications such as breast imaging. Computer-aided detection (CAD) is enhancing the value of screening mammography,

as is the use of CT laser mammography (CTLM). Tiny ultrasound transducers affixed to endoscopes are used to produce sonograms from inside the digestive tract. New contrast media are expanding the diagnostic scope of both ultrasound imaging and PET scanning. Three-dimensional images from various modalities are increasing the speed and accuracy of surgical procedures, while angiographic and endoscopic procedures that were once exclusively diagnostic are now also used for treatment, often eliminating the need for surgery. These advances in imaging provide challenges and avenues of specialization for technologists. We hope that this information will encourage you to conduct additional research and explore these areas further.

CARDIOVASCULAR AND INTERVENTIONAL RADIOGRAPHY
Angiography
Conventional catheter angiography

Radiographic procedures that demonstrate vessels are collectively known as **angiography**. A cerebral angiogram, for example, demonstrates the vessels of the brain (Fig. 12-1), while renal angiograms demonstrate the renal arteries and veins. An **angiocardiogram** is a contrast study that visualizes the

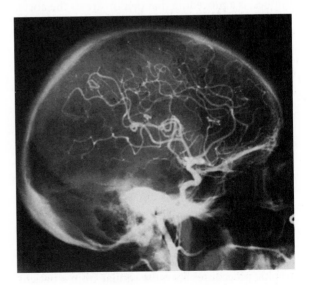

FIG. 12-1 Cerebral angiogram.

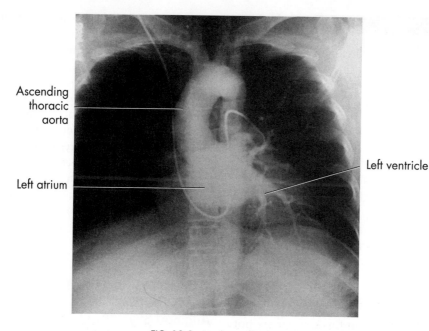

Ascending
thoracic
aorta

Left atrium

Left ventricle

FIG. 12-2 Angiocardiogram.

interior of the heart chambers and the great vessels that enter and exit the heart (Fig. 12-2). Selective angiocardiography can be used to demonstrate the coronary arteries. An **aortogram,** as the name implies, is a procedure that demonstrates the aorta. An arch aortogram demonstrates the thoracic portion and the branches that provide circulation to the head and the arms (Fig. 12-3); an abdominal aortogram demonstrates the portion between the diaphragm and the iliac bifurcation (Fig. 12-4). **Arteriograms** are studies of specific arteries (Fig. 12-5), and **venograms** are studies of veins (Fig. 12-6).

For all of these examinations, water-soluble iodine compounds are used for radiographic contrast and a rapid series of images is taken using highly specialized equipment. The contrast medium used for angiography is chosen according to the requirements of the specific procedure (see Table 10-1). Some diversity of technical methods exists among imaging departments, but it is not necessary to explore these variations here since all angiographic procedures are quite similar from a patient care standpoint.

Direct **percutaneous** (through the skin) injection may be used for some angiographic studies, such as those of the extremities, but the preferred injection method for angiocardiography, aortography, and most arteriography is to use a catheter. Angiographic catheters are radiopaque for visibility under the fluoroscope and come in a variety of lengths, gauges, and tip configurations. Catheter insertion is accomplished by the Seldinger technique (Fig. 12-7). A large artery, usually the femoral or brachial, is entered percutaneously with a large-bore needle. The needle is fitted with a stylet of equal length, which prevents blood from flowing back through the needle. When the needle is situated in the artery, the stylet is removed and a guide wire is threaded through the needle and into the artery under fluoroscopic control. The needle is then removed, the guide wire is left in the vessel, and the catheter is threaded over the wire. The wire is then removed, and the catheter remains in the artery for the duration of the procedure. Further manipulation of the catheter may be needed to ensure correct placement in the vessel before injection. For selective

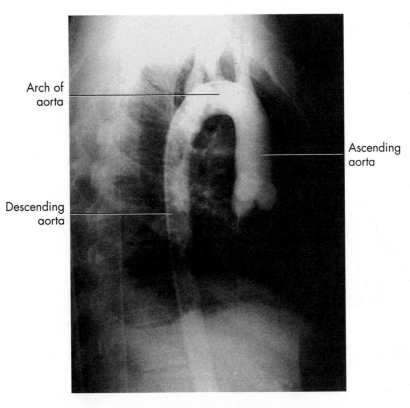

Arch of
aorta

Ascending
aorta

Descending
aorta

FIG. 12-3 Arch aortogram.

catheterization of smaller vessels, the catheter tip is maneuvered into the root of the vessel of interest, such as the coronary, celiac, renal, or carotid artery (Fig. 12-8).

A timed sequence of images is obtained during and after injection of the contrast medium, usually with the aid of an automatic power injector that is electronically coordinated with a programmable film changer and automated exposure control. Digital receptors are replacing the use of film and film changers in many imaging centers, and for some studies such as angiocardiograms, digital fluoroscopy equipment may be used to record the images.

Patients are usually given sedative medications before angiography, so apprehension and anxiety are seldom problems at the time of examination. The patient usually is alert enough to cooperate with positioning but must not be left alone on the table.

The radiographer's role, as in any injection procedure, is to be familiar with the radiologist's needs for equipment and supplies, to perform the skin preparation, and to assist with sterile technique (see Chapter 5). Because of the highly specialized nature of the procedures and equipment, specific training is needed to perform these functions, but the basic principles of patient care and aseptic technique are the same as for other sterile injections and must be followed meticulously (Fig. 12-9). Some angiography departments are staffed with nurses or cardiovascular technicians who assist the physician and handle patient care duties. When this is the case, the technologist's duties are mainly technical.

Follow-up care is very important after angiography to avoid the possibility of hemorrhage or hematoma at the puncture site. After any arterial puncture, firm, continuous pressure is applied to the injection site

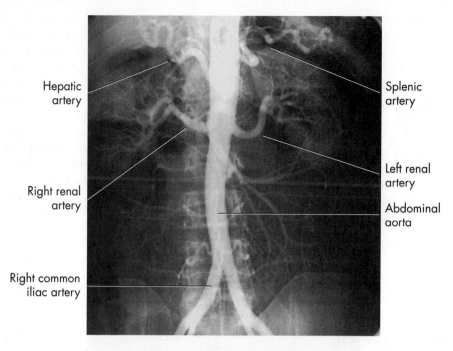

Hepatic artery

Splenic artery

Right renal artery

Left renal artery

Abdominal aorta

Right common iliac artery

FIG. 12-4 Abdominal aortogram.

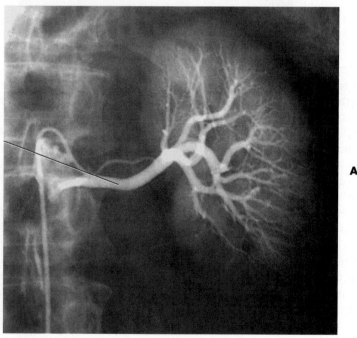

Left renal artery

A

FIG. 12-5 Arteriograms. **A,** Selective renal arteriogram.

for 5 to 10 minutes, followed by the application of a pressure dressing, which is monitored by the nursing service. A pressure dressing is also applied after studies that involve puncture of a vein.

Conventional angiography is not without risk. Potential complications include damage to the artery during manipulation of the guide wire or catheter, reaction to contrast media, hemorrhage or hematoma at the puncture site, and thrombosis of the vessel following the procedure. Because of these risks, as well as the differential in cost, angiography has been supplanted to some degree by technological advances in Doppler ultrasound, nuclear medicine, magnetic resonance angiography (MRA), and computed tomography angiography (CTA). Despite these advances, angiography continues to be used extensively because it provides the best anatomical demonstration of structures within the circulatory system and also offers the opportunity for immediate therapeutic interventions to treat the problems identified.

Digital subtraction angiography

Computerized imaging equipment is used in many imaging centers to perform digital subtraction angiography (DSA). Angiographic images are recorded in digital format on a computer rather than on film. The images can then be manipulated, using the computer to enhance contrast and decrease the visibility of superimposing structures. The resulting computer images can also be reproduced on film using a special camera or managed by a picture archiving and communication system (PACS) as

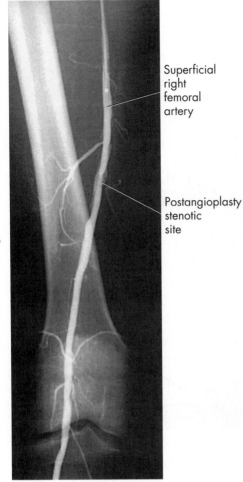

B

Superficial right femoral artery

Postangioplasty stenotic site

FIG. 12-5—cont'd **B,** Femoral arteriogram.

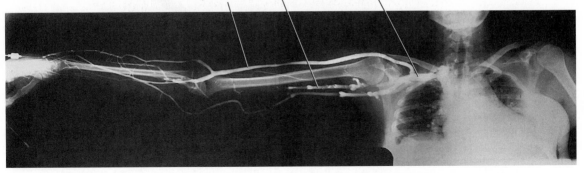

Cephalic vein   Basilic vein   Subclavian vein

FIG. 12-6 Venogram, normal upper extremity.

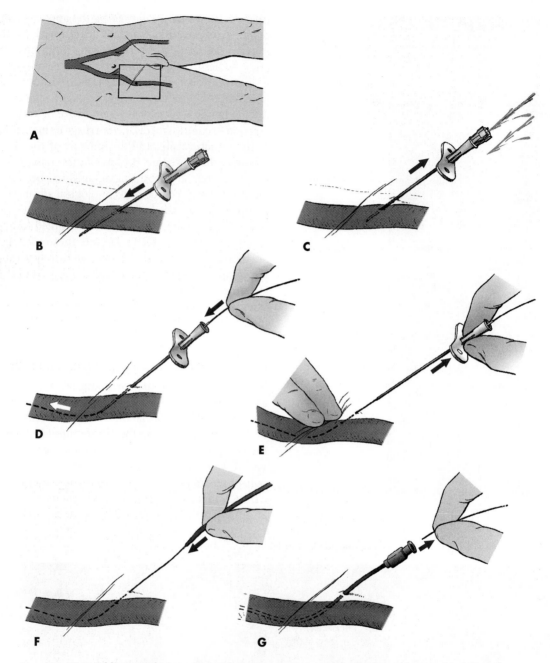

FIG. 12-7 Seldinger technique. **A,** An ideal arteriotomy occurs in the femoral artery just below the inguinal ligament. **B,** A beveled compound needle containing an inner cannula pierces through the artery. **C,** The needle's solid inner cannula is removed, and the needle is retracted until blood flow indicates placement of the tip within the lumen of the artery. **D,** A flexible guide wire is inserted into the artery through the needle. **E,** The needle is removed; pressure fixes the wire and reduces hemorrhage. **F,** The catheter is slipped over the wire and into the artery. **G,** The guide wire is removed, leaving the catheter in the artery.

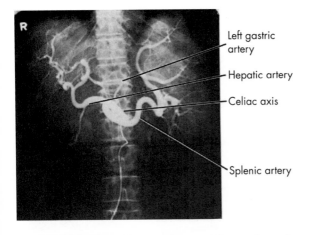

Left gastric artery

Hepatic artery

Celiac axis

Splenic artery

FIG. 12-8 Selective celiac arteriogram. Note catheter in abdominal aorta.

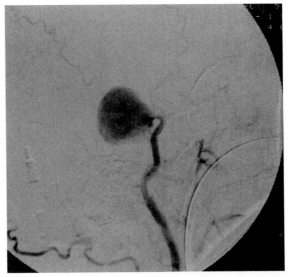

FIG. 12-10 Digital subtraction angiogram illustrates a large carotid aneurysm and demonstrates vessels with absence of superimposing bony structures.

with other digital images. In the subtraction process, two images in the same projection are used, one with contrast and one without. The computer then eliminates structures from the contrast image that are common to both images, leaving only the image of the contrast-enhanced vessels (Fig. 12-10). In some departments DSA has completely replaced

conventional film-screen angiography, especially for the cerebral vasculature.

DSA can be performed using either conventional arterial catheterization or IV contrast injection. IV administration is less invasive than arterial

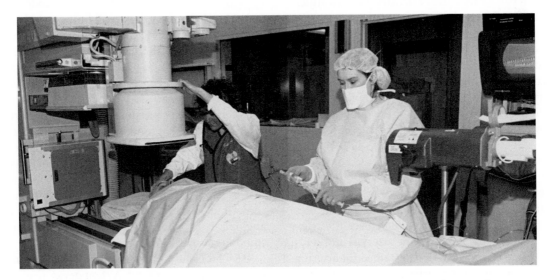

FIG. 12-9 Technologist assists radiologist with sterile technique during angiography procedure.

catheterization and is therefore less hazardous. It is relatively painless and can be safely used in patients at high risk for arterial catheterization. IV contrast is used less often, however, because of the relatively poor anatomical detail obtained compared with arterial injections.

Interventional Radiology

While the use of angiography for diagnosis has decreased somewhat due to the increased use of other modalities, the use of angiographic techniques for interventional radiology is expanding. Interventional radiology refers to the nonsurgical treatment or correction of a vascular problem, often at the time it is diagnosed and/or located radiographically. When the nature and precise location of a vascular constriction or bleed have been established using angiography and a specialized catheter is in place within the vessel, the catheter can be utilized to provide treatment. Most interventional radiology is performed in the angiography suite by the angiography team, usually in conjunction with a diagnostic angiographic procedure.

Percutaneous transluminal angioplasty

Percutaneous transluminal angioplasty (PTA) is an interventional technique that is commonly associated with arteriography. The term **angioplasty** means "vessel repair." PTA is used extensively as a treatment for **atherosclerosis,** narrowing or blockage of an artery due to the buildup of fatty plaque. Arteries may also become constricted due to calcium deposits and/or **thrombi** (blood clots; singular, **thrombus**). When arterial **stenosis** (narrowing) is localized on an arteriogram or with another imaging modality, a variety of nonsurgical techniques can be utilized to open the constricted area and increase blood flow.

Balloon angioplasty is a technique commonly used to treat atherosclerosis. A balloon-tipped catheter with a double lumen is used. The balloon is inflated with a dilute contrast medium, and the pressure from the expanding balloon extends the artery wall, enlarging the lumen of the artery (Fig. 12-11). Patient care is similar to that described for arteriography in the preceding section. Similar techniques

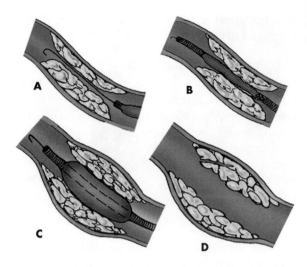

FIG. 12-11 Balloon angioplasty of atherosclerotic stenosis. **A,** Guide wire advanced through stenosis. **B,** Balloon across stenosis. **C,** Balloon inflated. **D,** Stenotic area postangioplasty.

can be used to dilate veins, ureters, bile ducts, and portions of the gastrointestinal (GI) tract.

Laser technology has been adapted for use in PTA. In laser-tipped angioplasty, the **atheroma** (mass of fatty material forming the blockage) is vaporized with laser energy delivered by a special catheter. Thermal angioplasty uses a laser-heated probe to reopen blocked vessels. Both laser methods leave a smoother surface on the vessel lining than balloon angioplasty, decreasing the likelihood of restenosis.

Percutaneous atherectomy is a PTA method in which the blocking plaque material is cut away. The term **atherectomy** refers to the removal of an atheroma. There are two basic types of special catheters for this purpose. One is fitted with a rotational head that functions with a liquid spray to pulverize the atheromatous material; the other type has a directional blade mechanism that cuts the material and captures it in a cylindrical housing that is a part of the catheter. Balloon angioplasty is sometimes used in combination with either laser angioplasty or atherectomy to provide a wider and smoother lumen in the vessel.

PTA procedures may also involve placement via catheter of a vascular stent. A stent device is a flexible plastic or wire tube that is permanently situated within a vessel or other tubular structure to keep it open.

Transcatheter embolization

Unlike PTA, whose purpose is to increase blood flow in a vessel, transcatheter embolization is an interventional technique used to decrease or stop blood flow. There are three principal reasons for performing transcatheter embolization: (1) to stop hemorrhage at active bleeding sites, for example, a bleeding ulcer; (2) to cut off the flow of blood to diseased or malformed areas such as tumors or arteriovenous malformations (AVMs); and (3) to reduce blood flow to a specific area to minimize blood loss during surgery. A variety of liquid, gel, and solid materials can be used to accomplish embolization, and the choice depends on the site and the duration of embolization desired. For example, polyvinyl alcohol (Ivalon), silicone beads, or stainless steel coils may be used to provide permanent vessel occlusion, whereas a special product called Gelfoam or a vasoconstricting drug such as vasopressin (Pitressin) provides temporary vessel closure. A catheter is placed using Seldinger technique, and angiography may be used to diagnose hemorrhage, locate the exact site for embolization, and/or to confirm the success of the procedure.

Sclerotic therapy and radiofrequency ablation

In the past, vein problems such as occlusion, stenosis, varicosity, and inflammation were treated surgically. The veins were either ligated (tied off) or stripped (surgically removed). Nonsurgical therapies such as chemical injection and interventional radiology now offer minimally invasive treatment options for these types of problems.

Sclerotic therapy involves injections that cause thickening and occlusion of the vein and is useful for treating "spider veins" and other small veins of the lower legs. Larger veins, such as the greater saphenous and the accessory saphenous vein systems, can now be treated with a method called radiofrequency (RF) ablation. Until recently this technology was utilized only for the treatment of tumors. When using RF ablation to treat veins, a special device is used that consists of a tiny RF generator associated with a sterile catheter and a collapsible electrode. The length of the vein is anesthetized with local injections of lidocaine, and the catheter is positioned in the vein over a guide wire using Seldinger technique under fluoroscopic control. The treatment is continuously monitored by color Doppler ultrasound to confirm reduction of blood flow in the vein. Patient care procedures include preparation for injection of lidocaine over the course of the vein to be treated, maintaining hemostasis at the puncture site following the procedure, and providing patient instruction for follow-up care. Care following RF ablation of the larger veins usually entails wearing compression stockings, following a prescribed walking regimen, and avoiding standing for prolonged periods. The patient is usually seen again in 72 hours, after which normal activity is resumed.

COMPUTED TOMOGRAPHY

Computed tomography (CT) is the same modality formerly called computer-assisted tomography (CAT) scanning. CT produces axial images, slicelike sections in the transverse plane that may be "reconstructed" by the computer to display the anatomical structures in other planes as well. Image characteristics such as brightness and contrast can be manipulated on the computer. The images may be viewed in different formats called "windows" that are designed to enhance visualization of specific tissues (Fig. 12-12). Institutions with PACS digital image management will include CT examinations in this system so that images can be viewed at PACS monitors.

Equipment

The CT scanner (Fig. 12-13) consists of a moveable table with remote control, a circular **gantry** structure that supports the x-ray tube and detectors, an operator console with a monitor and supporting computer system, plus hardware and software to archive and manage data and produce hard copies of the images.

During a scan, the x-ray tube (and sometimes also the detectors) rotates around the patient to collect the data. In conventional CT units the tube

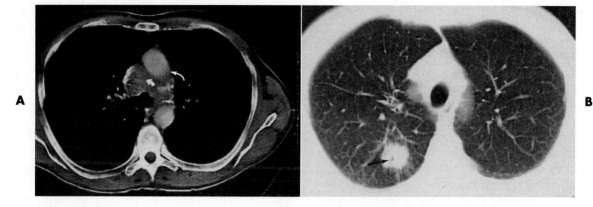

FIG. 12-12 Two CT windows demonstrate different structures of the chest from the same image. **A,** Mediastinal structures are demonstrated in the center of the field, but the lungs are not well seen. **B,** "Lung window" demonstrates the blood vessels of the lungs and a lung tumor *(arrow)*.

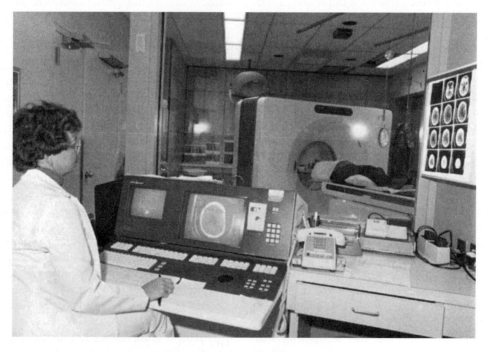

FIG. 12-13 Technologist operates CT scanner and monitors patient from control console.

makes a complete rotation to gather data for each slice. The table then moves and the tube rotates again to obtain the next slice. A newer generation of scanner, designated as spiral or helical, scans a spiral path around the patient and can collect data on a larger volume of tissue (Fig. 12-14). This system permits scanning of a relatively large area during a single breathhold and reduces scanning time compared to conventional units. The advanced software that supports spiral/helical CT can provide data reconstruction of volume information and render three-dimensional (3-D) images. The most recent generation of scanners, designated as multislice spiral/helical, creates multiple slices with each rotation of the tube, greatly speeding the process of image acquisition.

Applications

The versatility of CT is illustrated by its wide range of applications, including studies of the brain, spine, abdomen, pelvis, chest, neck, and paranasal sinuses, plus orthopedic examinations of the extremities and contrast-enhanced vascular studies known as CT angiography (CTA). CT is useful in localizing both lesions and needle position during needle aspiration biopsy, a nonsurgical method of obtaining cells for laboratory examination. Since CT is also a valuable tool for emergency use, especially in the detection of intracerebral or intra-abdominal hemorrhage, trauma centers often have a CT scanner in the emergency department.

Most CT examinations are noninvasive and are not uncomfortable for the patient. The equipment may cause apprehension, however, and careful explanations are necessary for patient cooperation and a satisfactory study.

Contrast CT Examinations

While many CT examinations do not require enhancement with contrast media, the use of contrast agents vastly increases the scope of CT imaging. Studies of the abdomen (Fig. 12-15) usually employ oral contrast to help differentiate the GI tract from the surrounding tissues. A special barium compound (e.g., E-Z-Cat) or an oral aqueous iodine medium (e.g., Gastrografin mixed with water and flavoring) is ingested by the patient over a specified period before the study. The amount of contrast and the time vary depending on whether the examination includes only the upper abdomen or the entire abdomen and pelvis. For these studies the patient is instructed to fast and to come early to drink the contrast preparation. Some departments have the patient take the contrast home with instructions to drink it before reporting for the appointment.

Intravenous (IV) injection of a water-soluble iodinated contrast medium may also be employed to increase the contrast level of the patient's tissues. This is advantageous for studies of the chest, abdomen, and soft tissues of the neck, since it highlights blood vessels and enhances visualization of vascular organs such as the liver and spleen. The contrast defines the renal collecting system, ureters, and bladder as it is excreted in the urine. In selected cases, IV contrast agents are employed in head CT scans to demonstrate brain lesions (Fig. 12-16).

IV contrast is essential in CT angiography. These procedures use spiral/helical scanners to create volumetric 3-D images of the arteries and veins of the head and trunk. CTA displays the vessels clearly in relation to the surrounding bone and soft tissues. This feature is especially advantageous for visualizing particular structures such as the renal circulation (Fig. 12-17) and the arteries at the base of the brain.

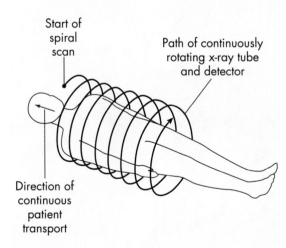

FIG. 12-14 Spiral CT scanners gather volume data as x-ray source and detectors trace a spiral path around the patient.

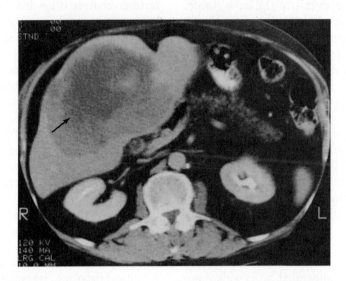

FIG. 12-15 Contrast-enhanced axial CT image of abdomen shows large liver lesion *(arrow)* and opacification of kidneys (lateral to spine).

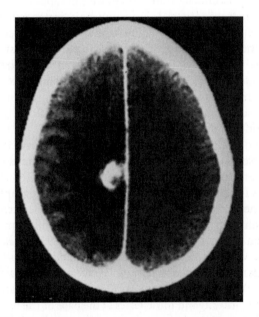

FIG. 12-16 CT brain scan with contrast enhancement.

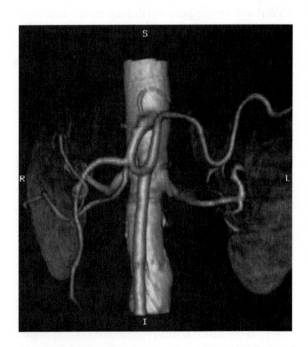

FIG. 12-17 Three-dimensional CTA image of abdominal aorta and renal arteries.

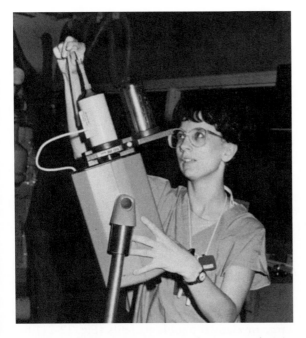

FIG. 12-18 Automatic injector controls contrast administration for CT examinations.

CTA involves less risk than conventional catheter angiography but also provides less image resolution for small vessels.

Intravenous contrast administration often consists of a bolus of the medium injected rapidly at the start of the procedure and a continuation of the injection at a much slower rate as the examination proceeds. The initial bolus of contrast may be injected with a syringe and followed by a drip infusion. The approach most often used is to connect the IV set to an automatic injector (Fig. 12-18) that is loaded with the contrast medium and programmed to provide the desired flow rates.

The IV line is usually established with an intravenous catheter and then connected to the syringe, IV tubing, or injector tubing. An intermittent injection port (saline lock) or an established IV line with an injection port may be used. An 18-gauge needle or needleless connector is attached to the injector tubing or syringe and is used to penetrate the port. Once situated, the attachment is secured with tape. If other IV fluids are being administered through the IV line, the tubing must be clamped off to stop the flow during the injection and released to restore the flow afterwards. The IV line is flushed before and after the contrast injection to avoid mixing the contrast with medication in the tubing or injection port.

The high volume of contrast used (often 200 ml) and the remote location of the technologist during the scan can create significant problems in the event of extravasation of the contrast medium. The use of a powerful automatic injector compounds this hazard. The following precautions will help minimize this risk:

- Select an IV site other than an antecubital vein to avoid the possibility that elbow flexion will compromise the IV line. If an antecubital vein must be used, prevent elbow flexion with an arm board.
- When using an intermittent injection port, flush before connecting the injection tubing to be sure the IV catheter is properly situated in the vein and contains no residual medication.
- Double-check the IV site for possible extravasation at the time the automatic injector is started.
- Instruct the patient to immediately report any sensation of burning, pressure, or other discomfort in the area of the IV site.

Review Chapter 7 for additional procedures and precautions related to IV injections. As with all contrast media injections, you must take a pertinent history in advance, identify signs of an adverse reaction, and be prepared to respond if a reaction occurs.

Computed Tomography Myelography

CT imaging can greatly expand the information obtained with myelography by demonstrating the dural sac and nerve roots in the transverse plane. As soon as the routine myelogram is completed (see Chapter 10), the patient is brought to the CT scanner for axial contrast-enhanced images of the spinal canal (Fig. 12-19). It is important to minimize delay between the fluoroscopic procedure and the CT examination because the contrast agent is rapidly absorbed from the spinal fluid into the bloodstream and will not be sufficiently concentrated for good visualization if too much time is lost.

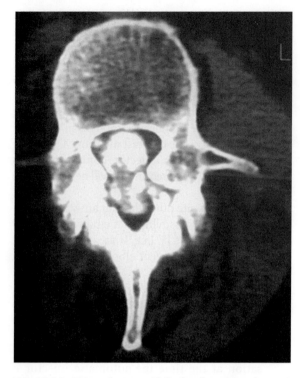

FIG. 12-19 CT myelogram of the lumbar spine demonstrating subarachnoid space narrowing *(arrows)*.

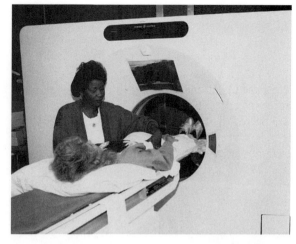

FIG. 12-20 Patient receives reassurance before entering conventional MRI gantry.

MAGNETIC RESONANCE IMAGING

Magnetic resonance imaging (MRI) is a noninvasive diagnostic modality that does not use ionizing radiation. A powerful magnetic field and RF pulses are combined to produce a radio signal in the body that can be detected and processed electronically to provide images on the computer monitor. The computer image is digitized and may be managed by a PACS. It can also be stored on magnetic tape and photographed with a special camera to produce film copies.

Equipment

MRI equipment includes a patient table, gantry, and console-monitor combination with computer support. The gantry houses the magnet. A conventional gantry is tubular, 5 to 8 feet long, and surrounds most of the patient's body during the scanning process (Fig. 12-20). An open configuration in

gantry design provides better accommodation for large or claustrophobic patients (Fig. 12-21) but does not always provide image quality equal to that produced by conventional units.

Radio frequency coils are essential components of the MR imaging system. The coils transmit pulses

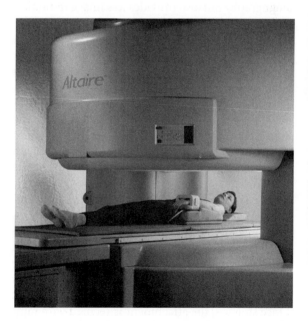

FIG. 12-21 Open-gantry MRI unit.

of RF energy to the patient's body and receive the RF signal emitted by the resonating tissue. The information associated with this signal is digitized, stored in the computer, and used to form the image. Depending on the application, the same or different coils are used for transmitting the RF pulses and receiving the RF signal. The three basic types of coils are body, head, and surface coils. The body coil is a permanent part of the scanner; it completely surrounds the patient's body in conventional, tubular-gantry scanners. The body coil transmits RF pulses for all scans and serves as a receiving coil for RF signals when scanning the trunk of the body. The helmet type of head coil completely surrounds the patient's head and is a receiver coil only; the body coil is used to transmit the RF pulses. Surface coils can be placed directly on or around the anatomical area of interest. They are designed with different shapes that correspond to the requirements of different body parts. Like the head coil, surface coils are receiver coils only.

Applications

MRI provides excellent imaging of the soft tissues of the nervous system (Fig. 12-22) and is useful in the diagnosis of many types of pathology, including brain and spinal cord tumors and diseases such as multiple sclerosis. MRI is being used extensively in place of myelography for diagnosis of herniated intervertebral disks. This modality is also effective in imaging the soft tissue components of joints (Fig. 12-23), providing an alternative to arthrography of the knee, shoulder, and temporomandibular joint.

Typical scan time for a series of slicelike images ranges from 1 to 10 minutes, and several series demonstrating different body planes and using a variety of RF pulse sequences may be included in an examination. It is critically important that the patient remain still during a scan series and that the initial position be maintained throughout the study. Some pulse sequences allow images to be made in the space of a breathhold, providing clear visualization of areas such as the lungs and the liver that would otherwise be blurred because of respiratory motion.

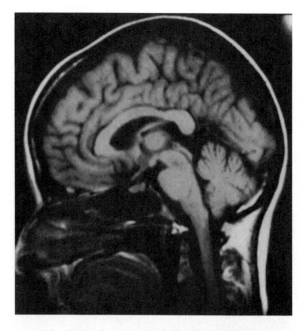

FIG. 12-22 Center sagittal MRI image of brain.

Magnetic Resonance Imaging Contrast Media

Although contrast media are not required for most MRI studies, paramagnetic agents such as gadopentetate dimeglumine (Magnevist) and gadoteridol (ProHance), made from the rare-earth element gadolinium, are sometimes injected intravenously. These agents provide contrast enhancement of certain lesions, particularly brain and spinal cord tumors, and aid in differentiating disk material from scar tissue in postoperative spine examinations. Allergic reactions to gadolinium contrast agents have been reported, but they are very rare. As with any contrast medium, a history is taken and emergency supplies must be readily available. See Chapter 8 for emergency response to contrast reactions.

Magnetic Resonance Angiography

A more recent advance in MRI is MRA, using magnetic resonance technology to study the cardiovascular system. MRA is used to detect, diagnose, and aid in the treatment of heart disorders, stroke, and blood vessel diseases. It can be used to confirm

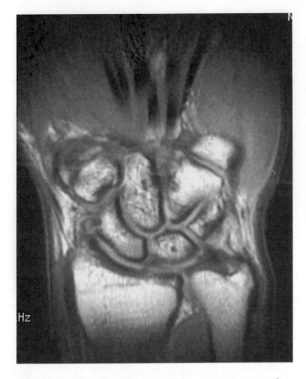

FIG. 12-23 Coronal MRI scan of the wrist using a surface coil is an example of an MRI joint study.

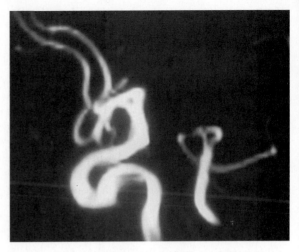

FIG. 12-24 Sagittal MRA image of cerebral circulation obtained using a three-dimensional, phase-contrast pulse sequence.

the diagnosis of vascular problems detected by Doppler ultrasound methods and is used as a screening tool for patients at risk of aneurysm. Although MRA can provide detailed images of blood vessels without using contrast media, gadolinium contrast usually is given during a portion of the study to enhance image detail. MRA encompasses a group of MR methods that involve special RF pulse sequences to highlight blood flow and suppress the images of surrounding structures (Fig. 12-24).

Magnetic Resonance Spectroscopy and Spectroscopic Imaging

Magnetic resonance spectroscopy (MRS) is a specialized MR technique that involves the scanning of a volume of tissue to identify and measure the quantities of specific chemicals in the tissue. Chemical and physiological information obtained with MRS makes it a particularly useful research tool for the investigation of brain function, but MRS also provides diagnostic information about biochemical and metabolic pathways in the central nervous system. The speed and precision of MRS analyses permit access to unique and transient biochemical events. The most prevalent uses of this technique include differential diagnosis of coma, multiple sclerosis, and human immunodeficiency virus (HIV), prognosis in cases of head injury and cerebrovascular accident (CVA), and investigation of neonatal hypoxia and congenital errors in metabolism. MRS also aids in surgical planning for patients with temporal lobe epilepsy and is being used in the investigation of muscle disorders.

Magnetic resonance spectroscopic imaging (MRSI) uses phase encoding methods to obtain spectra from multiple regions across the field of view. Instead of the volume information obtained with MRS, MRSI provides an image that maps the location and quantity of specific chemicals. MRSI holds great promise for the future but is still limited by technical problems that cause it to be currently somewhat less reliable than MRS for many applications.

MRS and MRSI are also referred to as functional MRI studies or fMRI.

MRI Safety

The unique MRI environment requires special safety precautions. Conditions affecting patient safety involve both the powerful magnetic field within the gantry and the thermal effects of RF pulses on certain materials that could overheat and possibly burn the patient. The RF energy used is a form of nonionizing radiation that can heat the tissues of the body. For this reason, the U.S. Food and Drug Administration (FDA) has established limits on exposure to RF energy that vary according to the anatomy being imaged.

The principal means of ensuring patient safety during an MRI is careful patient screening prior to the procedure. The magnetic field and/or the rapid RF gradients may be hazardous for patients with artificial heart valves, aneurysm clips, neurostimulators, middle ear prostheses, or intrauterine devices (IUDs). Special reference directories can be used to determine the safety of specific devices with respect to MRI. Cardiac pacemakers are a particular hazard, and *patients with pacemakers must not enter the scan room,* as the magnetic field may cause the device to malfunction. A few fatalities have resulted from overheating of these implanted devices when patients with pacemakers were scanned. Individuals with pacemakers who come within the influence of the magnetic field should see their cardiologists immediately for a pacemaker evaluation because the magnetic field may damage the pacemaker, causing it to fail without warning, even though the damage may not be immediately apparent.

Other conditions that merit assessment before entering the magnetic field include hemolytic anemia, orthopedic pins and screws, and metal fragments or shrapnel in the soft tissues. Most orthopedic hardware is safe in the magnet, although it may cause significant compromise of MRI image quality in the region. Metalworkers who might have steel slivers in their tissues must have a screening radiographic or CT head examination to detect fragments that could damage their eyes or brain, because the pull of the magnetic field is so strong that it could cause these fragments to move. Although the energies involved in MRI have not been demonstrated to cause complications with pregnancy, the prevailing philosophy is to avoid examination of pregnant patients during the first trimester.

Before the scan begins, the technologist places MRI-safe padding strategically to ensure that the patient's skin does not touch the magnet bore and is well insulated from the potential thermal effects of the RF pulses. Patients are instructed to report any unusual sensation of warmth immediately.

In addition to the magnetic field within the gantry, a significant magnetic field exists throughout the room and may affect anyone who enters. A lesser fringe field extends for some distance into the surrounding area. The magnetic field is present all the time, not just during a scan. All individuals entering the scan room should first be interviewed to determine if they have surgical implants or metallic foreign bodies that could cause harm.

Loose metal objects must never be carried into the room. A pair of scissors, for instance, may fly from a pocket when entering the magnetic field, endangering bystanders and damaging the gantry. Small metal objects such as hairpins or paperclips may be pulled into inaccessible portions of the magnet housing, where they distort the magnetic field and cause image degradation. *Never enter the scanning room with stretchers, wheelchairs, or crutches that are not made specifically for use with MRI,* since the magnetic field is strong enough to pull these items out of control, causing a serious accident. Steel oxygen tanks pose a lethal hazard and must never be taken into the scan room. (Oxygen is available from a wall outlet.)

Individuals entering the scanning area should be cautioned not to bring watches, credit cards, hearing aids, or neurostimulators because the magnet will damage them. No one should enter the scan room without the permission of the person responsible for controlling access. Personnel whose work requires that they enter the scan room must receive an orientation that includes safety instruction specific to this area.

Claustrophobia and Pain Management

The MRI technologist's duties include patient preparation for the examination and assistance in dealing with both physical and emotional discomfort.

Few people are completely comfortable for any length of time in a tightly enclosed space. Even patients with no history of claustrophobia may feel anxious when entering a conventional tubular MRI gantry. Occasionally this anxiety is so severe that it creates panic, preventing the patient from continuing the examination.

It is important for the patient to know in advance that the table will move into the gantry, that plenty of air is available and that no physical discomfort will occur other than the need to lie still. The machine will make a loud "knocking" noise during the scanning process. Earplugs or earphones with recorded music may be offered. Patients may be reassured to know that they can communicate with the technologist through an intercom and that the technologist is watching them and listening to them at all times during the procedure. Since no radiation danger exists, a friend or family member may be allowed to accompany the patient into the room and to stay throughout the procedure if desired. Remember that everyone who enters the scan room must be screened for pacemakers, pregnancy, loose metal objects, and items that could be damaged by the magnet.

A severely claustrophobic patient may be rescheduled at a facility with an open-gantry MRI or may be given an antianxiety medication. Medications may also be needed for patients whose pain makes it impossible to lie still for the duration of the study. For patients who require medication, an IV catheter with an intermittent injection port is established first. This provides access throughout the procedure in case it is needed for repeat doses, contrast administration, or emergency drug administration. The radiologist selects and administers the drug(s), and the technologist assists.

Diazepam is frequently used to treat claustrophobia, and morphine or meperidine may be used for analgesia. Remember that these drugs act as respiratory depressants. The patient must be monitored with a pulse oximeter during the procedure, because it is not possible to monitor the patient directly. Be certain that antagonists to reverse the effects of these drugs are available, as well as emergency supplies in the event of adverse reaction. (Review Chapter 7 for information on medication administration and sedation and Chapter 8 for responses to emergency situations.)

DIAGNOSTIC MEDICAL SONOGRAPHY

Diagnostic medical sonography is a noninvasive procedure that is considered to be very safe for the patient. This imaging modality, often referred to as diagnostic ultrasound, uses high-frequency sound waves to produce echoes within the body. As the echoes return to the sending point, or **transducer,** their strength and timing are interpreted by a computer to produce a map or graphic image of the echo distribution. The transducer is moved over the surface of the body, and the image is viewed in real time on the computer monitor (Fig. 12-25). Special transducer probes can be inserted into body cavities such as the rectum and the vagina to obtain more detailed examinations of the prostate gland and the uterus. Any interface between substances or tissues of varying density produces an ultrasound echo, making sonography an effective technique to visualize the shape, size, and condition of organs such as the heart, spleen, gallbladder, or pancreas (Fig. 12-26). Since sonography permits differentiation of fluid from adipose tissue, the presence of an abscess, cyst,

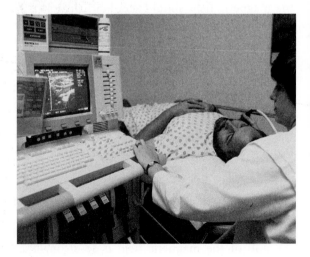

FIG. 12-25 Images are viewed in real time during sonography scanning procedure.

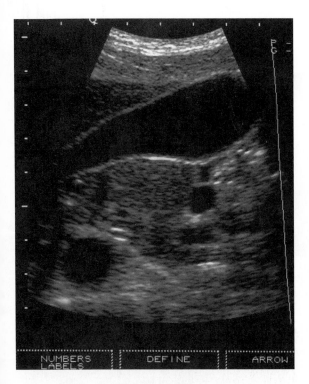

FIG. 12-26 Abdominal sonogram.

or tumor, or abnormal fluid such as ascites, can be demonstrated.

Recent technological advances in ultrasound technology include computer integration of data obtained in multiple planes to produce three-dimensional images that are more lifelike than conventional two-dimensional images (Fig. 12-27). Special contrast agents containing microscopic bubbles are available for use in cardiac imaging but have not been approved by the FDA for other applications. These agents transmit echoes from within tissues that would otherwise lack image detail. The recent invention of harmonic scanners permits acquisition of secondary sound vibrations in addition to the primary echoes. The computer uses this additional information to clarify the image. These harmonic scanners used with contrast agents present an exciting new frontier in ultrasound imaging.

Doppler ultrasound methodology allows recording of flow phenomena in color and permits demonstration of both arteries and veins. Doppler ultrasound is used extensively to detect vascular disease, particularly atherosclerosis in the carotid arteries and venous thrombosis of the lower extremities.

Among the more familiar uses of diagnostic sonography are the obstetrical applications. Sonography is the principal method used for fetal imaging because of its high level of safety compared to procedures that involve x-rays. A wide range of obstetrical information is obtainable using ultrasound methods; the most common studies are done to determine gestational size for age of the fetus and to localize needle placement for **amniocentesis** (sampling of amniotic fluid).

For pelvic and obstetrical studies, the patient is requested to force fluids and not to void for 1 to 2 hours preceding the examination. This preparation provides a full bladder, which is the best "sonic window" for ultrasound imaging in the pelvic region.

NUCLEAR MEDICINE

The term *nuclear medicine* refers to the medical use of radioactive isotopes or **radionuclides,** unstable isotopes that give off radiation in their attempt to reach stability. These nuclear materials are used to create **tracers,** radioactive substances that can be ingested or injected into the bloodstream. The isotopes enter into the same chemical reactions as their stable counterparts and are metabolized by the body in a similar way. The isotopes used in nuclear medicine decay quickly and are eliminated in urine or feces. Nuclear medicine examinations generally result in lower radiation doses than most x-ray examinations.

Nuclear medicine differs from most other imaging methods in that it provides information about the *function* of organs and tissues. Depending on the isotope used, it will be taken up in the target organ within a period that ranges from 30 minutes to a few days. It can then be detected and its location recorded by a gamma camera (Fig. 12-28). Abnormal tissues are demonstrated on the image because the isotope is metabolized at a different rate, at a different location, or to a greater or lesser extent than in normal tissue. Where no suitable isotope exists to

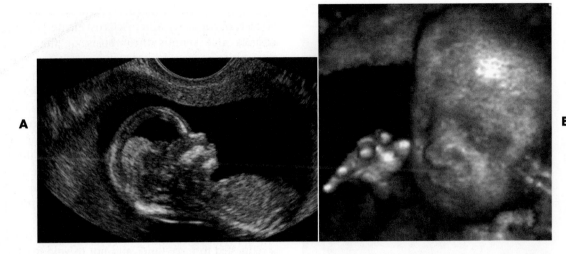

FIG. 12-27 Comparison of sonograms of a fetus using two-dimensional (**A**) and three-dimensional (**B**) techniques.

demonstrate a particular organ, a substance common to that organ can be "tagged" or "labeled" through a chemical process that binds it to a radioisotope. Technetium-99m (^{99m}Tc) is an isotope often used, alone or in combination with other substances, because it has a short half-life (6 hours) and is very versatile. It is commonly used for brain scans, bone scans, and a number of other examinations. In bone scanning, radioactive technetium is tagged to phosphorus, which is readily taken up by bone cells. The monitor screen image shows bright spots in areas of abnormally high metabolic activity and dark spots where there is low activity. Film copies of nuclear medicine images show reversal of the image characteristics seen on the screen, so areas of high activity will appear dark. Bone scanning is especially useful for detecting tumors, which generally have high metabolic activity.

Structures that can be demonstrated by nuclear medicine techniques include the thyroid gland, liver, lungs, brain, skeletal system (Fig. 12-29), kidneys, heart, and blood vessels. One form of tracer flows in the blood, allowing visualization of blood vessels to detect clots and other abnormalities. Gallium scans are used for diagnosis and follow-up of tumors and are used to evaluate organs suspected of involvement in inflammatory processes. Sentinel node scintigraphy

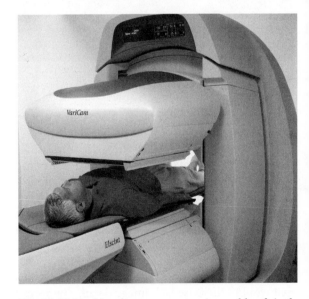

FIG. 12-28 Dual head gamma camera is capable of single photon emission computed tomography (SPECT) imaging and simultaneous posterior whole body and planar imaging.

(lymphoscintigraphy) is used to identify lymph drainage pathways and is valuable in staging cancer. Thallium stress studies of the heart are particularly useful in the evaluation of coronary artery disease.

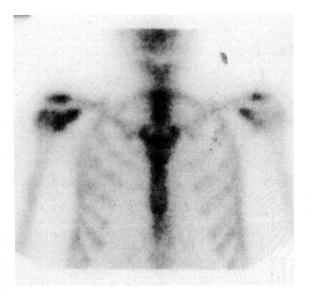

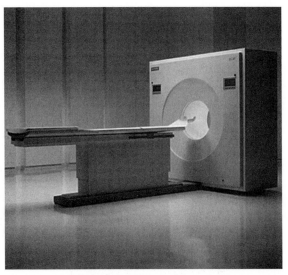

FIG. 12-30 PET scanner.

FIG. 12-29 Bone scan shows increased radionuclide uptake in right shoulder (image left), indicating inflammation due to joint impingement.

Special injection and disposal procedures required for the safe use of radioactive isotopes are beyond the scope of this text. For further information on this subject, consult a suitable nuclear imaging text.

Positron Emission Tomography

Positron emission tomography (PET) is a highly specialized nuclear medicine technique. Clinical use of PET is in its infancy, and research continues to expand the possibilities of this modality. It is similar to other nuclear medicine methods in that radioactive substances from within the body are detected and mapped by specialized equipment to obtain information about the function of organs, tissues, or systems. The PET scanner differs from the gamma camera, however, and is similar in appearance to a CT scanner (Fig. 12-30). A gamma detector array in the PET gantry surrounds the patient and obtains axial images that can be reconstructed by the computer to display the images in other planes (Fig. 12-31). The radioactivity level may be represented on the monitor screen in colors.

PET centers are not as accessible as other imaging modalities because they must be located near a

particle accelerator to obtain the short-lived radionuclides that are used with PET. These materials are quite different from those used in conventional nuclear medicine. Radioactive atoms such as ^{11}C (carbon), ^{13}N (nitrogen), ^{15}O (oxygen), and ^{18}F (fluorine) are made by bombarding normal chemicals with neutrons to produce radionuclides with

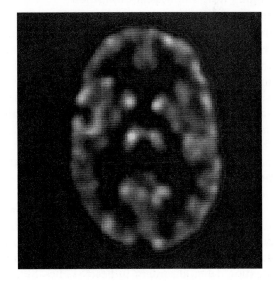

FIG. 12-31 PET image of brain.

very short half-lives. As they decay, they produce pairs of subatomic particles, each pair consisting of a positron and an electron. These particles interact with atoms in the body to produce simultaneous pairs of gamma rays called annihilation photons. The radionuclides used in PET are nearly identical to substances that are common in the body and are therefore capable of many chemical interactions and metabolic functions that are not possible with conventional radionuclides and tagged atoms. For example, a commonly used radiopharmaceutical for PET is a form of glucose, allowing measurement of the metabolism and distribution of sugar. PET is used extensively to study the brain and is also used routinely for measurements of metabolism and blood flow. These measurements may indicate tumor in tissues with abnormally increased metabolism, even when no abnormality can be seen with other imaging modalities. Scanners are designed to acquire data from the entire head and trunk, so studies can be performed on the brain, heart, lung, and abdominal structures. PET is a superior method for detecting and staging malignancies such as melanoma and tumors of the lung. Other types of tumors and organ transplants can also be studied using PET.

Single Photon Emission Computed Tomography

Single photon emission computed tomography (SPECT) is a nuclear medicine modality that is similar to PET but uses different radionuclides. The isotopes most commonly used with SPECT are ^{133}Xe (xenon), ^{99m}Tc (technetium), and ^{123}I (iodine). These tracers emit single gamma photons instead of pairs and have a longer decay time than those used in PET. The images provide less sensitivity and less detail than PET, but the procedure is less expensive and more accessible because SPECT centers do not have to be located near a particle accelerator.

The principal applications of SPECT imaging are studies of the brain and the heart. Brain perfusion studies have proven to be helpful in the diagnosis and classification of dementia and in evaluation of attention deficit disorders. In heart studies, SPECT provides information about blood flow levels and other indications of cardiac health such as aortic stenosis and the sufficiency of the heart valves. In some centers, SPECT scans are a routine aspect of evaluations for coronary artery disease. In the past, radioactive thallium has been used extensively for perfusion studies of the heart, but the latest tracer for cardiac studies is Cardiolite, a brand of **sestamibi,** a large synthetic molecule that can be labeled with ^{99m}Tc. The patient is scanned following exercise, and if abnormality is detected, the scan is repeated after a period of rest to evaluate the extent of the condition.

Gaseous tracers can be inhaled for SPECT studies of lung function, and lung scans using these tracers are also helpful in the early diagnosis of lupus erythematosus.

MAMMOGRAPHY

Mammography is a radiographic procedure that uses special equipment to produce images of high contrast and high resolution for diagnosis of breast lesions (Fig. 12-32). High-quality images are required to ensure that subtle but significant findings are not overlooked, because deficiencies in equipment, technique, or interpretation could result in failure to identify a life-threatening tumor. To assure patients and referring physicians that a facility meets the necessary quality requirements, the American College of Radiology (ACR) and the FDA cooperate to provide certification of mammography departments that demonstrate adherence to high standards of excellence. To qualify for this certification, the facility must be staffed by radiographers who have received specialized training and are certified in mammography by the American Registry of Radiologic Technologists (ARRT).

The American Cancer Society now recommends a baseline mammogram for women between the ages of 35 and 40, examination every 1 to 2 years between the ages of 40 and 50, and annual studies after age 50. Recommendations sometimes vary among organizations and agencies and may be controversial.

In preparation for mammography, patients are instructed not to use underarm deodorant and not to apply powder or lotions on the breasts or axillary and whether the patient has noticed any breast pain, breast lump(s), or nipple discharge. The precise locations of tenderness or lumps may be indicated on breast diagrams. When previous mammograms are available, every effort must be made to obtain them, because comparative evaluation is often significant in the radiologic diagnosis.

Some departments include manual breast examinations during the mammography appointment. Mammography also provides an opportunity for patient instruction in breast self-examination (BSE). Although this instruction may be provided for patients on DVD or videotape, mammographers must be familiar with the content to provide instruction and answer questions when necessary.

Since the breasts must be uncovered for this examination, a comfortable temperature must be maintained in the radiographic room. To protect the patient's modesty, drape the upper torso with a gown or sheet except during actual positioning and radiographic exposure (Fig. 12-33). Care must also be taken to avoid accidental intrusion by others during

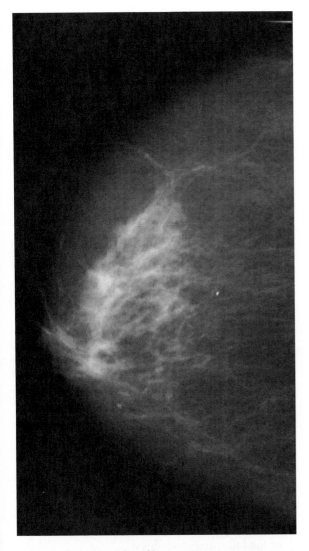

FIG. 12-32 Low-dose film-screen mammogram.

areas. These products may contain ingredients that produce artifacts on mammographic images. This is especially true of antiperspirants that contain aluminum salts.

Before the study, the mammographer obtains a pertinent patient history. This usually includes the date of the last menstrual period, number of pregnancies, date of last pregnancy, whether the patient takes any hormones (including birth control tablets),

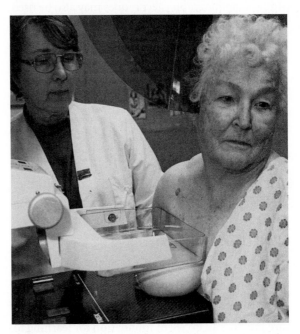

FIG. 12-33 Positioning patient and applying compression for mammography.

the examination. A simple door sign reading, "Examination in Progress: Do Not Enter," is very helpful.

Mammography units include a compression device that briefly presses the breast tightly against the film holder during each exposure. Firm compression greatly improves image quality, allowing more accurate interpretation and a reduction in the amount of radiation needed for an adequate exposure. Breast compression may cause patients discomfort and apprehension, but it does not usually cause pain. Patients with very tender breasts, often from fibrocystic breast disease, may experience pain during compression or during the 24 hours that follow. Aspirin or acetaminophen is recommended for the treatment of postmammography pain and may also be taken in advance of the examination to minimize discomfort. Premenopausal patients may be scheduled during the first 2 weeks of the menstrual cycle, as the breasts are less likely to be tender during this period.

In addition to routine screening examinations and studies for the evaluation of known breast lumps, mammographic techniques may also be used to localize needle placement for breast biopsies.

Digital units now provide filmless mammography systems, offering the ability to manipulate, archive and read these images electronically with a PACS. Mammography is not the only modality used for breast imaging. When lumps are identified, ultrasound studies are useful in differentiating tumors from cysts and may also provide localization for biopsies. CT laser techniques, MRI, and nuclear medicine studies are also used to supplement mammograms in breast evaluation and diagnosis.

CONCLUSION

Computer imaging in a wide variety of forms is adding to the diagnostic capability of major imaging centers everywhere. A radiographer's background in physics, imaging principles, anatomy, and patient care provides an excellent foundation for learning to make images with these advanced techniques. The radiologists you work with will be involved with at least some of these modalities, and your patients may also need examinations in these specialty areas. As part of the larger diagnostic imaging team, it is important for you to have at least a general understanding of the functions, roles, and possibilities that exist outside your immediate area.

REVIEW QUESTIONS

1. Which of the following procedures is NOT useful in the diagnosis of atherosclerosis?
   A. Doppler ultrasound
   B. DSA
   C. MRA
   D. CT myelography
   E. CTA
2. Which of the following procedures must be done in order to treat a stenosis with angioplasty?
   A. Doppler ultrasound of the carotid artery
   B. arteriogram
   C. MRI spectroscopy
   D. amniocentesis
   E. CTLM
3. Which of the following is NOT a nuclear medicine procedure?
   A. bone scan
   B. PET scan
   C. SPECT scan
   D. CT scan
   E. thallium stress test
4. A contrast agent that contains microscopic bubbles is used to enhance visualization in which of the following modalities?
   A. CT
   B. sonography
   C. MRI
   D. PET
   E. mammography
5. Which of the following modalities is useful for imaging the soft tissue structures of joints?
   A. CT
   B. MRI
   C. sonography
   D. nuclear medicine
   E. mammography

CRITICAL THINKING EXERCISES

1. Marjorie Nolan became lost on her way to the diagnostic sonography department and arrived in the radiography suite by mistake. Marjorie is 5 months pregnant and is very anxious about having an obstetrical ultrasound procedure. What can you say to Marjorie to reassure her as you show her the way to her appointment?

2. Dr. MacDougal, the radiologist, has not answered his page, and your supervisor has told you to go to the MRI department and ask him to return to the x-ray department. When you arrive in MRI, the scan room door is closed. Through the window you can see Dr. MacDougal inside visiting with a patient. What should you do?

3. Today your clinical assignment is to assist the technologist in the mammography department. Mrs. Georgia Bates is 73 and has just had her first mammogram. She complains that the procedure was very painful and that her breasts still hurt. She wants to know why the technologist would hurt her like that. What should you say to Mrs. Bates?

Radiography Practice Standards

INTRODUCTION TO RADIOGRAPHY PRACTICE STANDARDS

The complex nature of disease processes involves multiple imaging modalities. Although an interdisciplinary team of radiologists, radiographers and support staff plays a critical role in the delivery of health services, it is the radiographer who performs the radiographic examination that creates the images needed for diagnosis. Radiography integrates scientific knowledge and technical skills with effective patient interaction to provide quality patient care and useful diagnostic information.

Radiographer

Radiographers must demonstrate an understanding of human anatomy, physiology, pathology and medical terminology.

Radiographers must maintain a high degree of accuracy in radiographic positioning and exposure technique. He or she must maintain knowledge about radiation protection and safety. Radiographers prepare for and assist the radiologist in the completion of intricate radiographic examinations. They prepare and administer contrast media and medications in accordance with state and federal regulations.

Radiographers are the primary liaison between patients and radiologists and other members of the support team. They must remain sensitive to the physical and emotional needs of the patient through good communication, patient assessment, patient monitoring and patient care skills.

Radiographers use professional and ethical judgment and critical thinking when performing their duties. Quality improvement and customer service allow the radiographer to be a responsible member of the health care team by continually assessing professional performance. Radiographers embrace continuing education for optimal patient care, public education and enhanced knowledge and technical competence.

Education and Certification

Radiographers prepare for their role on the interdisciplinary team by satisfactorily completing an accredited educational program in radiologic technology. Two-year certificate, associate degree and four-year baccalaureate degree programs exist throughout the United States.

Accredited programs must meet specific curricular and educational standards. The Joint Review Committee on Education in Radiologic Technology (JRCERT) is the accrediting agency for radiologic technology programs recognized by the U.S. Department of Education.

Upon completion of a course of study in radiologic technology, individuals may apply to take the national certification examination. The American Registry of Radiologic Technologists (ARRT) is the recognized certifying agency for radiographers.

Those who successfully complete the certification examination in radiography may use the credential R.T.(R) following their name; the R.T. signifies registered technologist and the (R) indicates radiography.

To maintain ARRT certification, a level of expertise and awareness of changes and advances in practice, radiographers must complete 24 hours of appropriate continuing education every two years.

Practice Standards

The practice standards define the practice and establish general criteria to determine compliance. Practice standards are authoritative statements enunciated and promulgated by the profession for judging the quality of practice, service and education. They include desired and achievable levels of performance against which actual performance can be measured.

Professional practice constantly changes and actual practice varies from state to state as determined by local law and community custom. Recognizing this, the profession has adopted standards that are general in nature. The general format was favored over a "cookbook" style or "step-by-step" approach that would be difficult to maintain in a changing environment and confining for those practitioners with an expanded practice.

The standards focus on the dynamic nature of the health care delivery system. The standards are adaptable not only to the area of practice but also the locality of practice and institutional needs. While a minimum standard of acceptable performance is appropriate and should be followed by all practitioners in a specific area, it is unrealistic and highly inappropriate to assume that professional practice is the same in all regions of the United States.* State statue or regulation may dictate practice parameters.

---

*The term "practitioner" is used in all areas of the standards in place of the various names used in medical imaging and radiation therapy, such as radiologic technologist, sonographer or radiation therapist. Practitioner is defined as any individual practicing in a specific area or discipline. The profession believes that any individual practicing in one of the defined disciplines or specialties should be held to a minimum standard of performance to protect the patients who receive professional services.

To conduct an appropriate review of the standards, one must look to the professional standard as well as local or state law that may impact the nature and scope of practice.

Format — ASRT

The cohesive nature and inherent differences of medical imaging and radiation therapy are recognized in the general format of the standards. The standards are divided into three sections: clinical performance, quality performance and professional performance.

Clinical Performance Standards. The clinical performance standards define the activities of the practitioner in the care of patients and delivery of diagnostic or therapeutic procedures and treatments. The section incorporates patient assessment and management with procedural analysis, performance and evaluation.

Quality Performance Standards. The quality performance standards define the activities of the practitioner in the technical areas of performance including equipment and material assessment, safety standards and total quality management.

Professional Performance Standards. The professional performance standards define the activities of the practitioner in the areas of education, interpersonal relationships, personal and professional self-assessment and ethical behavior.

Each section of the standards is subdivided into individual standards. The standards are numbered and followed by a term or set of terms that identify the standards, such as "assessment" or "analysis/determination." The next statement is the expected performance of the practitioner when performing the procedure or treatment. A rationale statement follows and explains why a practitioner should adhere to the particular standard of performance.

Criteria. Criteria are used in evaluating a practitioner's performance. Each set of criteria is divided into two parts, the general criteria and the specific criteria. Both the measurement and specific criteria should be used when evaluating performance.

General Criteria. General criteria are written in a general style that applies to either medical imaging or radiation therapy practitioners. These criteria are the same in all sections of the standards and should be used for the appropriate area of practice. For example, a radiographer should use good professional judgment to make decisions concerning the adaptation of equipment and technical variables for a diagnostic procedure. Under these circumstances, the evaluation of the decision-making process concerning radiation therapy procedures would not be appropriate and should not be applied unless the procedure is diagnostic in nature, such as simulation.

Specific Criteria. Specific criteria meet the needs of the practitioners in the various areas of professional performance. While many areas of performance within medical imaging and radiation therapy are similar, others are not. The specific criteria are drafted with these differences in mind. For example, a criterion that calls for daily review of patient treatment records and doses to ensure that treatment does not exceed prescribed dose or normal tissue tolerance is imperative for those who practice in radiation therapy yet is not applicable to those who practice in the imaging professions.

A profession's practice standards serve as a guide for appropriate practice. Standards provide role definition for practitioners that can be used by individual facilities to develop job descriptions and practice parameters. Those outside the medical imaging and radiation therapy community can use the standards as an overview of the role and responsibilities of the practitioner as defined by the profession.

RADIOGRAPHY CLINICAL PERFORMANCE STANDARDS

Standard One—Assessment

The practitioner collects pertinent data about the patient and about the procedure.

Rationale

Information about the patient's health status is essential in providing appropriate imaging and therapeutic services.

General Criteria

The practitioner:
1. Uses consistent and appropriate techniques to gather relevant information from the medical record, significant others and health care providers. The collection of information is determined by the patient's needs or condition.
2. Reconfirms patient identification and verifies the procedure requested or prescribed.
3. Verifies the patient's pregnancy status when appropriate.
4. Determines whether the patient has been appropriately prepared for the procedure.
5. Assesses factors that may contraindicate the procedure, such as medications, insufficient patient preparation or artifacts.

Specific Criteria

The practitioner:
1. Identifies artifact-producing objects such as dentures, chest leads, jewelry and hearing aids.

Standard Two—Analysis/Determination

The practitioner analyzes the information obtained during the assessment phase and develops an action plan for completing the procedure.

Rationale

Determining the most appropriate action plan enhances patient safety and comfort, optimizes diagnostic and therapeutic quality and improves cost effectiveness.

General Criteria

The practitioner:
1. Selects the most appropriate and cost-effective action plan after reviewing all pertinent data and assessing the patient's abilities and condition.

2. Uses his or her professional judgment to adapt imaging and therapeutic procedures to improve diagnostic quality and therapeutic outcome.
3. Consults appropriate medical personnel to determine a modified action plan when necessary.
4. Determines the needs for accessory equipment.

Specific Criteria

The practitioner:
1. Evaluates lab values prior to administering contrast media and beginning interventional procedures.
2. Selects appropriate shielding devices.
3. Selects appropriate patient immobilization devices.
4. Determines appropriate type and dose of contrast agent to be administered, based on the patient's age, weight and medical/physical status.
5. Reviews the patient's chart and the physician's request to determine optimal imaging procedure for suspected pathology.

Standard Three—Patient Education

The practitioner provides information about the procedure to the patient, significant others and health care providers.

Rationale

Communication and education are necessary to establish a positive relationship with the patient, significant others and health care providers.

General Criteria

The practitioner:
1. Verifies that the patient has consented to the procedure and fully understands its risks, benefits, alternatives and follow-up. Verifies that written consent has been obtained when appropriate.
2. Provides accurate explanations and instructions at an appropriate time and at a level the patient can understand. Addresses and documents patient questions and concerns regarding the procedure when appropriate.
3. Refers questions about diagnosis, treatment or prognosis to the patient's physician.
4. Provides appropriate information to any individual involved in the patient's care.

Specific Criteria

The practitioner:
1. Consults with other departments, such as patient transportation and anesthesia, for patient services.
2. Instructs patients regarding preparation prior to imaging procedures, including providing information about oral or bowel preparation and allergy preparation.
3. Ensures that all procedural requirements are in place to achieve a quality diagnostic examination.
4. Explains precautions regarding administration of contrast agents to nursing mothers.

Standard Four—Implementation

The practitioner implements the action plan.

Rationale

Quality patient services are provided through the safe and accurate implementation of a deliberate plan of action.

General Criteria

The practitioner:
1. Implements an action plan that falls within established protocols and guidelines.
2. Elicits the cooperation of the patient to carry out the action plan.
3. Uses an integrated team approach as needed.
4. Modifies the action plan according to changes in the clinical situation.
5. Administers first aid or provides life support in emergency situations.
6. Uses accessory equipment when appropriate.
7. Assesses and monitors the patient's physical and mental state.

Specific Criteria

The practitioner:

1. Performs venipuncture, IV patency and maintenance procedures according to established guidelines.
2. Administers contrast agents according to established guidelines.
3. Monitors the patient for reactions to contrast agent.
4. Uses appropriate radiation safety devices.
5. Monitors the patient's physical condition during the procedure.
6. Applies appropriate patient immobilization devices when necessary.

Standard Five—Evaluation

The practitioner determines whether the goals of the action plan have been achieved.

Rationale

Careful examination of the procedure is necessary to determine that all goals have been met.

General Criteria

The practitioner:

1. Evaluates the patient and the procedure to identify variances that may affect patient outcome. The evaluation process should be timely, accurate and comprehensive.
2. Measures the procedure against established protocols and guidelines.
3. Identifies any exceptions to the expected outcome.
4. Documents any exceptions clearly and completely.
5. Develops a revised action plan to achieve the intended outcome if necessary.
6. Disseminates reasons for revisions to all team members.

Specific Criteria

The practitioner:

1. Reviews images to determine if additional images will enhance the diagnostic value of the procedure.

Standard Six—Implementation

The practitioner implements the revised action plan.

Rationale

It may be necessary to make changes to the action plan to achieve the intended outcome.

General Criteria

The practitioner:

1. Bases the revised action plan on the patient's condition and the most appropriate means of achieving the intended outcome.
2. Takes action based on patient and procedural variances.
3. Measures and evaluates the results of the revised action plan.
4. Notifies appropriate health provider when immediate clinical response is necessary based on procedural findings and patient condition.

Specific Criteria

None added.

Standard Seven—Outcomes Measurement

The practitioner reviews and evaluates the outcome of the procedure.

Rationale

To evaluate the quality of care, the practitioner compares the actual outcome with the intended outcome.

General Criteria

The practitioner:

1. Reviews all diagnostic or therapeutic data for completeness and accuracy.
2. Determines whether the actual outcome is within the established criteria.
3. Evaluates the process and recognizes opportunities for future changes.
4. Assesses the patient's physical and mental status prior to discharge from the practitioner's care.

Specific Criteria

None added.

Standard Eight—Documentation

The practitioner documents information about patient care, the procedure and the final outcome.

Rationale

Clear and precise documentation is essential for continuity of care, accuracy of care and quality assurance.

General Criteria

The practitioner:
1. Documents diagnostic, treatment and patient data in the appropriate record. Documentation must be timely, accurate, concise and complete.
2. Documents any exceptions from the established criteria or procedures.
3. Records diagnostic or treatment data.

Specific Criteria

None added.

QUALITY PERFORMANCE STANDARDS
Standard One—Assessment

The practitioner collects pertinent information regarding equipment, the procedures and the work environment.

Rationale

The planning and provision of safe and effective medical services relies on the collection of pertinent information about equipment, procedures and the work environment.

General Criteria

The practitioner:
1. Ensures that services are performed in a safe environment in accordance with established guidelines.
2. Ensures that equipment maintenance and operation comply with established guidelines.
3. Assesses equipment to determine acceptable performance based on established guidelines.
4. Ensures that protocol and procedure manuals include recommended criteria and are reviewed and revised on a regular basis.

Specific Criteria

The practitioner:
1. Maintains controlled access to restricted area during radiation exposure to ensure safety of patients, visitors and hospital personnel.

Standard Two—Analysis/Determination

The practitioner analyzes information collected during the assessment phase and determines whether changes need to be made to equipment, procedures or the work environment.

Rationale

Determination of acceptable performance is necessary for the provision of safe and effective services.

General Criteria

The practitioner:
1. Assesses whether services, procedures and the work environment meet or exceed established guidelines. If not, the practitioner develops an action plan.
2. Evaluates equipment to determine if it meets or exceeds established standards. If not, the practitioner develops an action plan.
3. Analyzes information collected during the assessment phase to determine whether optimal services are being provided. If not, the practitioner develops an action plan.

Specific Criteria

None added.

Standard Three—Education

The practitioner informs patients, the public and other health care providers about procedures, equipment and facilities.

Rationale

Open communication promotes safe practices.

General Criteria
The practitioner:
1. Elicits confidence and cooperation from the patient, the public and health care providers by providing timely communication and effective instruction.
2. Presents explanations and instructions at the learner's level of understanding and learning style.

Specific Criteria
The practitioner:
1. Instructs health care providers and students regarding radiographic procedures and radiation safety.
2. Educates the public about radiographic procedures and radiation safety.

Standard Four—Performance
The practitioner performs quality assurance activities or acquires information on equipment and materials.

Rationale
Quality assurance activities provide valid and reliable information regarding the performance of materials and equipment.

General Criteria
The practitioner:
1. Performs quality assurance activities based on established quality protocols.
2. Provides evidence of ongoing quality assurance activities.

Specific Criteria
The practitioner:
1. Monitors image production to determine variance from established quality standards.

Standard Five—Evaluation
The practitioner evaluates quality assurance results and establishes an appropriate action plan.

Rationale
Materials, equipment and procedure safety depend on ongoing quality assurance activities that evaluate performance based on established guidelines.

General Criteria
The practitioner:
1. Compares quality assurance results to established acceptable values.
2. Verifies quality assurance testing conditions and results.
3. Formulates an action plan following verification of testing.

Specific Criteria
None added.

Standard Six—Implementation
The practitioner implements the quality assurance action plan.

Rationale
Implementation of a quality assurance action plan is imperative for quality diagnostic and therapeutic procedures and patient care.

General Criteria
The practitioner:
1. Obtains assistance from appropriate personnel to implement the quality assurance action plan.
2. Implements the quality assurance action plan.

Specific Criteria
None added.

Standard Seven—Outcomes Measurement
The practitioner assesses the outcome of the quality assurance action plan in accordance with established guidelines.

Rationale
Outcomes assessment is an integral part of the ongoing quality assurance plan to enhance diagnostic and therapeutic services.

General Criteria
The practitioner:
1. Reviews the implementation process for accuracy and validity.

2. Determines whether the performance of equipment and materials is safe for practice based on outcomes assessment.
3. Develops and implements a modified action plan when testing results are not in compliance with guidelines.

Specific Criteria

None added.

Standard Eight—Documentation

The practitioner documents quality assurance activities and results.

Rationale

Documentation provides evidence of quality assurance activities designed to enhance the safety of patients, the public and health care providers during diagnostic and therapeutic services.

General Criteria

The practitioner:
1. Maintains documentation of quality assurance activities, procedures and results in accordance with established guidelines.
2. Provides timely, concise, accurate and complete documentation.
3. Provides documentation that adheres to current protocol, policy and procedures.

Specific Criteria

None added.

PROFESSIONAL PERFORMANCE STANDARDS
Standard One—Quality

The practitioner strives to provide optimal care to all patients.

Rationale

All patients expect and deserve optimal care during diagnosis and treatment.

General Criteria

The practitioner:
1. Works with others to elevate the quality of care.
2. Participates in quality assurance programs.
3. Adheres to the accepted standards, policies and procedures adopted by the profession and regulated by law.
4. Provides the best possible diagnostic study or therapeutic treatment for each patient by applying professional judgment and discretion.
5. Anticipates and responds to the needs of the patient.

Specific Criteria

None added.

Standard Two—Self-Assessment

The practitioner evaluates personal performance, knowledge and skills.

Rationale

Self-assessment is an important tool in professional growth and development.

General Criteria

The practitioner:
1. Monitors personal work ethics, behaviors and attitudes.
2. Monitors and evaluates orientation guidelines and recommends improvements or changes as needed.
3. Evaluates performance and recognizes opportunities for improvement.
4. Recognizes his or her strengths and uses them to benefit patients, coworkers and the profession.
5. Performs procedures only after receiving appropriate education and training.
6. Recognizes and takes advantage of opportunities for educational growth and improvement in technical and problem-solving skills.
7. Actively participates in professional societies and organizations.

Specific Criteria

None added.

STANDARD THREE—EDUCATION

The practitioner acquires and maintains current knowledge in clinical practice.

Rationale

Advancements in medical science require enhancement of knowledge and skills through education.

General Criteria

The practitioner:
1. Maintains appropriate credentials and certification related to clinical practice.
2. Demonstrates completion of the appropriate education related to clinical practice.
3. Participates in educational activities to enhance knowledge, skills and performance.
4. Shares knowledge and expertise with others.

Specific Criteria

None added.

Standard Four—Collaboration and Collegiality

The practitioner promotes a positive, collaborative practice atmosphere with other members of the health care team.

Rationale

To provide quality patient care, all members of the health care team must communicate effectively and work together efficiently.

General Criteria

The practitioner:
1. Shares knowledge and expertise with colleagues, peers, students and all members of the health care team.
2. Develops collaborative partnerships with other health care providers in the interest of diagnostic and therapeutic quality and cost effectiveness and safety.

Specific Criteria

None added.

Standard Five—Ethics

The practitioner adheres to the profession's accepted Code of Ethics.

Rationale

All decisions and actions made on behalf of the patient are based on a sound ethical foundation.

General Criteria

The practitioner:
1. Provides health care services with respect for the patient's dignity and age-specific needs.
2. Acts as a patient advocate to support patients' rights.
3. Takes responsibility for professional decisions.
4. Delivers patient care and service without bias based on personal attributes, nature of the disease, sex, race, creed, religion or socioeconomic status.
5. Respects the patient's right to privacy and confidentiality.
6. Adheres to the established practice standards of the profession.

Specific Criteria

None added.

Standard Six—Exploration and Investigation

The practitioner participates in the acquisition, dissemination and advancement of the professional knowledge base.

Rationale

Scholarly activities such as research, scientific investigation, presentation and publication advance the profession and thereby improve the quality and efficiency of patient services.

General Criteria

The practitioner:
1. Reads and critically evaluates research in diagnostic and therapeutic services.
2. Investigates new, innovative methods and applies them in practice.

3. Shares information with colleagues through publication, presentation and collaboration.
4. Pursues lifelong learning.
5. Participates in data collection.

Specific Criteria

None added.

Informed Consent Form*

Southwest Washington Medical Center
VANCOUVER, WA

SPECIAL CONSENT TO OPERATION, POST OPERATIVE CARE, MEDICAL TREATMENT, ANESTHESIA, OR OTHER PROCEDURE

Patient: _____ Patient No. _____

Washington State law guarantees that you have both the <u>right</u> and <u>obligation</u> to make decisions concerning your health care. Your physician can provide you with the necessary information and advice, but as a member of the health care team, you must enter into the decision making process. This form has been designed to acknowledge your acceptance of treatment recommended by your physician.

1. I hereby authorize Dr. _____
and/or such associates or assistants as may be selected by said physician to treat the following condition(s) which has (have) been explained to me: (Explain the nature of the condition(s) in professional and lay language.)

_____
_____
_____

2. The procedures planned for treatment of my condition(s) have been explained to me by my physician. I understand them to be: (Describe procedures to be performed in professional and lay language.)

_____
_____
_____
_____

At: _____
(NAME OF HOSPITAL OR MEDICAL FACILITY)

3. I recognize that, during the course of the operation, post operative care, medical treatment, anesthesia or other procedure, unforeseen conditions may necessitate additional or different procedures than those above set forth. I therefore authorize my above named physician, and his or her assistants or designees, to perform such surgical or other procedures as are in the exercise of his, her or their professional judgment necessary and desirable. The authority granted under this paragraph shall extend to the treatment of all conditions that require treatment and are not known to my physician at the time the medical or surgical procedure is commenced.

4. I have been informed that there are significant risks such as severe loss of blood, infection and cardiac arrest that can lead to death or permanent or partial disability, which may be attendant to the performance of any procedure. I acknowledge that no warranty or guarantee has been made to me as to result or cure.

IMPORTANT: HAVE PATIENT SIGN FULL OR LIMITED DISCLOSURE BOX AND SIGNATURE LINE AT BOTTOM.

Full Disclosure

I certify that my physician has informed me of the nature and character of the proposed treatment, of the anticipated results of the proposed treatment, of the possible alternative forms of treatment; and the recognized serious possible risks, complications, and the anticipated benefits involved in the proposed treatment and in the alternative forms of treatment, including non-treatment.

PATIENT/OTHER LEGALLY RESPONSIBLE PERSON SIGN
IF APPLICABLE

Limited Disclosure

I certify that my physician has explained to me that I have the right to have clearly described to me the nature and character of the proposed treatment; the anticipated results of the proposed treatment; the alternative forms of treatment; and the recognized serious possible risks, complications, and anticipated benefits involved in the proposed treatment, and in the alternative forms of treatment, including non-treatment.

I do not wish to have these risks and facts explained to me.

PATIENT/OTHER LEGALLY RESPONSIBLE PERSON SIGN
IF APPLICABLE

Any sections below which do not apply to the proposed treatment may be crossed out. All sections crossed out must be initialed by both physician and patient.

5. I consent to the administration of anesthesia by my attending physician, by an anesthesiologist, or other qualified party under the direction of a physician as may be deemed necessary. I understand that all anesthetics involve risks of complications and serious possible damage to vital organs such as the brain, heart, lung, liver and kidney and that in some cases may result in paralysis, cardiac arrest and/or brain death from both known and unknown causes. I understand there is a risk of dental injury during airway management.

6. I consent to the use of transfusion of blood and blood products as deemed necessary, and potential complications associated with this procedure have been explained by my physician.

7. Any tissues or parts surgically removed may be disposed of by the hospital or physician in accordance with accustomed practice.

I certify this form has been fully explained to me, that I have read it or have had it read to me, that the blank spaces have been filled in, and that I understand its contents.

DATE: _____ TIME: _____ A.M. P.M.

PATIENT/OTHER LEGALLY RESPONSIBLE PERSON SIGN

WITNESS: _____

RELATIONSHIP OF LEGALLY RESPONSIBLE PERSON TO PATIENT

*Courtesy Southwest Washington Medical Center.

Abbreviated List of Spanish Phrases With Guides to Pronunciation*

1. Hello, my name is _____. I am the technician.

   Buenos dias, me llamo _____. Soy el technico.

   Boo-**ay**-nohs **dee**-ahs. May **yah**-moh _____. Soy el **teck**-nee-koh.

2. What is your name?

   Como se llama?

   Coh-moh say **yah**-mah?

3. Please come with me.

   Favor de venir conmigo.

   Fah-**vore** day vay-**neer** cone-**me**-goh.

4. Please remove all your clothing and put on the gown.

   Favor de quitar toda la ropa y vestirse en la bata.

   Fah-**vore** day key-**tar** **toh**-dah lah **roh**-pah ee vess-**teer**-say en lah **bah**-tah.

5. Please remove your clothing to the waist and put on the gown.

   Favor de quitar la ropa hasta la cintura y vestirse en la bata.

   Fah-**vore** day key-**tar** lah **roh**-pah **ah**-stah lah sin-**too**-rah ee vess-**teer**-say en lah **bah**-tah.

6. Stand here, please.

   Parese aqui por favor.

   Pah-**ray**-say ah-**key** pore fah-**vore**.

7. Lift your arms.

   Levante los brazos.

   Lay-**vahn**-tay los **brah**-sohs.

8. Don't move.

   No se mueva.

   Noh say moo-**ay**-vah.

9. When I tell you, hold your breath.

   Cuando le avise, no respire.

   Kwan-doh lay ah-**vee**-say, noh ray-**spee**-ray.

---

*Modified from Joyce EV, Villanueva, ME: *Say it in Spanish*, ed 2, St Louis, 2000, Mosby.

10. Stop breathing.

    No respire.

    Noh   ray-**spee**-ray.

11. You can breathe now.

    Ya puede respirar ahora.

    Yah   poo-**ay**-day   ray-spee-**rahr**   ah-**ohr**-ah.

12. Please lie down on the table.

    Acuestese en la mesa por favor.

    Ah-**quest**-ay-say en lah **may**-sah, pore fah-**vore**.

13. I will return shortly.

    Regresarse en seguida.

    Ray-gray-**sahr**-say   en   say-**ghee**-dah.

14. I am finished. That's all.

    Ya termine. Es todo.

    Yah   tare-**mee**-nay.   Ace   **toh**-doh.

15. Now you can get dressed.

    Ahora se puede ponar su ropa.

    Ah-**ohr**-ah   say   poo-**ay**-day   poh-**nahr** soo   **roh**-pah.

16. Thank you. Goodbye.

    Gracias. Adios.

    Grah-see-ahs.   Ah-dee-**ohs**.

17. Please sit here.

    Sientese aqui por favor.

    See-**en**-tay-say   ah-**key**   pore   fah-**vore**.

18. Are you pregnant?

    Esta embarazada?

    Ess-**tah**   em-bah-rah-**sah**-dah?

19. One time more.

    Uno vez mas.

    Oo-noh   vase   mahs.

20. Remain here.

    Quedese aqui.

    Kay-**day**-say   ah-**key**.

21. The doctor will talk to you.

    El doctor hablara con usted.

    Ell   dock-**tohr**   hah-**blah**-rah   cone   oo-**sted**.

Accepted Abbreviations and Descriptive Terms for Charting

ABBREVIATIONS TYPICALLY USED IN CHARTING

Abbreviation	Word or Phrase
abd	abdomen
ac	before meals
ad lib	freely, as desired
AED	automatic external defibrillator
amt	amount
AP	apical pulse
aq	water
b i d *or* 2 i d	2 times a day
BP	blood pressure
BRP	bathroom privileges
C	centigrade, celsius
c̄	with
caps	capsule
cc	cubic centimeter
CHF	congestive heart failure
cm	centimeter
CPR	cardiopulmonary resuscitation
DC	discontinue
ECG *or* EKG	electrocardiogram
ED	emergency department
EEG	electroencephalogram
EENT	eye, ear, nose, and throat
ENT	ear, nose, and throat
ER	emergency room or emergency department
fld	fluid
GB	gallbladder
GI	gastrointestinal
Gm *or* gm	gram
gtt	drop, drops
GU	genitourinary
gyn	gynecology
(H)	hypodermically
H *or* hrs	hour, hours
H₂O	water
HA	headache
Hgb *or* Hb	hemoglobin
HS	bedtime
I&O	intake and output
IM	intramuscular
IV	intravenous
Kg *or* kg	kilogram
KUB	kidneys, ureters, and bladder
L	left
L or l	liter
lab	laboratory
LBP	low back pain
LLQ	left lower quadrant—abdomen
LP	lumbar puncture
LUQ	left upper quadrant—abdomen
MI	myocardial infarction
mcg *or* μg	microgram
mg	milligram
ml *or* mL	milliliter
MVA	motor vehicle accident
noct	at night
NPO	nothing by mouth
NS	normal saline solution
OB *or* obs	obstetrics
OD	right eye

389

OJ	orange juice	Rx	therapy
OPC	outpatient clinic	s̄	without
OR	operating room	SOB	short of breath
OS	left eye	spec	specimen
P or p̄	after	SQ	subcutaneous
pc	after meals	s̄s̄	one half
pH	hydrogen ion concentration	stat	at once
PO	by mouth	t i d or 3 i d	3 times a day
PP	postprandial, after meals	TPR	temperature, pulse, respiration
prn	when necessary, as needed	URI	upper respiratory infection
qh	every hour	UTI	urinary tract infection
q 2 h	every 2 hours	WBC	white blood cells or white blood cell count
q i d or 4 i d	4 times a day		
qs	sufficient quantity	WC	wheelchair
RBC	red blood cells or red blood cell count	wt	weight
RLQ	right lower quadrant—abdomen	×	times
RUQ	right upper quadrant—abdomen		

DESCRIPTIVE TERMS TYPICALLY USED IN CHARTING

Area of Concern	Factor to Be Charted	Suggested Terms to Use
Abdomen	Hard, boardlike	Hard, rigid
	Appears swollen, rounded	Distended
	Soft, flabby, flat	Relaxed, flaccid, flat
	Region	

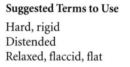

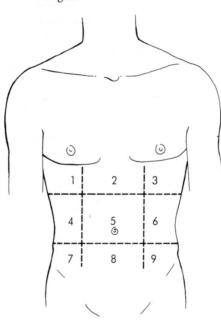

1. Right hypochondriac

2. Epigastric

3. Left hypochondriac

4. Right lumbar

5. Umbilical

6. Left lumbar

7. Right iliac

8. Hypogastric

9. Left iliac region

Abdomen	Area or region	

1. Right upper quadrant

2. Left upper quadrant

3. Right lower quadrant

4. Left lower quadrant

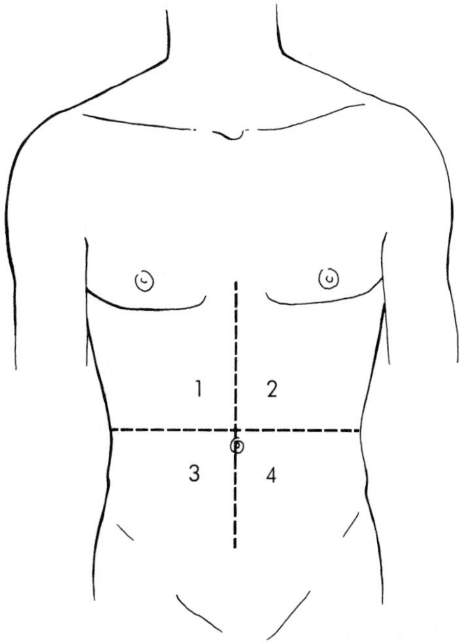

Amounts	Large amount	Excessive, profuse, copious
	Moderate amount	Moderate, usual
	Small amount	Scanty, slight
Appearance, general	Thin and undernourished	Emaciated
	Fat, greatly overweight	Obese
	Seems very sick	Acutely ill
Appetite	Loss of appetite	Anorexia
	Would not eat	Refused food (state reason)
Attitude (mental state)	Has "don't care" attitude	Apathetic
	Afraid, worried	Anxious, apprehensive
	Feeling blue, sad	Depressed
	Other characteristic terms:	Anxiety, defiance, anger, pain, boredom, happiness, dissatisfaction, irritability, worry
Back regions	Upper back	Thoracic region, dorsal region
	Small of the back	Lumbar region
	Lower spine	Sacral region
	Buttocks	Gluteal area
Bleeding	Very little	Oozing
	Abnormal bleeding	Hemorrhage
	Nosebleed	Epistaxis
	Blood in vomitus	Hematemesis
	Blood in urine	Hematuria

	Coughing or spitting up blood	Hemoptysis
	Bleeding stopped	Hemorrhage controlled
Breathing	Breathing	Respiration
	Act of inhaling	Inspiration
	Act of exhaling	Expiration
	Difficulty in breathing	Dyspnea, dyspneic
	Unable to breathe lying down	Orthopnea
	Cessation of breathing for short periods	Apnea
	Rapid breathing	Hyperpnea
	Increasing dyspnea with periods of apnea	Cheyne-Stokes respiration
	Large amount of air inspired or expired	Deep breathing
	Small amount of air inspired or expired	Shallow breathing
	Abnormal variations in rhythm	Irregular respiration
Chill	Blanket applied to keep warm	External heat applied
	Severity (degree of)	Severe, moderate, slight
	Long lasting	Persistent, long duration
	Lasting only briefly	Short duration
	Came on suddenly	Sudden onset
Level of consciousness	Fully conscious, aware of surroundings	Alert, fully conscious
	Only partly conscious	Stuporous
	Unconscious, but can be aroused	Semicomatose
	Unconscious, cannot be aroused	Comatose

Incident Report Form

Redland Valley Hospital INCIDENT REPORT	(Patient ID Imprint)

(Not a part of medical record)

Incident date _____ Time _____

Affected person ☐ Patient ☐ Employee ☐ Visitor ☐ Other _____

Name _____ Gender _____ Address _____

Phone _____

Location of incident: _____

_____

_____

_____

Description of occurrence: _____

_____

Condition of victim:

  Before incident: _____

  After incident: _____

Seen by physician: ☐ Yes ☐ No Physician name: _____

Date _____ Time _____

Action taken: _____

_____

_____

Name: _____	Witness: _____
Signature: _____	Signature: _____
Title: _____	Witness: _____
	Signature: _____

Facility copy original (White)   Attorney copy (Blue)   Insurance copy (Yellow)

Radiology Department Infection Control Procedures

ROUTINE DEPARTMENTAL CLEANING

Counters and Surfaces Frequently Contacted by Personnel Who Handle Patients

- Any hospital-grade disinfectant-detergent registered by the U.S. Environmental Protection Agency (EPA) may be used for cleaning counters and surfaces. Additionally, the use of a dilute bleach solution* or commercially prepared germicide-impregnated disposable cloths may be used.
- Wipe down twice daily using disinfectant, dilute bleach,* or germicide cloths. (**Note:** These surfaces are to include counters and work areas in radiography rooms, counters surrounding reception desk, image processing counters, and counters in image-viewing areas.)

Closed Storage Areas Containing Linen and Nonsterile Medical Supplies

- Wipe shelves and doors weekly with disinfectant, dilute bleach,* or germicide cloths.

Storage Areas Containing Sterile Supplies

- Dust daily, and remove all items from shelves weekly and wash surfaces using disinfectant.

---

*Use a solution of 5.25% sodium hypochlorite (household bleach) diluted 1:10 with water.

- Check expiration dates on all sterile supplies at time of weekly cleaning. Resterilize or replace items as needed.

Lead Aprons and Gloves

- Clean weekly using disinfectant, dilute bleach,* or germicide cloths.
- Clean following contact with blood or body fluids, using recommended disinfectant.

Mobile X-Ray Machines

- Clean weekly using a disinfectant, dilute bleach,* or germicide cloth. Pay particular attention to the x-ray tube, tube arm, and collimator, which are suspended over the patient, as well as those parts that contact the floor, such as cables and wheels.
- Wipe thoroughly with a disinfectant, dilute bleach,* or germicide cloth before entering surgery, newborn nursery, or patient room designated for protective precautions.

X-Ray Machines, Tables, Vertical Buckys

- Thoroughly wash radiography table top and vertical bucky with a disinfectant, dilute bleach,* or germicide cloth after patient contact.
- Change pillowcases, using clean linen for each patient.
- Dust daily the overhead tube, spot film devices, image intensifiers, and television monitors.

- Dust weekly the overhead tracks for ceiling-mounted equipment using a vacuum cleaner.
- Wash weekly the control stands, spot film devices, and the entire radiography table with disinfectant.

Wheelchairs and Stretchers

- Thoroughly wash/clean entire surface of wheelchair and stretcher with a disinfectant, dilute bleach,* or germicide cloth weekly.
- Wipe down patient contact areas at least once daily.
- Wash down wheelchairs or stretchers used for isolation patients with disinfectant immediately following use.
- Wash down wheelchairs or stretchers contaminated with patient secretions or excretions with a disinfectant or dilute bleach* before being reused.

PERSONNEL PRACTICES
Hand Hygiene

Personnel are instructed to wash hands with either a nonantimicrobial soap or antimicrobial soap and water in the following clinical situations:

- When hands are visibly dirty or contaminated with blood or body fluids
- Before eating and after using a restroom
- After blowing or wiping your nose
- If exposure to *Bacillus anthracis* is suspected or proven, because the physical action of washing and rinsing hands helps remove spores

An alcohol-based hand rub, or alternatively handwashing, may be used in these clinical situations:

- On reporting for duty
- Between examinations of patients
- Before donning sterile gloves

- Before inserting indwelling urinary catheters
- Following contact with patient's intact skin (e.g., taking a pulse, blood pressure, lifting a patient)
- Following contact with inanimate objects (including medical equipment) in the immediate vicinity of the patient
- Following removal of gloves
- On entering and leaving isolation areas or handling articles for isolation areas
- After handling dressings, sputum containers, urinals, catheters, or bedpans (use handwashing if hands are visibly contaminated)
- If moving from a contaminated-body site to a clean-body site during patient care
- On completing duty

Standard Precautions

All personnel are to observe Standard Precautions (see Chapter 5 and Appendix G) whenever contact with blood or body fluids is possible.

Good Personal Hygiene

Personnel are directed to practice the following.

- Bathe and wash hair regularly.
- Wear clean uniforms/scrubs and duty shoes.
- Pay particular attention to frequently overlooked items of personal cleanliness, such as fingernails, watchbands, intricate jewelry, and shoelaces.
- Change clothing that is soiled in the process of patient care before continuing work.
- Do not report for duty when affected by the following:
  Contagious skin diseases
  Acute upper respiratory infections
  Any other communicable diseases

Isolation Guidelines*

STANDARD PRECAUTIONS

Use Standard Precautions for the care of all patients.

A. Handwashing
1. Wash hands after touching blood, body fluids, secretions, excretions, and contaminated items, whether or not gloves are worn. Wash hands immediately after gloves are removed, between patient contacts, and when otherwise indicated to avoid transfer of microorganisms to other patients or environments. It may be necessary to wash hands between tasks and procedures on the same patient to prevent cross-contamination of different body sites.
2. Use a plain (nonantimicrobial) soap for routine handwashing.
3. Use an antimicrobial agent or a waterless antiseptic agent for specific circumstances (e.g., control of outbreaks or hyperendemic infections), as defined by the infection control program.

B. Gloves
1. Wear gloves (clean, nonsterile gloves are adequate) when touching blood, body fluids, secretions, excretions, and contaminated items.
2. Put on clean gloves just before touching mucous membranes and nonintact skin.
3. Change gloves between tasks and procedures on the same patient after contact with material that may contain a high concentration of microorganisms.
4. Remove gloves promptly after use, before touching noncontaminated items and environmental surfaces, and before going to another patient, and wash hands immediately to avoid transfer of microorganisms to other patients or environments.

C. Mask, Eye Protection, Face Shield
Wear a mask and eye protection or a face shield to protect mucous membranes of the eyes, nose, and mouth during procedures and patient-care activities that are likely to generate splashes or sprays of blood, body fluids, secretions, and excretions.

D. Gown
1. Wear a gown (a clean, nonsterile gown is adequate) to protect skin and to prevent soiling of clothing during procedures and patient-care

*From Centers for Disease Control and Prevention: http://www.cdc.gov/ncidod/hip/isolat/isopart2.htm (Part II Recommendations for Isolation Precautions in Hospitals); http://www.cdc.gov/ncidod/hip/isolat/isotab_1.htm (Synopsis of Types of Precautions and Patients Requiring the Precautions).

activities that are likely to generate splashes or sprays of blood, body fluids, secretions, or excretions.

2. Select a gown that is appropriate for the activity and amount of fluid likely to be encountered.

3. Remove a soiled gown as promptly as possible, and wash hands to avoid transfer of microorganisms to other patients or environments.

E. Patient-Care Equipment

1. Handle used patient-care equipment soiled with blood, body fluids, secretions, and excretions in a manner that prevents skin and mucous membrane exposures, contamination of clothing, and transfer of microorganisms to other patients and environments.

2. Ensure that reusable equipment is not used for the care of another patient until it has been cleaned and reprocessed appropriately.

3. Ensure that single-use items are discarded properly.

F. Environmental Control

Ensure that the hospital has adequate procedures for the routine care, cleaning, and disinfection of environmental surfaces, beds, bedrails, bedside equipment, and other frequently touched surfaces, and ensure that these procedures are being followed.

G. Linen

Handle, transport, and process used linen soiled with blood, body fluids, secretions, and excretions in a manner that prevents skin and mucous membrane exposures and contamination of clothing, and that avoids transfer of microorganisms to other patients and environments.

H. Occupational Health and Bloodborne Pathogens

1. Take care to prevent injuries when using needles, scalpels, and other sharp instruments or devices; when handling sharp instruments after procedures; when cleaning used instruments; and when disposing of used needles.

2. Never recap used needles, or otherwise manipulate them using both hands, or use any other technique that involves directing the point of a needle toward any part of the body; rather, use either a one-handed "scoop" technique or a mechanical device designed for holding the needle sheath.

3. Do not remove used needles from disposable syringes by hand, and do not bend, break, or otherwise manipulate used needles by hand.

4. Place used disposable syringes and needles, scalpel blades, and other sharp items in appropriate puncture-resistant containers, which are located as close as practical to the area in which the items were used, and place reusable syringes and needles in a puncture-resistant container for transport to the reprocessing area.

5. Use mouthpieces, resuscitation bags, or other ventilation devices as an alternative to mouth-to-mouth resuscitation methods in areas where the need for resuscitation is predictable.

6. Refer to Chapters 5 and 7 for OSHA policy regarding safe medical devices.

I. Patient Placement

Place a patient who contaminates the environment, or who does not (or cannot be expected to) assist in maintaining appropriate hygiene or environmental control, in a private room. If a private room is not available, consult with infection control professionals regarding patient placement or other alternatives.

AIRBORNE PRECAUTIONS

In addition to Standard Precautions, use Airborne Precautions for patients known or suspected to have serious illnesses transmitted by airborne droplet nuclei.

Diseases Requiring Airborne Precautions

- Measles
- Varicella (including disseminated zoster)
- Tuberculosis

Precautions

- Wear respiratory protection (N95 respirator) when entering the room of a patient with known or suspected infectious pulmonary tuberculosis.
- Susceptible persons should not enter the room of patients known or suspected to have measles

(rubeola) or varicella (chickenpox) if other immune caregivers are available.
- If susceptible persons must enter the room of a patient known or suspected to have measles or varicella, they should wear respiratory protection (N95 respirator).
- Persons immune to measles (rubeola) or varicella need not wear respiratory protection.

DROPLET PRECAUTIONS

In addition to Standard Precautions, use Droplet Precautions, or the equivalent, for patients known or suspected to be infected with microorganisms transmitted by large particle droplets that can be generated by patients during coughing, sneezing, talking, or the performance of procedures.

Diseases Requiring Droplet Precautions

- Invasive *Haemophilus influenzae* type b disease, including meningitis, pneumonia, epiglottitis, and sepsis.
- Invasive *Neisseria meningitidis* disease, including meningitis, pneumonia, and sepsis.
- Other serious bacterial respiratory infections spread by droplet transmission, including:
  - Diphtheria (pharyngeal)
  - *Mycoplasma* pneumonia
  - Pertussis
  - Pneumonic plague
  - Streptococcal (group A) pharyngitis, pneumonia, or scarlet fever in infants and young children
- Serious viral infections spread by droplet transmission, including:
  - Adenovirus
  - Influenza
  - Mumps
  - Parvovirus B19
  - Rubella

Precautions

Wear a surgical mask when working within 3 ft of the patient. Some hospitals may implement the wearing of a mask to enter the room.

CONTACT PRECAUTIONS

In addition to Standard Precautions, use Contact Precautions, or the equivalent, for specified patients known or suspected to be infected or colonized with epidemiologically important microorganisms that can be transmitted by direct contact with the patient (hand or skin-to-skin contact that occurs when performing patient-care activities that require touching the patient's dry skin) or indirect contact (touching) with environmental surfaces or patient-care items in the patient's environment.

Diseases Requiring Contact Precautions

- Gastrointestinal, respiratory, skin, or wound infections or colonization with multidrug-resistant bacteria judged by the infection control program, based on current state, regional, or national recommendations, to be of special clinical and epidemiologic significance.
- Enteric infections with a low infectious dose or prolonged environmental survival, including:
  - Enterocolitis due to *Clostridium difficile.*
  - Enterohemorrhagic *Escherichia coli* 0157:H7, *Shigella,* hepatitis A and rotavirus for diapered or incontinent patients.
- Respiratory syncytial virus, parainfluenza virus, or enteroviral infections in infants and young children.
- Skin infections that are highly contagious or that may occur on dry skin, including:
  - Diphtheria (cutaneous)
  - Herpes simplex virus (neonatal or mucocutaneous)
  - Impetigo
  - Major (noncontained) abscesses, cellulitis, or decubiti
  - Pediculosis
  - Scabies
  - Staphylococcal furunculosis in infants and young children
  - Zoster (disseminated or in the immunocompromised host)
- Viral/hemorrhagic conjunctivitis
- Viral hemorrhagic infections (Ebola, Lassa, or Marburg)

Precautions

- Wear clean, nonsterile gloves.
- A clean nonsterile gown is also worn whenever you anticipate that your clothing will have substantial contact with the patient, environmental surfaces, or items in the patient's room, or if the patient is incontinent or has diarrhea, an ileostomy, a colostomy, or wound drainage not contained by a dressing.
- During the course of providing care for a patient, change gloves after having contact with infective material that may contain high concentrations of microorganisms (fecal material and wound drainage).
- Remove gown and gloves before leaving the patient's room and wash hands immediately with an antimicrobial agent or a waterless antiseptic agent.
- After glove and gown removal, ensure that clothing does not contact potentially contaminated environmental surfaces to avoid transfer of microorganisms to other patients or environments.

Remember to follow Standard Precautions in addition to the Transmission-Based Precautions described above. This includes practicing hand hygiene before and after patient contact, disinfecting equipment and supplies before use on other patients, and proper placement of contaminated disposable items and linen.

Urine Collection

PROCEDURE FOR COLLECTING A URINE SPECIMEN

Since improperly collected urine may yield incorrect test results, urine should always be collected using the *clean-catch midstream specimen (CCMS)* technique. This technique is based on the concept that the tissues adjacent to the urethral meatus must be cleansed with an appropriate cleansing solution prior to collection to avoid contamination of the specimen. Only the middle portion of the urine stream is collected for analysis. The initial and final portions of the urine stream are discarded.

Supplies

Urine specimen containers should be clean and dry and are used only once. A variety of collection containers is available. Some have pour spouts to facilitate filling the urinalysis tubes, and others have caps. Cups with caps should be used if the specimen will not be analyzed immediately following collection. This type is most practical for occasional use in the imaging department.

Gauze sponges moistened with an appropriate cleansing solution are used to cleanse the patient prior to urine collection. A variety of appropriate cleansing solutions is available, and standard 2 × 2-inch gauze sponges are adequate. Towelettes premoistened with an appropriate cleansing solution are also available and can be used in place of gauze sponges.

Specimen Collection

Female: A female patient spreads the labia and cleanses in an anterior-to-posterior direction with three separate gauze sponges or towelettes moistened with cleansing solution. A separate sponge is used to cleanse each side of the meatus, and a third sponge is wiped directly over the meatus. A dry sponge is then wiped directly over the meatus. Keeping the labia spread, a small amount of urine is passed into the toilet. At least 15 ml of urine is collected into an appropriate specimen container. The remaining urine in the bladder is then passed into the toilet.

Male: A circumcised male simply cleanses the glans penis using sponges moistened with cleansing solution, wiping from the center outward. An uncircumcised male must first retract the foreskin and keep it retracted during cleansing and collection. A dry sponge is used to wipe directly over the meatus. At least 15 ml of urine is collected into a specimen container from the middle portion of the urine stream.

Iodinated Contrast Media Products for Radiography

TRADE NAME	GENERIC NAME	IODINE (%WEIGHT/ VOLUME)	IONIC/ NONIONIC	OSMOLALITY	APPROVED USES
Conray	Iothalamate meglumine	28.2	Ionic	High	Multipurpose
Conray-30	Iothalamate meglumine	14.1	Ionic	High	Excretory urography, CT
Conray-43	Iothalamate meglumine	20.2	Ionic	High	Excretory urography, venography, CT, DSA
Conray-400	Iothalamate sodium	40	Ionic	High	Angiography
Cysto-Conray II	Iothalamate meglumine	8.1	Ionic	High	Retrograde cystourethrography
Cystografin	Diatrizoate meglumine	14.1	Ionic	High	Retrograde cystourethrography
Cystografin-Dilute	Diatrizoate meglumine	8.5	Ionic	High	Retrograde cystourethrography
Ethiodol	Ethiodized oil	37			Lymphography
Gastrografin	Diatrizoate meglumine and diatrizoate sodium	47.1	Ionic	High	Gastrointestinal studies, CT body scans (oral administration)
Hexabrix	Sodium meglumine ioxaglate	32	Ionic	Low	Angiography and multipurpose
Hypaque 76	Diatrizoate meglumine and diatrizoate sodium	34	Ionic	High	Multipurpose
Hypaque Meglumine 60%	Diatrizoate meglumine	30	Ionic	High	Multipurpose

Continued

TRADE NAME	GENERIC NAME	IODINE (%WEIGHT/ VOLUME)	IONIC/ NONIONIC	OSMOLALITY	APPROVED USES
Hypaque Sodium 50%	Diatrizoate sodium	25	Ionic	High	Multipurpose
Hypaque Sodium Oral Powder	Diatrizoate sodium	58	Ionic	High	Gastrointestinal studies
Hypaque-Cysto 30%	Diatrizoate meglumine	15	Ionic	High	Retrograde cystourethrography
Imagopaque 150 mg I/ml	Iopentol	15	Nonionic	Low	Femoral arteriography, ERCP
Imagopaque 200 mg I/ml	Iopentol	20	Nonionic	Low	Venography, ERCP
Imagopaque 250 mg I/ml	Iopentol	25	Nonionic	Low	Venography, ERCP, hysterosalpingography
Imagopaque 300 mg I/ml	Iopentol	30	Nonionic	Low	Angiography, aortography, excretory urography, venography, DSA, CT, arthrography, gastrointestinal studies (oral)
Imagopaque 350 mg I/ml	Iopentol	35	Nonionic	Low	Angiocardiography, excretory urography, DSA, CT, arthrography, gastrointestinal studies (oral)
Iomeron 150	Iomeprol	15	Nonionic	Low	Urography infusion, cystourethrography, CT, arterial DSA
Iomeron 200	Iomeprol	20	Nonionic	Low	Venography, CT, arterial DSA, arthrography, hysterosalpingography, ERCP, retrograde urography, ERCP
Iomeron 250	Iomeprol	25	Nonionic	Low	Excretory urography, venography, CT, IV and arterial DSA
Iomeron 300	Iomeprol	30	Nonionic	Low	Angiocardiography, excretory urography, venography, CT, IV and arterial DSA, arthrography, hysterosalpingography, discography, ERCP

TRADE NAME	GENERIC NAME	IODINE (%WEIGHT/ VOLUME)	IONIC/ NONIONIC	OSMOLALITY	APPROVED USES
Iomeron 350	Iomeprol	35	Nonionic	Low	Angiocardiography, coronary arteriography, excretory urography, CT, IV and arterial DSA, arthrography, ERCP, hysterosalpingography
Iomeron 400	Iomeprol	40	Nonionic	Low	Angiocardiography, coronary arteriography, excretory urography, CT, IV DSA
Isovue-200	Iopamidol	20	Nonionic	Low	Venography
Isovue-300	Iopamidol	30	Nonionic	Low	Peripheral arteriography
Isovue-370	Iopamidol	37	Nonionic	Low	Selective visceral arteriography
Isovue-M 200	Iopamidol	20	Nonionic	Low	Thoracic myelography
Isovue-M 300	Iopamidol	30	Nonionic	Low	Total column myelography
MD-76	Diatrizoate meglumine and diatrizoate sodium	37	Ionic	High	Excretory urography, angiography, CT
MD-Gastroview	Diatrizoate meglumine and diatrizoate sodium	37	Ionic	High	Gastrointestinal studies (oral administration)
Omnipaque 140	Iohexol	14	Nonionic	Low	Arterial DSA
Omnipaque 180	Iohexol	18	Nonionic	Low	Myelography
Omnipaque 240	Iohexol	24	Nonionic	Low	Multipurpose
Omnipaque 300	Iohexol	30	Nonionic	Low	Arteriography, aortography, CT (IV and intrathecal)
Omnipaque 350	Iohexol	35	Nonionic	Low	Aortography, angiocardiography, CT (IV), IV DSA
Optiray 160	Ioversol	16	Nonionic	Low	Arterial DSA
Optiray 240	Ioversol	24	Nonionic	Low	Cerebral arteriography, venography, excretory urography, CT
Optiray 300	Ioversol	30	Nonionic	Low	Arteriography, excretory urography, CT
Optiray 320	Ioversol	32	Nonionic	Low	Angiography
Optiray 350	Ioversol	35	Nonionic	Low	Angiography, excretory urography, IV DSA, CT
Oragrafin Calcium (granules)	Ipodate calcium	61.7			Cholecystography (oral administration)
Oragrafin Sodium capsules)	Ipodate sodium	61.4			Cholecystography (oral administration)

Continued

TRADE NAME	GENERIC NAME	IODINE (%WEIGHT/ VOLUME)	IONIC/ NONIONIC	OSMOLALITY	APPROVED USES
Renografin-60	Diatrizoate meglumine and diatrizoate sodium	29.25	Ionic	High	Multipurpose
Reno-30	Diatrizoate meglumine	14.1	Ionic	High	Retrograde urography
Reno-60	Diatrizoate meglumine and diatrizoate sodium	29.25	Ionic	High	Multipurpose
Reno-Dip	Diatrizoate meglumine	14.1	Ionic	High	Urography infusion, leg venography
Renovist	Diatrizoate meglumine and diatrizoate sodium	69.3			Multipurpose
Renovist II	Diatrizoate meglumine and diatrizoate sodium	57.6			Multipurpose
Renovue-65	Iodamide meglumine	65			Excretory urography
Renovue-Dip	Iodamide meglumine	24			Urography infusion
Sinografin	Diatrizoate meglumine and iodipamide meglumine	47.1	Ionic	High	Hysterosalpingography
Telepaque	Iopanoic acid	66.7			Cholecystography (oral administration)
Visipaque 270	Iodixanol	27	Nonionic	Very low	Angiography, cerebral angiography, IV and arterial DSA, excretory urography, venography, CT, arthrography, ERCP, hysterosalpingography
Visipaque 320	Iodixanol	32	Nonionic	Very low	Angiocardiography, peripheral arteriography, DSA, CT, arthrography, ERCP, hysterosalpingography

Molecular Structure of Some Typical Iodinated Contrast Media

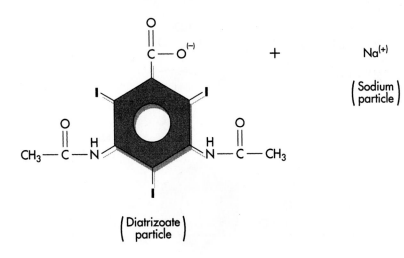

Diatrizoate
anion

Osmotically active
radiopaque anion
with 3 iodine atoms

Sodium
cation

Osmotically active
cation

$Na^{(+)}$

$\left(\begin{matrix} Sodium \\ particle \end{matrix} \right)$

$\left(\begin{matrix} Diatrizoate \\ particle \end{matrix} \right)$

Diatrizoate sodium

Representation of high-osmolar ionic contrast agent. Diatrizoate sodium contains one osmotically active negative particle (anion) and one osmotically active positive particle (cation), for a total of two osmotically active particles when in solution. Diatrizoate sodium contains three iodine (I) atoms per every two osmotically active particles, to constitute a ratio of 3:2, which equals 1.5.

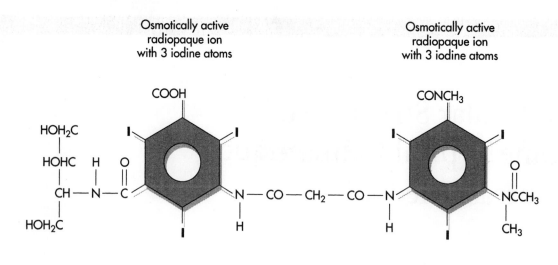

Ioxaglate

Representation of low-osmolar ionic contrast agent. Ioxaglate contains a total of six iodine atoms per every two osmotically active particles, to constitute a ratio of 6:2, which equals 3.0.

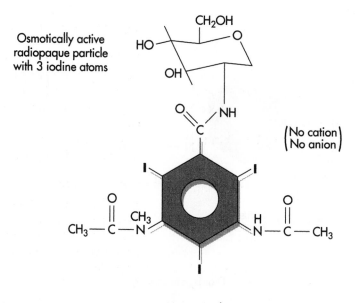

Metrizamide

Representation of nonionic contrast agent. Metrizamide does not dissociate into anions and cations in solution. It contains only one osmotically active particle to constitute a ratio of 3:1, which equals 3.0.

Catheterization Technique

For routine cystography (both male and female), size 14 or 16 Foley (retention) catheters are recommended. Review Chapter 5 for procedures involving sterile trays, gloving, and aseptic technique.

FEMALE CATHETERIZATION PROCEDURE
Prepare for Catheterization:
- Perform hand hygiene.
- Obtain and assemble equipment: catheter, antiseptic solution, cotton balls, sterile lubricant, specimen bottle, waste urine receptacle, drapes, forceps, syringe, needle, sterile water, and sterile gloves. (All are commercially available in a sterile, disposable tray.)
- Check patient identification, and explain the procedure. Provide privacy.
- Position patient supine with hips and knees flexed and legs separated, exposing perineum. Drape torso and legs.
- Place tray between patient's legs. Open tray and don gloves, using sterile technique (see Chapter 5).
- Position sterile drapes by first placing a drape under the buttocks. (Cuff drape around your hands to avoid contaminating gloves.) Place the fenestrated (window) drape over the pubis and genital area, exposing the labia.
- Pour antiseptic over cotton balls. Open lubricant and squeeze some onto the drape.

- Using nondominant hand, separate the labia to provide a clear view of the urethral orifice (Fig. K-1).

Note: This hand is now contaminated and will not be used to handle sterile objects.

Cleanse Genital Area:
- Using your fingers or the small forceps, grasp an antiseptic cotton ball with the dominant hand.
- With a single, firm, downward stroke, cleanse the far side of the labia from pubis to anus; discard cotton ball.
- Repeat the previous step for near side of labia.
- With a third cotton ball, cleanse down the center of the labia, directly over the urethral orifice.

To Insert Catheter:
- Place the distal (wide) end of the catheter in the drainage receptacle.
- With your dominant hand or the large forceps, grasp the catheter about 3 inches from its tip.
- Apply lubricant to the tip.
- Still exposing the orifice with the nondominant hand, gently insert the tip of the catheter into the orifice, guiding it posteriorly and superiorly about 2 inches (Fig. K-2). Slight resistance may be encountered at the internal urethral sphincter, which will relax when the patient exhales.

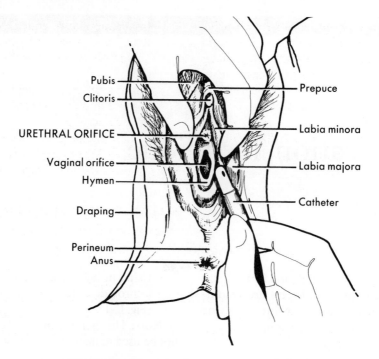

FIG. K-1 Female perineal anatomy, external view.

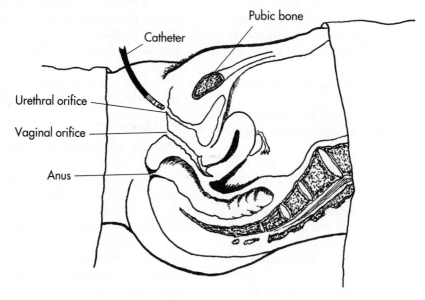

FIG. K-2 Female perineal anatomy, sagittal view.

- Release the pressure on the catheter. If urine does not flow, the catheter tip may be lodged against the bladder wall. Rotate the catheter between thumb and forefinger, and insert up to 1 inch farther.

If Specimen Is Needed:

- Clamp the catheter after a small amount of urine has drained into the receptacle.
- Transfer the distal end of the catheter into the specimen container.
- Release the forceps, allowing at least 30 ml (1 ounce) of urine to flow into the container; reclamp the catheter.
- Transfer the catheter end back to the drainage receptacle; unclamp.

Note: Normally the bladder is emptied completely in preparation for the cystogram. However, no more than 1000 ml should be removed at one time, since the patient may go into shock. (Some hospitals have policies that restrict the drainage of urine to fewer than 1000 ml of urine at one time. Be familiar with institutional policies that apply.)

When Catheter Is Situated and Bladder Is Empty:

- Inflate the retention balloon by using a syringe and needle to inject 5 ml of sterile water into the balloon valve on the catheter's distal end. The valve is self-sealing when the needle is removed.
- Tug gently on the catheter to be certain that it will be properly retained. Firm resistance indicates proper inflation of the balloon.
- Chart the amount of urine removed if the patient is under orders for the recording of intake and output (I&O). Patient is now ready for cystography.
- Remove gloves, and repeat hand hygiene.
- Discard tray, unless a combination catheterization and cystography tray has been used. In this case, change gloves and proceed with the cystogram.

To Remove Catheter:

- Perform hand hygiene, and don gloves.
- Deflate the retention balloon. This may be accomplished by using a scissors to snip off the balloon valve and allowing the water to drain into a basin, or by using a 10-ml syringe and needle to withdraw the water through the valve.
- Place paper towels under the catheter.
- Remove by pulling gently.
- Discard catheter.
- Cleanse the genital area with towel or cotton balls, and attend to patient's comfort.
- Remove gloves, and repeat hand hygiene.

MALE CATHETERIZATION PROCEDURE
Prepare for Catheterization:

- Perform hand hygiene.
- Obtain equipment: catheter, antiseptic solution, cotton balls, sterile lubricant, specimen bottle, waste urine receptacle, drapes, forceps, syringe, needle, sterile water, and sterile gloves. (All are commercially available in a sterile, disposable tray.)
- Check patient identification, and explain the procedure. Provide privacy.
- Place the patient in the supine position, with legs extended and relaxed.
- Drape the torso down to the pubis, and the legs up to the groin, leaving the penis exposed.
- Place tray adjacent to patient's hip on the side nearest you.
- Open tray, and don gloves using sterile technique (see Chapter 5).
- Position sterile drapes by first placing a drape under the buttocks. (Cuff drape around your hands to avoid contaminating gloves.) Place the fenestrated (window) drape over the penis.
- Pour antiseptic over cotton balls.
- Open lubricant, and squeeze some onto the drape.
- Place the penis in the palm of the nondominant hand, and grasp it with the third and fourth fingers.
- Holding the penis in a vertical position, use the thumb and forefinger to spread the urinary orifice (Fig. K-3).

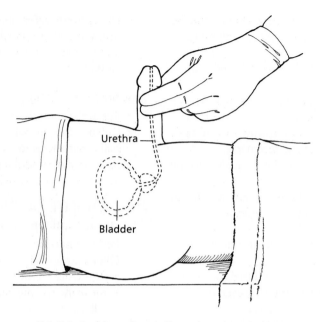

FIG. K-3 Position of penis for male catheterization.

Note: This hand is now contaminated.

Note: Handle the penis firmly, but not roughly. (Too gentle a touch may stimulate an erection.)

Cleanse Penis:

- Using the dominant hand, pick up an antiseptic cotton ball.
- Cleanse with a circular motion, and work toward the tip; discard cotton ball.
- Use second cotton ball to cleanse firmly but gently over the orifice; discard.

To Insert Catheter:

- Grasp the catheter with the large forceps about 4 inches from its tip, and place the distal end in drainage receptacle.
- Lubricate the catheter tip.
- Still holding the penis firmly in the nondominant hand, draw it forward and upward (60° to 90° degrees toward the legs), stretching it slightly. This action will straighten the urethra for easy insertion of the catheter.
- Insert gently and slowly about 7 inches. (This will require releasing the catheter and regrasping it about 4 inches distal to the original hold.)

Note: Resistance may be felt as the catheter passes the internal urethral sphincter. Use continuous, gentle pressure, and instruct the patient to try to void. Do not force insertion of the catheter. If there seems to be an obstruction or stricture, stop the procedure and call the physician.

If Specimen Is Needed:

- Clamp the catheter after a small amount of urine has drained into the receptacle.
- Transfer the distal end of the catheter into the specimen container.
- Release the forceps, allowing at least 30 ml (1 ounce) of urine to flow into the container; reclamp the catheter.
- Transfer the catheter end back to the drainage receptacle; unclamp.

Note: Normally the bladder is emptied completely in preparation for the cystogram. However, no more than 1000 ml should be removed at one time, since the patient may go into shock. (Some hospitals have policies that restrict the draining of urine to fewer than 1000 ml of urine at one time. Be familiar with the institutional policies that apply.)

When Catheter Is Situated and Bladder Is Empty:

- Inflate the retention balloon by using a syringe and needle to inject 5 ml of sterile water into the balloon valve on the catheter's distal end. The valve is self-sealing when the needle is removed.
- Tug gently on the catheter to be certain that it will be properly retained. Firm resistance indicates proper inflation of the balloon.
- Chart the amount of urine removed if the patient is under orders for the recording of intake and output (I&O). Patient is now ready for cystography.
- Remove gloves. Repeat hand hygiene.

- Discard tray, unless a combination catheterization and cystography tray has been used. In this case, change gloves and proceed with the cystogram.

To Remove Catheter:

- Perform hand hygiene, and don gloves.
- Deflate the retention balloon. This may be accomplished by using a scissors to snip off the balloon valve and allowing the water to drain into a basin, or by using a 10-ml syringe and needle to withdraw the water through the valve.
- Place paper towels under the catheter.
- Remove by pulling gently.
- Discard catheter.
- Cleanse the genital area with towel or cotton balls, and attend to the patient's comfort.
- Remove gloves, and repeat hand hygiene.

Glossary

Abdominal binder a bandage or elasticized wrap that is applied around the lower part of the torso to support the abdomen. It is sometimes applied after abdominal surgery to decrease discomfort.

Abdominal thrust subdiaphragmatic force applied as a treatment for choking. See also **Heimlich maneuver**.

Abduct, abduction to move away from the median plane of the body.

Abrasion a scraping or rubbing away of a surface, such as skin or teeth, by friction.

Acute beginning abruptly with marked intensity or sharpness, then subsiding after a relatively short period.

Adduct, adduction to move toward the median axis of the body.

Adult respiratory distress syndrome (ARDS) a respiratory disorder characterized by respiratory insufficiency and hypoxemia.

Aggravate to produce inflammation, to worsen.

Aggressiveness undesirable behavior characterized by anger or hostility.

Airborne contamination materials in the atmosphere that can affect the health of persons in the same or nearby environments.

ALARA principle a principle that states that all radiation exposure to humans should be limited to levels that are *as low as reasonably achievable.*

Allergen an agent that causes an allergic response.

Allergic reaction, allergic response an unfavorable physiological response to an allergen to which an organism has previously been exposed and to which it has developed antibodies.

Allergy, allergenic a hypersensitive reaction to intrinsically harmless antigens. Allergenic describes an individual prone to allergic response.

Alleviate to relieve or to partially remove or correct.

Alzheimer's disease a progressive mental deterioration characterized by confusion, memory failure, disorientation, restlessness, agnosia, speech disturbances, inability to carry out purposeful movement, and hallucinosis.

Ambulatory able to walk, hence describing a patient who is not confined to bed or designating a health service for people who are not hospitalized.

Ameba (also amoeba) a microscopic, single-celled, parasitic organism.

Amebiasis an infection of the intestine or liver by species of pathogenic amebas acquired by ingesting food or water contaminated with infected feces.

Amniocentesis an obstetrical procedure in which a small amount of amniotic fluid is removed for laboratory analysis.

Ampule a small, sterile glass or plastic container that usually contains a single dose of a solution.

Analgesic a drug that relieves pain.

Anaphylaxis, anaphylactic, anaphylactoid an exaggerated, life-threatening hypersensitivity reaction to a previously encountered antigen. Penicillin injection is the most common cause of anaphylactic shock.

Anastomosis a connection between two vessels or a surgical joining of two ducts, blood vessels, or bowel segments to allow flow from one to the other.

Anemia a decrease in hemoglobin in the blood to levels below the normal range of 4.2 million/mm³ to 6.1 million/mm³.

Anesthetic, anesthesia a drug or agent that is capable of producing a complete or partial loss of feeling (anesthesia).

Aneurysm a localized dilation of the wall of a blood vessel.

Angina pectoris a paroxysmal thoracic pain that usually radiates down the inner aspect of the left arm and is frequently accompanied by a feeling of suffocation and impending death.

Angiocardiogram a series of radiographic images demonstrating vessels of the heart.

Angioedema an acute, painless, dermal, subcutaneous, or submucosal swelling of short duration. It involves the face, neck, lips, larynx, hands, feet, genitalia, or viscera.

Angiogram, angiography a radiographic image/examination of a blood vessel into which contrast medium has been injected.

Angioplasty the reconstruction of blood vessels damaged by disease or injury.

Anode the electrode at which oxidation occurs. Also, the electrically positive end of an x-ray tube.

Anomaly deviation from what is regarded as normal; a congenital malformation, such as the absence of a limb or the presence of an extra finger.

Anorexia lack or loss of appetite, resulting in the inability to eat.

Anoxia an abnormal condition characterized by a lack of oxygen. It may result from an inadequate supply of oxygen to the respiratory system or from an inability of the blood to carry oxygen to the tissues or an inability of the tissues to absorb the oxygen.

Antecubital in front of the elbow; at the bend of the elbow.

Anthrax a disease affecting primarily farm animals caused by the bacterium *Bacillus anthracis*.

Antiallergic a medication used to treat allergies, or one administered in advance to patients who might be expected to have an allergic reaction.

Antibacterial pertaining to a substance that kills bacteria or inhibits their growth or replication.

Antibiotic an antimicrobial agent used to treat infections.

Antibody an immunoglobulin produced by lymphocytes in response to bacteria, viruses, or other antigenic substances. An antibody is specific to an antigen. Antibodies are responsible for acquired immunity and for allergic responses.

Anticholinergic pertaining to a blockade of acetylcholine receptors that inhibits the transmission of parasympathetic nerve impulses, thus inhibiting secretions.

Anticonvulsant pertaining to a substance or procedure that prevents or reduces the severity of epileptic or other convulsive seizures.

Antidote a drug or other substance that opposes the action of a poison.

Antifungal pertaining to a substance that kills fungi or inhibits their growth or reproduction.

Antigen a substance, usually a protein, that causes the formation of an antibody that reacts specifically with that antigen.

Antihistamine any substance capable of reducing the physiological and pharmacological effects of histamine. Antihistamines include a wide variety of drugs that block histamine receptors.

Antihypertensive a substance or procedure that reduces high blood pressure.

Antimicrobial an agent that kills or inhibits the growth or replication of microorganisms.

Antiseptic a substance that tends to inhibit the growth and reproduction of microorganisms.

Aortogram a radiographic image of the aorta made after the injection of a radiopaque contrast medium in the blood.

Apex, apical the top, the end, or the tip of a structure, such as the apex of the heart.

Aphasia, aphasic an abnormal neurological condition in which language function is defective or absent because of an injury to certain areas of the cerebral cortex.

Aqueous describing a solution prepared with water.

Arteriogram, arteriography an x-ray image/examination of an artery injected with a radiopaque medium.

Arthritis, arthritic an inflammatory condition of a joint.

Arthrography a method of radiographically visualizing the inside of a joint using a radiolucent or radiopaque contrast medium.

Arthropod a form of animal life that may cause allergic reactions and may serve as vectors for viruses and other disease-causing agents. Arthropods generally are distinguished by a jointed exoskeleton (shell) and paired, jointed legs. This group includes crustaceans, insects, and similar animal forms.

Asepsis the absence of microorganisms.

Aspirate, aspiration to withdraw fluid or air from a cavity, or to inhale fluid into the lungs.

Assault the threat of touching in an injurious way.

Assertiveness a desirable behavior characterized by a calm, firm expression of feelings or opinions.

Asthma, asthmatic a respiratory disorder characterized by recurring episodes of paroxysmal dyspnea, wheezing caused by constriction of the bronchi, coughing, and viscous mucoid bronchial secretions.

Asymptomatic without symptoms.

Asystole a life-threatening cardiac condition characterized by the absence of electrical and mechanical activity in the heart.

Atelectasis an abnormal condition characterized by the collapse of the alveoli, preventing the respiratory exchange of carbon dioxide and oxygen.

Atherectomy surgical removal of an atheroma in a major artery.

Atheroma an abnormal mass of fat or lipids, as in a sebaceous cyst or in deposits in an arterial wall.

Atherosclerosis a common disorder characterized by yellowish plaques of cholesterol, other lipids, and cellular debris in the inner layers of the walls of arteries.

Atrium a chamber or cavity, such as the right and left atria of the heart.

Atropine an alkaloid that blocks parasympathetic stimuli by raising the threshold of response of effector cells to acetylcholine.

Attenuate, attenuation the process of reduction, such as the reduction of x-ray beam intensity when it penetrates matter.

Aura a sensation, as of light or warmth, that may precede an attack of migraine or an epileptic seizure.

Autoclave an appliance used to sterilize medical instruments or other objects with steam under pressure.

Autonomy the quality of having the ability or tendency to function independently.

Axilla, axillary a pyramid-shaped space forming the underside of the shoulder between the upper arm and the side of the chest. Also called **armpit**.

Bacterium (plural, bacteria) small, unicellular microorganism.

Barbiturate a derivative of barbituric acid that acts as a sedative or hypnotic by depressing the respiratory rate, blood pressure, temperature, and central nervous system.

Barium impaction solidification of barium sulfate suspension in the intestine causing constipation and potential bowel obstruction.

Barium sulfate, "barium" a radiopaque medium used as a diagnostic aid in gastrointestinal radiography.

Base of support the portion of the body in contact with a horizontal surface, such as the floor.

Battery the unlawful use of force on a person.

B-cell a cell with the ability to produce an immune response induced by B-lymphocytes. Contact with a foreign antigen stimulates B-cells to differentiate into plasma cells that release antibodies.

Benign not recurrent or progressive, not malignant.

Benzodiazepine one of a group of psychotropic agents prescribed to alleviate anxiety or to treat insomnia.

Beta-blocker a popular term for beta-adrenergic blocking agents used to treat hypertension, rapid heart rate, and sometimes migraine headaches.

Bile a bitter, yellow-green secretion of the liver.

Biliary pertaining to bile or to the gallbladder and bile ducts, which transport bile.

Bilirubin the orange-yellow pigment of bile, formed principally by the breakdown of hemoglobin in red blood cells after termination of their normal lifespan. Also, a measurement of the bilirubin content of blood as a clinical test of biliary function.

Biopsy the removal of a small piece of living tissue from an organ or other part of the body for microscopic examination to confirm or establish a diagnosis, estimate prognosis, or follow the course of a disease.

Bismuth a reddish, crystalline, trivalent metallic element. It is combined with various other elements, such as oxygen, to produce numerous salts used in the manufacture of many pharmaceutical substances.

Bolus (injection) a quantity of undiluted contrast medium injected intravenously over a short period of time.

Bowel obstruction blockage of the intestine. Acute bowel obstruction is very painful and may be life threatening if untreated.

Bradycardia a heart condition in which the ventricles contract at a rate of less than 60 beats/min.

Bradypnea an abnormally low rate of breathing.

Bronchodilation an increase in the diameter of the bronchial lumen, allowing increased airflow to and from the lungs.

Bronchoscopy the visual examination of the tracheal and bronchial tree using a flexible fiberoptic bronchoscope.

Bronchospasm an abnormal contraction of the smooth muscle of the bronchi, resulting in an acute narrowing and obstruction of the respiratory airway, resulting in dyspnea.

Buccal pertaining to the inside of the cheek, the surface of a tooth, or the gum beside the cheek.

Bucky a moving grid that limits the amount of scattered radiation reaching a radiographic film, thereby increasing the image contrast.

BUN abbreviation for **blood urea nitrogen,** a clinical laboratory test of kidney function.

Cancer a neoplasm characterized by the uncontrolled growth of anaplastic cells that tend to invade surrounding tissue and to metastasize to distant body sites.

Cannula a flexible tube that may be inserted into a duct or cavity to deliver medication or drain fluid.

Carcinogenesis the process of initiating and promoting cancer.

Cardiac pertaining to the heart; pertaining to a person with heart disease.

Cardiac arrest a sudden cessation of cardiac output and effective circulation. It is usually precipitated by ventricular fibrillation or ventricular asystole.

Cardiac tamponade compression of the heart produced by the accumulation of blood in the pericardial sac. Also called **cardiac compression**.

Cardiogenic originating in the heart muscle.

Cardiopulmonary resuscitation (CPR) a basic emergency procedure for life support, consisting of artificial respiration and manual external cardiac massage.

Cardioversion the restoration of the heart's normal sinus rhythm through an electric shock delivered by a defibrillator.

Cassette a device used in radiography for holding a sheet of x-ray film and a set of intensifying screens. A cassette also may have a grid to absorb scattered radiation.

Cataractogenesis the process of initiating and promoting cataracts.

Cathartic a laxative preparation.

Catheter a hollow, flexible tube that can be inserted into a vessel or cavity of the body to withdraw or to instill fluids, monitor types of various information, and visualize a vessel or cavity.

Catheterize, catheterization the introduction of a catheter into a body cavity or organ to inject or remove a fluid.

Cathode the negative side of the x-ray tube, which consists of the focusing cup(s) and the filament(s).

Cathode ray tube (CRT) a vacuum tube that focuses a beam of electrons onto a spot on a screen coated with a phosphor, creating a visible image of information on the face of the tube. The CRT provides a means for graphically representing data processed by a computer.

CCU abbreviation for **coronary care unit** or **critical care unit**.

Center of gravity the midpoint or center of the weight of a body or object. In the standing adult human, the center of gravity is in the midpelvic cavity.

Central nervous system (CNS) one of the two main divisions of the nervous system, consisting of the brain and the spinal cord. The central nervous system processes information to and from the peripheral nervous system and is the main network of coordination and control for the entire body.

Central ray (CR) an imaginary photon in the center of the x-ray beam that is directed toward the center of the object being radiographed.

Cerebrovascular accident (CVA) an abnormal condition of the brain characterized by occlusion by an embolus, thrombus, or cerebrovascular hemorrhage, resulting in ischemia of the brain tissues normally perfused by the damaged vessels.

Chart, charting to note data in a patient record, usually at prescribed intervals.

Chemotherapy the treatment of infections and other diseases with chemical agents. In modern usage, chemotherapy entails the use of chemicals to destroy cancer cells on a selective basis, usually resulting in immunosuppression.

Cholangiogram, cholangiography image/examination of the biliary ducts after injection of a radiopaque contrast medium. It is usually performed before or after biliary tract surgery, and may be a part of the surgical procedure.

Cholecystectomy the surgical removal of the gallbladder.

Cholecystogram, cholecystography an x-ray image/examination of the gallbladder, made after the ingestion or injection of a radiopaque substance, usually a contrast material containing iodine.

Cholera an acute bacterial infection of the small intestine, characterized by severe diarrhea and vomiting, muscular cramps, dehydration, and depletion of electrolytes. The disease is spread by water and food that have been contaminated by feces of persons previously infected.

Chronic developing slowly and persisting for a long period.

Chronic obstructive pulmonary disease (COPD) a progressive and irreversible condition characterized by diminished inspiratory and expiratory capacity of the lungs.

Cilia (singular, cilium) small, hairlike processes on the outer surfaces of some cells, aiding metabolism by producing motion, eddies, or current in a fluid.

Circulating nurse an assistant to the scrub nurse and surgeon whose role is to provide necessary supplies, dispose of soiled supplies, and to keep an accurate count of instruments, needles, and sponges.

Claustrophobia, claustrophobic a morbid fear of being in or becoming trapped in enclosed or narrow places.

CNS abbreviation for **central nervous system**.

Coccidioidomycosis an infectious fungal disease caused by the inhalation of spores of the bacterium *Coccidioides immitis*, which is carried on windborne dust particles.

Coccus (plural, cocci) a bacterium that is round, spherical, or oval, as gonococcus, pneumococcus, staphylococcus, streptococcus.

Code a discreet signal used to summon a special team to resuscitate a patient, as in "Code zero, 3 west" announced over a public address system to summon the team to the west wing of the third floor without alarming patients or visitors.

Code team a specially trained and equipped team of physicians, nurses, and technicians that is available to provide cardiopulmonary resuscitation when summoned by a code set by the institution. A code team usually includes a physician, registered nurse, respiratory therapist, and pharmacist.

Collimator a device for limiting the size and shape of a radiation beam.

Colostomy surgical creation of an artificial anus (stoma) on the abdominal wall by incising the colon and drawing it out to the surface.

Coma, comatose pertaining to a state of **coma,** or abnormally deep sleep, caused by illness or injury.

Commode a toilet.

Computed radiography (CR) the method of using a digital computer for projecting radiographic images onto a video monitor.

Computed tomography (CT) a computerized radiographic technique that produces an image of a detailed cross section of tissue structure.

Concussion damage to the brain caused by a violent jarring or shaking, such as a blow or an explosion.

Congenital present at birth, as a congenital anomaly or defect.

Congenital megacolon the congenital absence of autonomic ganglia in the smooth muscle wall of the colon, which causes poor or absent peristalsis in the involved segment of the colon, accumulation of feces, and dilation of the bowel.

Congestive heart failure (CHF) an abnormal condition that reflects impaired cardiac pumping. It is caused by myocardial infarction, ischemic heart disease, or cardiomyopathy.

Conjunctiva (plural, conjunctivae) the mucous membrane lining the inner surfaces of the eyelids and anterior part of the sclera.

Contaminate, contamination to soil, stain, touch, or otherwise expose to harmful agents, making an object potentially unsafe for use as intended or without barrier techniques.

Contraindication the presence of a disease or physical condition that makes it impossible or undesirable to treat a particular client in the usual manner or to prescribe medicines that might otherwise be suitable.

Contrast medium (plural, contrast media), contrast agent a radiopaque substance that is injected into the body, introduced via catheter, or swallowed in order to facilitate radiographic imaging of internal structures that otherwise are difficult to visualize radiographically.

Controlled substance any drug defined in the five categories of the federal Controlled Substances Act of 1970. The categories, or schedules, cover opium and its derivatives, hallucinogens, depressants, and stimulants.

Contusion an injury that does not disrupt the integrity of the skin, caused by a blow to the body and characterized by swelling, discoloration, and pain. Also called a **bruise**.

Convulsion the hyperexcitation of neurons in the brain that leads to a sudden, involuntary series of contractions of a group of muscles. Also called a **seizure**.

COPD abbreviation for **chronic obstructive pulmonary disease**.

Coronary pertaining to encircling structures, such as the coronary arteries; pertaining to the heart.

Corticosteroid any one of the natural or synthetic hormones elaborated by the adrenal cortex (excluding the sex hormones of adrenal origin) that influence or control key processes of the body. A corticosteroid may be prescribed as an antiallergic medication.

Cortisone a glucocorticoid produced in the liver and made synthetically. It may be prescribed as an antiinflammatory.

Costal pertaining to a rib; situated near a rib or on a side close to a rib. Costal respirations involve movement of the rib cage.

Creatinine a substance formed from the metabolism of creatine, commonly found in blood, urine, and muscle tissue.

It is measured in blood and urine tests as an indicator of kidney function.

Creutzfeldt-Jakob disease the human variant of mad cow disease. A rare fatal condition of the structure and function of brain tissues caused by an unidentified slow virus or prion.

CRT abbreviation for **cathode ray tube,** a computer monitor.

CT abbreviation for **computed tomography**.

CVA abbreviation for **cerebrovascular accident**. See **stroke**.

Cyanosis, cyanotic bluish discoloration of the skin and mucous membranes caused by an excess of deoxygenated hemoglobin in the blood or a structural defect in the hemoglobin molecule.

Cyst, cystic pertaining to a **cyst,** a fluid-filled sac.

Cytomegalovirus a member of a group of large, species-specific herpes-type viruses with a wide variety of disease effects. It causes serious illness in persons with human immunodeficiency virus, in newborns, and in people being treated with immunosuppressive drugs and therapy, especially after organ transplantation.

Dacryocystography radiography of the lacrimal drainage system, the passage from the tear duct to the nasopharynx.

Debilitated feeble, weak, or otherwise disabled.

Decompression the removal of pressure caused by gas or fluid in a body cavity, as the stomach or intestinal tract.

Decubitus ulcers lesions that develop over bony prominences when pressure is exerted for any length of time. Also called **bedsores**.

Defecate, defecation the elimination of feces from the digestive tract through the rectum.

Defendant the party named in a plaintiff's complaint and against whom the plaintiff's allegations are made.

Defibrillate, defibrillation to terminate ventricular fibrillation by delivery of an electrical shock to the patient's precordium.

Defibrillator a device that delivers an electrical shock at a preset voltage to the myocardium through the chest wall.

Degenerative pertaining to or involving degeneration or change to a lower or dysfunctional form.

Dehiscence the separation of a surgical incision or rupture of a wound closure, typically an abdominal incision.

Dehydrate, dehydration to remove or lose water from a substance. Dehydration of the body is accompanied by a disturbance in the balance of essential electrolytes, particularly sodium, potassium, and chloride.

Dengue fever an acute arbovirus infection transmitted to humans by the *Aedes* mosquito and occurring in tropic and subtropic regions.

Dermatitis an inflammatory condition of the skin. Various cutaneous eruptions occur and may be unique to a particular allergen, disease, or infection.

Diabetes, diabetic clinical condition characterized by the excessive excretion of urine. The excess may be caused by a deficiency of antidiuretic hormone (ADH), as in diabetes insipidus, or it may be the polyuria resulting from the hyperglycemia that occurs in diabetes mellitus.

Diabetic coma a life-threatening condition occurring in persons with diabetes mellitus. It is caused by inadequate treatment, failure to take prescribed insulin, excessive food intake, or, most frequently, infection, surgery, trauma, or other stressors that increase the body's need for insulin.

Diagnosis, diagnostic identification of a disease or condition by a scientific evaluation of physical signs, symptoms, history, laboratory test results, and procedures.

Dialysis a medical procedure for the removal of certain elements from the blood or lymph by virtue of the difference in their rates of diffusion through an external semipermeable membrane or, in the case of peritoneal dialysis, through the peritoneum. Dialysis is a treatment for chronic kidney failure.

Diaphoresis, diaphoretic the secretion of sweat, especially the profuse secretion associated with an elevated body temperature, physical exertion, exposure to heat, and mental or emotional stress.

Diastole, diastolic pertaining to **diastole,** or the blood pressure at the instant of maximum cardiac relaxation.

Differentiation a process in development in which unspecialized cells or tissues are systemically modified and altered to achieve specific and characteristic physical forms, physiological functions, and chemical properties.

Digitalis a general term for cardiotonic glycosides used to treat congestive heart failure and atrial fibrillation.

Dilation the process of causing an increase in the diameter of a body opening, blood vessel, or tube.

Diluent a substance, generally a fluid, that makes a solution or mixture less concentrated, less viscous, or more liquid.

Diphtheria an acute contagious disease caused by the bacterium *Corynebacterium diphtheriae.* It is characterized by the production of a false membrane on mucosal surfaces and is usually accompanied by severe prostration.

Disinfectant liquid chemical applied to objects to eliminate many or all pathogenic microorganisms.

Distal away from or farthest from the point of origin or attachment.

Diuretic a drug or other substance that tends to promote the formation and excretion of urine.

Diverticulitis inflammation of one or more diverticula. The penetration of fecal matter through the thin-walled diverticula causes inflammation and abscess formation in the tissues surrounding the colon.

Diverticulosis the presence of pouchlike herniations through the muscular layer of the colon.

Diverticulum (plural, diverticula) a pouchlike herniation through the muscular wall of a tubular organ. A diverticulum may be present in the stomach, the small intestine, or, most commonly, the colon.

DNA abbreviation for **deoxyribonucleic acid,** the protein substance of genes.

Doppler a sonographic device that allows the measurement of flowing media, such as blood, by measuring the Doppler shift of the reflected ultrasound beam.

Dosimeter an instrument to detect and measure accumulated radiation exposure.

Down's syndrome a congenital condition characterized by varying degrees of mental retardation and multiple defects. Same as **Trisomy 21.**

Drip infusion the administration of diluted fluids or medications through an intravenous catheter.

Dysentery an inflammation of the intestine, especially of the colon, that may be caused by chemical irritants, bacteria, protozoa, or parasites and is characterized by diarrhea and abdominal cramping.

Dysphagia difficulty in swallowing, commonly associated with obstructive or motor disorders of the esophagus.

Dyspnea difficult or painful breathing that may be caused by certain heart conditions, strenuous exercise, or anxiety.

EDE limits a level of effective dose of radiation that has been recommended as an upper limit for employees who are exposed to radiation.

Edema the abnormal accumulation of fluid in interstitial spaces of tissues. Also called **swelling**.

Electrical ground the connection of an electric circuit to the earth, which becomes a part of the circuit. Grounding "drains off" excess charges, preventing electrical shocks and overheating of the circuit.

Electrocardiogram (ECG, EKG) a graphic record produced by an electrocardiograph, a device for recording electrical conduction through the heart.

Electrode a medium for conducting an electrical current from the body to physiological monitoring equipment.

Electrolarynx an electromechanical device that enables a person without a larynx to speak.

Electrolyte an element or compound that, when dissolved in water or another solvent, dissociates into ions and is able to conduct an electric current. An appropriate electrolyte balance in blood and body tissues, especially sodium, calcium, and chlorides, is essential to transmission of nerve impulses.

Electromagnetic energy pertaining to magnetism that is induced by an electric current. Also, energy in the form of electromagnetic waves, such as light, x-rays, and radio waves.

Emesis the act of vomiting, or a term for **vomit**.

Empathy the ability to recognize and to some extent share the emotions and states of mind of another and to understand the meaning and significance of that person's behavior.

Emphysema an abnormal condition of the pulmonary system characterized by overinflation and destructive changes of alveolar walls.

Endemic constantly present within a community. Endemic describes diseases and physical or mental disorders.

Endoscope an illuminated optical instrument for the visualization of the interior of a body cavity or organ.

Endospore a form assumed by certain bacteria in which they resist drying and can live for long periods without warmth, moisture, or nutrients.

Endotracheal within or through the trachea.

Enema the introduction of a solution into the rectum for cleansing or therapeutic purposes.

Enteral within the small intestine, or via the small intestine.

Enteric pertaining to the intestine.

Epidemic the appearance of an infectious disease or condition that affects many people at the same time in the same geographical area.

Epilepsy, epileptic a group of neurological disorders characterized by recurrent episodes of convulsive seizures, sensory disturbances, abnormal behavior, loss of consciousness, or all of these. Common to all types of epilepsy is an uncontrolled electrical discharge from the nerve cells of the cerebral cortex.

Epinephrine an endogenous adrenal hormone and synthetic adrenergic vasoconstrictor. An important emergency drug for the treatment of anaphylaxis.

Epistaxis a nosebleed.

Erythema "radiation burn," redness, or inflammation of the skin or mucous membranes caused by the dilation and congestion of superficial capillaries.

Estrogen one of a group of hormonal steroid compounds that promote the development of female secondary sex characteristics.

Ethics the science or study of moral values or principles, including ideals of autonomy, beneficence, and justice.

Ethnic of or relating to a large group of people classed according to common cultural or racial origin.

Euthanasia the deliberate causing of the death of a person suffering from an incurable disease or condition.

Evisceration the removal of the viscera from the abdominal cavity; disembowelment. Also, the removal of the contents from an organ or an organ from its cavity.

Exocrine gland any of the multicellular glands that open onto the skin surface through ducts in the epithelium, as the sweat glands and the sebaceous glands.

Expiratory pertaining to the expiration of air from the lungs.

Extracorporeal something that is outside the body.

Extravasation a passage or escape into the tissues, usually of blood, serum, or lymph. With respect to intravenous fluids, the same as **infiltration**.

False imprisonment the intentional unjustified, nonconsensual detention or confinement of a person for any length of time.

Fasting the act of abstaining from food for a specific period, usually for therapeutic or religious purposes.

Felony a crime declared by statute to be more serious than a misdemeanor and deserving a more severe punishment.

Fiberoptics the technical process by which an internal organ or cavity can be viewed, using glass or plastic fibers to transmit light through a specially designed tube and reflect a magnified image.

Fibrillation involuntary recurrent contraction of a single muscle fiber or of an isolated bundle of nerve fibers.

Fibrocystic breast disease the presence of single or multiple cysts that are palpable in the breasts. The cysts are benign and fairly common, yet must be considered potentially malignant and observed carefully for growth or change.

Fistula, fistulous tract abnormal passage from an internal organ to the body surface or between two internal organs, often the result of infection.

Flail chest a thorax in which multiple rib fractures cause instability in part of the chest wall and paradoxical breathing, with the lung underlying the injured area contracting on inspiration and bulging on expiration.

Flavivirus a genus of a family of Flaviviridae single-stranded positive-sense ribonucleic acid viruses, including species that cause yellow fever, dengue, and St. Louis encephalitis.

Flora microorganisms that live on or within a body to compete with disease-producing microorganisms and provide a natural immunity against certain infections.

Fluid overload an excessive accumulation of fluid in the body caused by excessive parenteral infusion or deficiencies in cardiovascular or renal fluid volume regulation. Same as **hypervolemia.**

Fluorescence the emission of light of one wavelength (usually ultraviolet) when exposed to energy of a different, usually shorter wavelength.

Fluoroscope a device used for the immediate projection of a radiographic image on a fluorescent screen for visual examination.

Flushing, flushed a prolonged reddening of the face such as that caused by a reaction to certain drugs.

Fomite nonliving material such as bed linen that may transmit microorganisms.

Forceps any of a large variety of surgical instruments, all of which have two handles or sides, each attached to dull blades that move in opposition to each other like scissors.

Fungus (plural, fungi) a type of organism that requires an external carbon source.

Gadolinium an element that is a component of certain intensifying screen phosphors and of paramagnetic contrast agents.

Gamma camera a device that uses the emission of light from a crystal struck by gamma rays to produce an image of the distribution of radioactive material in a body organ. The light is detected by an array of light-sensitive electronic tubes and is converted to electric signals for further processing.

Gantry assembly a subsystem of an MRI or CT unit that surrounds the patient, emits imaging energy, and detects information needed for image formation.

Gas gangrene necrosis (tissue death) accompanied by gas bubbles in soft tissue after surgery or trauma. It is caused by anaerobic organisms. Gas gangrene causes toxic delirium and is rapidly fatal if untreated.

Gastrointestinal (GI) pertaining to the organs of the alimentary tract, from mouth to anus.

Gastroscopy the visual inspection of the interior of the stomach by means of a special fiberoptic instrument, a **gastroscope,** inserted through the mouth and esophagus.

Generic pertaining to a substance, product, or drug that is not protected by trademark.

Germicide, germicidal a drug that kills pathogenic microorganisms.

Gestation, gestational in viviparous animals, the period from the fertilization of the ovum until birth. Gestation varies with the species; in humans the average duration is 266 days, or approximately 280 days from the onset of the last menstrual period.

Giardiasis an inflammatory intestinal condition. The source of infection is usually untreated water contaminated with *Giardia lamblia* cysts. Also called **traveler's diarrhea.**

Glucose a simple sugar found in certain foods, especially fruits, and a major source of energy present in human and animal body fluids.

Grand mal seizure a seizure characterized by loss of consciousness and a rigid arching of the back followed by alternate relaxation. Same as **major motor seizure.**

Granule a particle, grain, or other small, dry mass capable of free movement. Unlike powders, granules are usually free flowing because of small surface forces involved.

Grid a device used during a radiographic examination to absorb radiation that is not heading along a straight line from the x-ray source to the film.

Half-life the time required for a radioactive substance to lose 50% of its activity through decay.

Hallucinogen a substance that causes excitation of the central nervous system, characterized by hallucination, mood change, anxiety, sensory distortion, delusion, depersonalization; and increased pulse, temperature, and blood pressure; and dilation of the pupils.

Hantavirus a genus of viruses in the Bunyaviridae family. *Hantavirus* is the cause of several different forms of hemorrhagic fever with renal syndrome.

Heimlich maneuver an emergency procedure for dislodging food or other obstruction from the trachea to prevent asphyxiation. Also called **abdominal thrust.**

Hematoma a collection of extravasated blood trapped in the tissues of the skin or in an organ, resulting from trauma or incomplete hemostasis after surgery.

Hemodynamics the physical aspects of blood circulation, including cardiac function and peripheral vascular physiological characteristics.

Hemoglobin a complex protein-iron compound in the blood that carries oxygen to the cells from the lungs and carbon dioxide away from the cells to the lungs.

Hemolytic uremia syndrome a rare kidney disorder marked by renal failure, microangiopathic hemolytic anemia, and platelet deficiency. The syndrome, the cause of which is unknown, usually occurs in infancy.

Hemorrhage, hemorrhagic a loss of a large amount of blood in a short period, either externally or internally. Hemorrhage may be arterial, venous, or capillary.

Hemorrhoids a varicosity in the lower rectum or anus caused by congestion in the veins of the hemorrhoidal plexus.

Hemostat a procedure, device, or substance that arrests the flow of blood. Common term for small forceps used to clamp blood vessels or tubing.

Hemothorax an accumulation of blood and fluid in the pleural cavity, between the parietal and visceral pleura, usually the result of trauma.

Heparin an anticoagulant that prevents intravascular clotting.

Heparin lock a small adapter with a diaphragm that is attached to an intravenous (IV) catheter when more than one injection is anticipated. Same as **intermittent injection port.**

Hepatic pertaining to the liver.

Hepatitis an inflammatory condition of the liver, characterized by jaundice, hepatomegaly (liver enlargement), anorexia, abdominal and gastric discomfort, abnormal liver function, clay-colored stools, and tea-colored urine.

Herniation a protrusion of a body organ or portion of an organ through an abnormal opening in a membrane, muscle, or other tissue.

Herpes a category of virus, which includes herpes simplex virus (HSV), herpes simplex virus 1 (oral herpes, herpes labialis) and herpes simplex virus 2 (herpes genitalis).

Hiatal hernia protrusion of a portion of the stomach upward through the diaphragm. The condition occurs in about 40% of the population, and most people display few, if any, symptoms.

Histamine a compound, found in all cells, produced by the breakdown of histidine. It is released in allergic and inflammatory reactions and causes dilation of capillaries, decrease in blood pressure, increase in secretion of gastric juice, and constriction of smooth muscles of the bronchi and uterus.

Histoplasmosis an infection caused by inhalation of spores of the fungus *Histoplasma capsulatum.*

Hives blotchy reddening of the skin with itching. Same as **urticaria**.

Human immunodeficiency virus (HIV) a retrovirus that causes acquired immunodeficiency syndrome (AIDS). It is transmitted through contact with an infected individual's blood, semen, breast milk, cervical secretions, cerebrospinal fluid, or synovial fluid. HIV infects T-helper cells of the immune system and causes infection with a long incubation period, averaging 10 years.

Hydration a chemical process in which water is taken up without disrupting the rest of the molecule.

Hydrostatic pressure the pressure exerted by a liquid.

Hyperextension a position of maximum extension of a joint.

Hypertension a common, often asymptomatic disorder characterized by elevated blood pressure persistently exceeding 140/90 mm Hg.

Hyperthermia a much higher than normal body temperature.

Hyperventilation a pulmonary ventilation rate that is greater than that metabolically necessary for pulmonary gas exchange. It is the result of an increased frequency of breathing, an increased tidal volume, or a combination of both and causes excessive intake of oxygen and elimination of carbon dioxide.

Hypervolemia an abnormal increase in the amount of intravascular fluid, particularly in the volume of circulating blood or its components. Same as **fluid overload**.

Hypodermic pertaining to the area below the skin, such as a hypodermic injection.

Hypoglycemia a less than normal amount of glucose in the blood, usually caused by administration of too much insulin, excessive secretion of insulin by the islet cells of the pancreas, or dietary deficiency.

Hypotension an abnormal condition in which the blood pressure is not adequate for normal perfusion and oxygenation of the tissues. See also **shock**.

Hypothalamus a portion of the diencephalon of the brain. It activates, controls, and integrates the peripheral autonomic nervous system, endocrine processes, and many somatic functions, such as body temperature, sleep, and appetite.

Hypovolemia an abnormally low circulating blood volume.

Hypoxemia, hypoxia insufficient oxygenation of the blood.

Hysterosalpingography a method of producing radiographic images of the uterus and fallopian tubes as part of the diagnosis of abnormalities in the reproductive tract of a nonpregnant woman.

ICU abbreviation for **intensive care unit**.

Ileostomy surgical formation of an opening of the ileum onto the surface of the abdomen, through which fecal matter is emptied.

Image intensifier an electronic device used to produce a fluoroscopic image with a low-radiation exposure. A beam of x-rays passing through the patient is converted in a special vacuum tube into a pattern of electrons. The electrons are accelerated and concentrated onto a small fluorescent screen, where they present a bright image, which is generally displayed on a television monitor.

Immunosuppressant an agent that significantly interferes with the ability of the immune system to respond to antigenic stimulation by inhibiting cellular and humoral immunity.

Incision a cut produced surgically by a sharp instrument that creates an opening into an organ or space in the body.

Incontinence inability to control urination or defecation.

Inert (of a chemical substance) not taking part in a chemical reaction; (of a medication ingredient) not active pharmacologically; serving only as a bulking, binding, or sweetening agent or other excipient in a medication.

Infectious mononucleosis an acute herpes virus infection caused by the Epstein-Barr virus. It is characterized by fever, sore throat, swollen lymph glands, atypical lymphocytes, splenomegaly, hepatomegaly, abnormal liver function, and bruising. The disease is usually transmitted by droplet infection but is not highly or predictably contagious.

Infiltration the process whereby a fluid passes into the tissues, such as when a local anesthetic is administered or an intravenous infusion infiltrates.

Inflammation, inflammatory the protective response of body tissues to irritation, infection or injury, characterized by redness, swelling, pain, and loss of function.

Influenza highly contagious infection of the respiratory tract caused by a myxovirus and transmitted by airborne droplet infection.

Informed consent permission obtained from a patient to perform a specific test or procedure. Informed consent is required before performing most invasive procedures and before admitting a patient to a research study. The document used must be written in a language understood by the patient and be dated and signed by the patient and at least one witness.

Ingest, ingestion to take substances into the body through the mouth.

Inpatient a patient who has been admitted to a hospital or other health care facility for at least an overnight stay.

Insulin a naturally occurring hormone secreted by the beta cells of the islets of Langerhans in the pancreas in response to increased levels of glucose in the blood.

Intercostal space the space between two ribs.

Interferon a natural cellular protein formed when cells are exposed to a virus or another foreign particle of nucleic acid.

Intermammillary line a horizontal anatomical line drawn between the nipples.

Intermittent injection port a small adapter with a diaphragm that is attached to an IV catheter when more than one injection is anticipated. Same as **heparin lock** or **saline lock.**

Intern a physician in the first postgraduate year, learning medical practice under supervision before beginning a residency program or practice.

Intradermal within the dermis layer of the skin.

Intramuscular within muscle tissue.

Intrathecal pertaining to a structure, process, or substance within a sheath, such as within the spinal canal.

Intrauterine device (IUD) a contraceptive device. It consists of a bent strip of radiopaque plastic with a fine monofilament tail and is placed within the uterus.

Intravascular within a blood vessel.

Intravenous (IV) pertaining to the inside of a vein, as of a thrombus or an injection, infusion, or catheter.

Intubate, intubation passage of a tube into a body aperture, specifically the insertion of a breathing tube through the mouth or nose into the trachea to ensure a patent airway for the delivery of anesthetic gases or oxygen or both.

Invasive characterized by a tendency to spread, infiltrate, and intrude. Invasive procedures involve penetration of the body wall (e.g., surgery or angiography).

Iodinated refers to types of contrast media prepared with iodine compounds, which absorb radiation to a greater degree than blood or soft tissues and therefore produce a more clearly visible white or light shadow on the radiograph.

Ion, ionic a charged particle, an atom or group of atoms that has acquired an electrical charge through the gain or loss of an electron or electrons.

Ionize, ionization to separate or change into ions (charged particles).

Irrigate, irrigation to flush with a fluid, usually with a slow steady pressure on a syringe plunger. It may be done to cleanse a wound or to clear tubing.

Ischemia a decreased supply of oxygenated blood to a body organ or part.

Isolette trademark for a self-contained incubator unit that provides a controlled heat, humidity, and oxygen micro-environment for the isolation and care of premature and low-birth-weight neonates.

Ketoacidosis acidosis accompanied by an accumulation of ketones in the body, resulting from extensive breakdown of fats because of faulty carbohydrate metabolism.

Kilovolt (kv), kilovoltage measure of electrical potential, 1000 volts.

Kilovoltage peak (kVp) potential difference measured at the peak of the electrical cycle. An x-ray control setting that determines the penetrating power of the x-ray beam.

Kyphosis, kyphotic posterior curvature of the spine, characteristic of the thoracic spinal segments. When abnormally exaggerated, kyphosis results in protrusion of the upper back.

Laceration a torn, jagged wound.

Laparoscope a type of fiberoptic instrument consisting of an illuminated tube with an optical system. It is inserted through the abdominal wall for examining the peritoneal cavity.

Laryngectomy surgical removal of the larynx performed to treat cancer of the larynx.

Larynx, laryngeal the organ of voice that is part of the air passage connecting the pharynx with the trachea.

Lesion a wound, injury, or pathological change in body tissue. Also, any visible, local abnormality of the tissues of the skin, such as a wound, sore, rash, or boil. A lesion may be described as benign, cancerous, gross, occult, or primary.

Leukemia a broad term given to a group of malignant diseases affecting the bone marrow.

Level of consciousness (LOC) degree of cognitive function involving arousal mechanisms of the reticular formation of the brain.

Libel a false accusation written, printed, or typewritten, or presented in a picture or a sign that is made with malicious intent to defame the reputation of a person who is living or the memory of a person who is dead, resulting in public embarrassment, contempt, ridicule, or hatred.

Lidocaine a local anesthetic agent, also given intravenously to treat ventricular tachycardia.

Line of gravity an imaginary line that extends from the center of gravity to the base of support.

Lipoprotein a conjugated protein in which fats or oils form an integral part of the molecule.

Lithotripsy a procedure for eliminating a calculus in the renal pelvis, ureter, bladder, or gallbladder.

Lordosis, lordotic anterior curvature of the spine, characteristic of both the cervical and lumbar spinal segments.

Lumbar puncture (LP) the introduction of a hollow needle and stylet into the subarachnoid space of the lumbar part of the spinal canal. Same as **spinal tap.**

Lumen (plural, lumina) the interior canal of an organ or catheter.

Lyme disease an acute recurrent inflammatory infection transmitted by a tickborne spirochete, *Borrelia burgdorferi*.

Lymphocyte small agranulocytic leukocyte (white blood cell) originating from fetal stem cells and developing in the bone marrow.

Lymphomas types of neoplasms of lymphoid tissue that originate in the reticuloendothelial and lymphatic systems. They are usually malignant but in rare cases may be benign.

Lysozyme an enzyme with antiseptic actions that destroys some foreign organisms.

Magnetic resonance imaging (MRI) a noninvasive computerized diagnostic modality that uses a magnetic field and pulses of radio waves to produce an image on a computer monitor.

Major motor seizure a seizure characterized by loss of consciousness and a rigid arching of the back followed by alternate relaxation. Same as **grand mal seizure**.

Malaria a severe infectious illness caused by one or more of at least four species of the protozoan genus *Plasmodium*. The disease is transmitted from human to human by a bite from an infected *Anopheles* mosquito. Malarial infection can also be spread by blood transfusion from an infected patient or by the use of an infected hypodermic needle.

Malpractice professional negligence that is the proximate cause of injury or harm to a patient, resulting from a lack of professional knowledge, experience, or skill that can be expected in others in the profession or from a failure to exercise reasonable care or judgment in the application of professional knowledge, experience, or skill.

Mammogram, mammography an x-ray image/examination of the soft tissues of the breast to allow identification of various benign and malignant neoplastic processes.

Manometer a device for measuring the pressure of a fluid, consisting of a tube marked with a scale and containing a relatively incompressible fluid, such as mercury.

Mastectomy surgical removal of one or both breasts, usually to remove a malignant tumor. It may include breast tissue, chest muscle, and axillary lymph nodes.

Medication pump a pump that automatically delivers measured amounts of drugs through an intravenous catheter.

Meningitis any infection or inflammation of the membranes covering the brain and spinal cord.

Metabolism the aggregate of all chemical processes that take place in living organisms, resulting in growth, generation of energy, elimination of wastes, and other body functions as they relate to the distribution of nutrients in the blood after digestion.

Metabolite a substance produced by metabolic action or necessary for a metabolic process.

Microbe, microbial a microorganism, pertaining to a living organism too small to be seen by the naked eye.

Microbial dilution the process of reducing the total number of microorganisms, which is accomplished at three levels: cleanliness measures, disinfection, and sterilization.

Microorganism any tiny, usually microscopic, entity capable of carrying on living processes.

Milliampere seconds (mAs) the product obtained by multiplying the electric current in milliamperes by the exposure time in seconds. It is used to describe the exposure setting of a radiography machine and determines the density of the radiographic image.

Milliampere, milliamperage (mA) a unit of electric current that is one thousandth of an ampere.

Miscible able to be mixed or blended with another substance.

Misdemeanor an offense that is considered less serious than felony and carries a lesser penalty, usually a fine or imprisonment for less than 1 year.

Mission statement the role of a hospital or health care facility stated in a one- or two-paragraph declaration of the institution's basic philosophy and primary goals. This statement provides guidance for the decisions that govern the activities of the facility.

Mitosis, mitotic a type of cell division that occurs in somatic cells and results in the formation of two genetically identical daughter cells containing the diploid number of chromosomes characteristic of the species.

Moral agent the one responsible for implementing an ethical decision.

Motile, motility capable of spontaneous but unconscious or involuntary movement.

Mucocutaneous pertaining to the mucous membrane and the skin.

Mucosa, mucosal, mucous membrane any one of four major kinds of thin sheets of tissue that cover or line various parts of the body. Mucous membrane lines cavities or canals of the body that open to the outside.

Mutation an unusual change in genetic material occurring spontaneously or by induction.

Myelogram, myelography an x-ray image/examination after the injection of a radiopaque medium into the subarachnoid space to demonstrate any distortions of the spinal cord, spinal nerve roots, and subarachnoid space.

Narcotic pertaining to a substance that produces insensibility or stupor.

Nasoenteric (NE) tube a kind of tube that can penetrate farther into the intestinal tract than a nasogastric tube. It is used to aspirate gas and fluid that may cause distention postoperatively.

Nasogastric (NG) tube a tube placed to allow feeding of a patient directly into the stomach. May also be connected to a suction device to empty the stomach.

Nebulizer a device for producing a fine spray. Intranasal and respiratory medications are often administered by a nebulizer. Also called **atomizer**.

Negligence the commission of an act that a prudent person would not have done or the omission of a duty that a prudent person would have fulfilled, resulting in injury or harm to another person.

Neonate, neonatal an infant from birth to 28 days of age.

Nephrogram a radiograph of the kidney; usually refers to an image of the parenchyma of the kidney in the early postinjection phase of an excretory urogram.

Neurogenic pertaining to the formation of nervous tissue, originating from the nervous system.

Neurology, neurological the field of medicine that deals with the nervous system and its disorders.

Neurostimulator an electronic device worn by patients to control pain and muscle spasm.

Noninvasive pertaining to a diagnostic or therapeutic technique that does not require the skin to be broken or a cavity or organ of the body to be entered.

Nonionic pertaining to compounds that do not dissociate into charged particles when in solution.

Normal saline a 0.9% weight per volume (w/v) sterile solution of sodium chloride in water that is isotonic with blood and injectable intravenously.

Nosocomial pertaining to a hospital.

Nosocomial infection refers to hospital-acquired disease.

NPO (nil per os, nothing by mouth) a patient care instruction advising that the patient is prohibited from ingesting food, beverage, or medicine.

Nurse practitioner a registered nurse who has advanced education in nursing and clinical experience in a specialized area of nursing practice.

Occlude, occlusion (in anatomy) a blockage in a canal, vessel, or passage of the body.

Oncology the branch of medicine concerned with the study of malignancy.

Opaque, opacify, opacification pertaining to a substance or surface that neither transmits nor allows the passage of light. See also **radiopaque**.

Open reduction a surgical procedure for realigning a fracture or dislocation by exposing the skeletal parts involved.

Ophthalmology the branch of medicine concerned with the study of the physiology, anatomy, and pathology of the eye and the diagnosis and treatment of disorders of the eye.

Opiate a narcotic drug that contains opium, derivatives of opium.

Opioid pertaining to natural and synthetic chemicals that have opiumlike effects although they are not derived from opium.

Opportunistic infection an infection caused by normally nonpathogenic organisms in a host whose resistance has been decreased by disorders such as diabetes mellitus, human immunodeficiency virus (HIV) infection, or cancer.

Orthopedic pertaining to the locomotor system of the body, including the skeleton, muscles, and joints.

Orthopnea an abnormal condition in which a person must sit or stand to breathe deeply or comfortably.

Orthostatic hypotension a transient state of cerebral anoxia and low blood pressure occurring when an individual assumes a standing posture. Same as **postural hypotension**.

Osmolality the osmotic pressure of a solution expressed in osmoles or milliosmoles per kilogram of water. Normal adult blood osmolality is 285 to 295 mOsm/kg H_2O.

Osseous consisting of or resembling bone; **bony**.

OTC abbreviation for **over the counter**, a drug available to the consumer without a prescription.

Outpatient a patient, not hospitalized, who is being treated in an office, clinic, or other ambulatory care facility.

Pacemaker an electric device used in most cases to increase the heart rate in severe bradycardia by electrically stimulating the heart muscle.

PACU abbreviation for **postanesthesia care unit**, an area designed and staffed to provide close observation and care of patients following operative procedures requiring an anesthetic agent. Also called a **recovery room**.

Palliative a substance or treatment that soothes or relieves.

Pallor an unnatural paleness or absence of color in the skin.

Paralysis the loss of muscle function, loss of sensation, or both.

Paramagnetic agents agents with a small but positive magnetic susceptibility, the small addition of which may greatly reduce the MRI relaxation times of a substance and used as a contrast medium in MRI.

Parenteral pertaining to treatment introduced into the body other than through the digestive system.

Parietal pertaining to the outer wall of a cavity or organ (e.g., the parietal pleura lines the walls of the thoracic cavity).

Patent, patency a state of being open or exposed.

Pathogen any microorganism capable of producing disease.

Pediatric pertaining to health care and treatment of children and the study of childhood diseases.

Penicillin any one of a group of antibiotics derived from cultures of species of the fungus *Penicillium* or produced semisynthetically.

Percutaneous performed through the skin, such as a biopsy.

Perforated ulcer an ulcer (sore) that penetrates the thickness of a wall or membrane.

Pericardium a fibroserous sac that surrounds the heart and the roots of the great vessels.

Peristalsis the coordinated, rhythmic serial contraction of smooth muscle that forces food through the digestive tract, bile through the bile duct, and urine through the ureter.

Peritonitis inflammation of the membrane lining the abdominal cavity (peritoneum). It is produced by bacteria or irritating substances introduced into the abdominal cavity by a penetrating wound or perforation of an organ in the gastrointestinal tract or the reproductive tract.

Permeability the degree to which one substance allows another substance to pass through it.

Pertussis an acute, highly contagious respiratory disease characterized by paroxysmal coughing that ends in a loud whooping inspiration. Also called **whooping cough**.

Phagocytosis the process by which certain cells engulf and destroy microorganisms and cellular debris.

Pharmacodynamics the study of how a drug acts on a living organism, including the pharmacological response and the duration and magnitude of response observed.

Pharmacokinetics the study of how drugs enter the body, are absorbed, reach their site of action, are metabolized, and exit the body.

Pharmacology the study of the preparation, properties, uses, and actions of drugs.

Pharyngitis inflammation or infection of the throat.

Phlebitis inflammation of a vein.

Phlebotomist a person with special training in the practice of drawing blood.

Phosphors fluorescent crystals that give off light when exposed to x-rays.

Photomultiplier tube a device used in many radiation detection applications that converts low levels of light into electrical pulses.

Photon the smallest quantity of electromagnetic energy. It has no mass and no charge and travels at the speed of light. Photons may occur in the form of light rays, x-rays, gamma rays, and other electromagnetic energies.

Photosensitive reactive to light.

Plaintiff a person who files a lawsuit initiating a legal action.

Pleura, pleural a delicate serous membrane covering the lung and lining the thoracic cavity.

Pleural effusion an abnormal accumulation of fluid between the visceral and parietal pleura.

Pleurisy inflammation of the pleura, sometimes resulting in adhesion of pleural membranes and causing dyspnea.

Pneumatic pertaining to air or gas.

Pneumonia an acute inflammation of the lungs, often caused by inhaled pneumococci of the species *Streptococcus pneumoniae*.

Pneumothorax a collection of air or gas in the pleural space causing the lung to collapse.

Positron emission tomography (PET) a computerized nuclear medicine scanning modality involving the injection of radionuclides that emit ion pairs.

Postictal the immediate period following a seizure.

Postural hypotension a transient cerebral anoxia that occurs when a patient is bedridden for an extended period of time and blood pools in the extremities when the torso is elevated. Same as **orthostatic hypotension**.

Potent, potency active, powerful, or strong.

Precipitate to cause a substance to separate or to settle out of solution; a substance that has separated from or settled out of a solution.

Premedication any sedative, tranquilizer, hypnotic, or anticholinergic medication administered before anesthesia or other procedure.

Primary health care a basic level of health care that includes programs directed at the promotion of health, early diagnosis of disease or disability, and prevention of disease.

Prognosis a prediction of the probable outcome of a disease based on the condition of the person and the usual course of the disease as observed in similar situations.

Proprietary medications medicinal substance that is protected from commercial competition because its ingredients or method of manufacture is kept secret or is protected by trademark or patent.

Prosthesis (plural, prostheses) an artificial replacement for a missing body part, or a device designed and applied to improve function, such as a hearing aid.

Protocol a written plan specifying the procedures to be followed in giving a particular examination, in conducting research, or in providing care for a particular condition.

Protozoan (plural, protozoa) single-celled microorganism of the subkingdom Protozoa.

Proximal nearer to a point of reference or attachment, usually the trunk of the body, than other parts of the body.

Psychomotor pertaining to or causing voluntary movements usually associated with neural activity. Psychomotor skill is the ability to move purposefully.

Pulmonary pertaining to the lungs or the respiratory system.

Pulmonary edema the accumulation of extravascular fluid in lung tissues and alveoli, caused most commonly by congestive heart failure.

Pulse oximeter a digital monitor connected to the patient by means of a cable and a small probe attached to a finger or earlobe.

Pyloric stenosis a narrowing of the pyloric sphincter at the outlet of the stomach, causing an obstruction that blocks the flow of food into the small intestine.

Pylorospasm a spasm of the pyloric sphincter of the stomach, as occurs in pyloric stenosis.

Pyrexia the abnormal elevation of body temperature above 37° Celsius (98.6° Fahrenheit). Same as **fever**.

Qualitative pertaining to the quality, value, or nature of something.

Quality factor (QF) a term that expresses the biological damage that radiation can produce.

Quantitative capable of being measured.

Quantum (plural, quanta) a group or "bundle" of photons.

Rad abbreviation for **radiation absorbed dose,** the basic unit of absorbed dose of ionizing radiation. One rad is equal to the absorption of 100 ergs of radiation energy per gram of matter.

Radiation field the cross section of the x-ray beam at the point where it is utilized.

Radiograph an x-ray image.

Radiographer an allied health professional who performs diagnostic examinations on patients using a variety of modalities, including radiography, computed tomography, magnetic resonance imaging, mammography, and cardiovascular interventional technology.

Radiography the production of images using ionizing radiation.

Radioisotope a radioactive isotope of an element, used for therapeutic and diagnostic purposes.

Radiologic technologist a person who, under the supervision of a physician radiologist, operates diagnostic imaging equipment and assists radiologists and other health professionals.

Radiologist a physician who specializes in medical imaging.

Radiolucent pertaining to materials that allow x-rays to penetrate with a minimum of absorption.

Radionuclide an isotope that undergoes radioactive decay. Same as **radioisotope**.

Radiopaque not permitting the passage of x-rays or other radiant energy.

Rapport a sense of harmony and understanding underlying a relationship between two persons, which is an essential bond between a therapist and patient.

RBE abbreviation for **relative biological effectiveness,** a measure of the cell-killing ability of a particular radiation compared with a reference radiation. The reference is 250 keV x-rays.

Rectal pertaining to the distal portion of the large intestine, about 12 cm long, between the sigmoid colon and the anus.

Recumbent lying down or leaning backward.

Regimen a strictly regulated therapeutic program such as a diet or exercise schedule.

Remnant radiation the radiation that passes through an object to produce an image.

Renal pertaining to the kidney.

Resident a physician in one of the postgraduate training (often specialized) after the first, or 1

Residual pertaining to the part of something th removing the bulk of the substance.

Respiration, respiratory the process of th exchange of oxygen and carbon dioxide within tissues, from the lungs to cellular oxidation.

Respiratory arrest the cessation of breathing.

Respite care short-term health services to the dependen adult to provide relief for the primary caregiver.

Resuscitation the process of sustaining the vital function person in respiratory or cardiac failure while reviving him her, using techniques of artificial respiration and cardi massage, correcting acid-base imbalance, and treating th cause of failure.

Retention catheter a type of rectal or urinary catheter with an inflatable cuff that holds the catheter securely in place.

Retrograde moving backward; moving or flowing in the opposite direction to that which is considered normal.

Retrovirus any of a family of ribonucleic acid (RNA) viruses containing an enzyme, reverse transcriptase, in the virion.

Rickettsia (plural, rickettsiae) a genus of microorganisms that combine aspects of both bacteria and viruses.

Rocky Mountain spotted fever (RMSF) a serious tickborne infectious disease occurring throughout the temperate zones of North and South America, caused by *Rickettsia rickettsii.*

Roentgen (R or r) the traditional unit of radiation exposure, it is a measurement of radiation intensity in the air. The roentgen is equal to the quantity of radiation that will produce 2.08×10^9 ion pairs in a cubic centimeter of dry air.

Sclerosis, sclerotic a condition characterized by hardening of tissue resulting from any of several causes, including inflammation, the deposit of mineral salts, and infiltration of connective tissue fibers.

Secondary health care an intermediate level of health care that includes diagnosis and treatment, performed in a hospital having specialized equipment and laboratory facilities.

Sedation an induced state of quiet, calmness, or sleep, as by means of a **sedative** or hypnotic medication.

Seizure a hyperexcitation of neurons in the brain leading to a sudden, violent involuntary series of contractions of a group of muscles.

Senile, senility pertaining to or characteristic of old age or the process of aging.

Sepsis, septic infection, contamination.

Sestamibi a radiopharmaceutical used in nuclear imaging to create contrast in tissues.

Sharps any needles, scalpels, or other articles that could cause wounds or punctures to personnel.

Shock an abnormal condition of inadequate blood flow to the body's peripheral tissues, with life-threatening cellular dysfunction.

Shunt to redirect the flow of a body fluid from one cavity or vessel to another, or a device for accomplishing this.

Side effect any reaction to or consequence of a medication or therapy other than the therapeutic effect.

Sigmoidoscope a fiberoptic instrument used to examine the lumen of the sigmoid colon.

Single photon emission computed tomography (SPECT) a computerized nuclear medicine scanning modality similar to PET imaging but involving the injection of radionuclides that emit single photons as opposed to ion pairs as in PET.

Sinus rhythm a cardiac rhythm stimulated by the sinus (sinoatrial) node. A rate of 60 to 100 beats/min is normal.

Sinus tachycardia a rapid heartbeat generated by discharge of the sinoatrial pacemaker. The rate is generally 100 to 180 beats/min in the adult.

Siphon using atmospheric pressure to withdraw fluid from a cavity through a tube, or the tube used for this purpose.

Slander any words spoken with malice that are untrue and prejudicial to the reputation, professional practice, commercial trade, office, or business of another person.

Solution a mixture of one or more substances dissolved in another substance. The molecules of each of the substances disperse homogenously and do not change chemically.

Sonography the process of imaging deep structures of the body by measuring and recording the reflection of pulsed or continuous high-frequency sound waves.

Source-image distance (SID) the distance between the x-ray tube target and the image receptor, measured along the central ray.

Spasm, spasmodic an involuntary muscle contraction of sudden onset.

Sphygmomanometer an instrument for indirect measurement of blood pressure. It consists of an inflatable cuff that fits around the arm, a bulb for controlling air pressure within the cuff, and a mercury or aneroid manometer.

Spinal tap a procedure that involves the insertion of a needle into the subarachnoid space to withdraw spinal fluid. May be performed to inject a contrast medium for myelography. Same as **lumbar puncture.**

Spontaneous abortion a termination of pregnancy before the twentieth week of gestation as a result of abnormalities of the conceptus or maternal environment. Also called **miscarriage.**

Spontaneous combustion an explosion that occurs when a chemical reaction in or near a flammable material causes sufficient heat to generate a fire.

Spore a reproductive unit of some genera of fungi or protozoa. Also, a common term for **endospore,** a form assumed by some bacteria that is resistant to heat, drying, and chemicals.

Standing order a written document containing rules, policies, procedures, regulations, and orders for the conduct of patient care in various stipulated clinical situations.

Stat immediately, at once.

Status epilepticus a medical emergency characterized by continuous seizures occurring without interruptions.

Stenosis an abnormal condition characterized by the constriction or narrowing of an opening or passageway in a body structure.

Stent a tubular device for supporting hollow structures during surgical anastomosis or for holding arteries open during angioplasty.

"Sterile conscience" the awareness of sterile technique and the responsibility for notifying those in charge whenever contamination occurs.

Sterile field a specified area, such as within a tray or on a sterile towel, that is considered free of microorganisms.

Sterile, sterilization free of living microorganisms, the process of destroying all microorganisms.

Steroid any of a large number of hormonal substances with a similar basic chemical structure, produced mainly in the adrenal cortex and gonads, may be used to treat inflammatory conditions or as antiallergic medication.

Stoma a pore, orifice, or opening on a surface; the external opening of a colostomy or ileostomy.

Stridor an abnormal high-pitched sound caused by an obstruction in the trachea or larynx, usually heard during inspiration.

Stroke an abnormal condition of the brain characterized by a rupture or obstruction of an artery of the brain. Same as **cerebrovascular accident (CVA).**

Stupor, stuporous a state of unresponsiveness in which a person seems unaware of the surroundings.

Subcellular of less than a cellular structure or function.

Subcutaneous beneath the skin.

Subdiaphragmatic beneath the diaphragm.

Subliminal taking place below the threshold of sensory perception or outside the range of conscious awareness.

Sublingual pertaining to the area beneath the tongue.

Suppository an easily melted medicated mass for insertion into the rectum, urethra, or vagina.

Surgical resection partial removal of a structure or organ by surgery.

Suspension a liquid in which small particles of a solid are dispersed, but not dissolved, and in which the dispersal is maintained by stirring or shaking the mixture. If left standing, the solid particles settle at the bottom of the container.

Syncope a brief lapse in consciousness caused by transient cerebral hypoxia, **fainting.**

Synergistic effect the acting or working together of a number of components, as when medications produce a combined effect.

Syphilis a sexually transmitted disease caused by the spirochete *Treponema pallidum,* characterized by distinct stages of effects over a period of years.

Systemic effect pertaining to the whole body rather than to a localized area or regional part of the body.

Systolic pertaining to systole, or the blood pressure resulting from a ventricular contraction.

Tachycardia a condition in which the myocardium contracts at a rate greater than 100 beats/min.

Tachypnea an abnormally rapid rate of breathing (more than 20 breaths per minute), as seen with hyperpyrexia.

Tepid moderately warm to the touch, "lukewarm."

Tertiary health care a specialized, highly technical level of health care that includes diagnosis and treatment of disease and disability in sophisticated, large research and teaching hospitals.

Tetanus an acute, potentially fatal infection of the central nervous system caused by an exotoxin, tetanospasmin, elaborated by an anaerobic bacillus, *Clostridium tetani.*

Therapeutic effect the desired benefit of a medication, treatment, or procedure.

Therapy, therapeutic the treatment of any disease or pathological condition.

Thoracotomy a surgical opening into the thoracic cavity.

Thready an abnormal pulse that is weak, somewhat difficult to palpate, and often fairly rapid; the artery does not feel full, and the rate may be difficult to count.

Thrombus (plural, thrombi) an aggregation of platelets, fibrin, clotting factors, and the cellular elements of the blood attached to the interior wall of a vein or artery.

Thrombosis an abnormal vascular condition in which a clot (**thrombus**) develops within a blood vessel of the body.

Topical medication applied to the surface of a part of the body.

Tort a civil wrong, including negligence, false imprisonment, assault, and battery.

Tourniquet a device, usually a wide, constricting band of elastic material, wrapped around a limb to restrict blood flow. It is applied to a limb to control hemorrhage or to enhance accessibility of veins for venipuncture.

Toxicity, toxic effect resulting from an excess amount of medication in the blood, these effects may be caused by excessive use of medications, overdose, impaired excretion, or an idiosyncratic reaction to the medication.

Toxin, toxic a poison, having a poisonous effect.

Tracer a radioactive isotope that is used in diagnostic nuclear medicine techniques to allow a biological process to be seen.

Tracheostomy an opening through the neck into the trachea through which an indwelling tube may be inserted to ventilate the patient.

Tracheotomy an incision made into the trachea through the neck below the larynx, performed to gain access to the airway below a blockage with a foreign body, tumor, or edema of the glottis.

Traction the process of putting a limb, bone, or group of muscles under tension by means of weights and pulleys to align or immobilize the part or to relieve pressure on it.

Tranquilizer a drug prescribed to calm anxious or agitated people, ideally without decreasing their consciousness. A common term for **benzodiazepines**.

Transducer a hand-held device, used in diagnostic sonography, that sends and receives a sound wave signal. It changes electrical impulses into sound waves, receives the reflected sound wave, and converts it back into electrical energy.

Transient ischemic attack (TIA) an episode of cerebrovascular insufficiency, usually associated with partial occlusion of an artery by an atherosclerotic plaque or an embolism.

Trauma physical injury caused by violent or disruptive action or by the introduction into the body of a toxic substance.

Tremor rhythmic, purposeless movements resulting from the involuntary alternating contraction and relaxation of opposing groups of skeletal muscles.

Trichomoniasis a vaginal infection caused by the protozoan *Trichomonas vaginalis.*

Trisomy 21 see **Down's Syndrome**.

Trocar a sharp, pointed rod that fits inside a tube. It is used to pierce the skin and the wall of a cavity or canal in the body to aspirate fluids, to instill a medication or solution, or to guide the placement of a soft catheter.

Tubercle, tuberculin a nodule or a small eminence, such as that on a bone or the nodules caused by tuberculosis. Tuberculin means referring to or related to a tubercle or to tuberculosis.

Tuberculosis (TB) a chronic granulomatous infection caused by an acid-fast bacillus, *Mycobacterium tuberculosis.* It is generally transmitted by the inhalation or ingestion of infected droplets and usually affects the lungs, although infection of multiple organ systems occurs.

Tungsten a metallic element. It has the highest melting point of all metals and is used as a target material in x-ray tubes and as filaments in both x-ray tubes and incandescent light bulbs.

Tympanic membrane a thin semitransparent membrane in the middle ear that transmits sound vibrations to the internal ear by means of the auditory ossicles, the **ear drum**.

Typhoid fever a bacterial infection usually caused by *Salmonella typhi,* transmitted by contaminated milk, water, or food.

Typhus fever any of a group of acute infectious diseases caused by various species of *Rickettsia* and usually transmitted from infected rodents to humans by the bites of lice, fleas, mites, or ticks.

Ulcerative colitis a chronic, episodic, inflammatory disease of the large intestine and rectum.

Urogram, urography a radiograph/examination of the urinary tract, obtained using a radiopaque substance.

Urticaria a pruritic skin eruption characterized by transient wheals of varying shapes and sizes with well-defined erythematous margins and pale centers. Same as **hives**.

Vaccine, vaccination a suspension of attenuated or killed microorganisms administered intradermally, intramuscularly, orally, or subcutaneously to induce active immunity to infectious disease.

Valid choice a selection of options, all of which are acceptable. Offering valid choices to patients increases their sense of autonomy.

Valsalva maneuver any forced expiratory effort against a closed airway, such as when an individual holds the breath and tightens the muscles in a concerted, strenuous effort to move a heavy object.

Value a personal belief about the worth of a given idea or behavior.

Vascular pertaining to a blood vessel.

Vasoconstriction a narrowing of the lumen of any blood vessel, especially the arterioles and the veins in the blood reservoirs of the skin and the abdominal viscera.

Vasodilation an increase in the diameter of a blood vessel.

Vasovagal reflex a stimulation of the vagus nerve by reflex in which irritation of the larynx or the trachea results in slowing of the pulse rate.

Vector (of infection) an animal in whose body a pathogen multiplies or develops before becoming infective to a new host.

Vehicle (of infection) any substance, such as food or water, that can serve as a mode of transmission for infectious agents.

Venipuncture the transcutaneous puncture of a vein by a sharp, rigid stylet or cannula carrying a flexible plastic catheter or by a steel needle attached to a syringe or catheter.

Venogram, venography a radiographic image/study of the veins. Same as **phlebogram**.

Ventilation the process by which gases are moved into and out of the lungs.

Ventilator any of several devices used in respiratory therapy to provide assisted respiration and intensive positive-pressure breathing.

Ventricle small cavity, such as the right and the left ventricles of the heart or one of the cavities filled with cerebrospinal fluid in the brain.

Vertigo a sensation of instability, loss of equilibrium, or rotation, caused by a disturbance in the semicircular canal of the inner ear or the vestibular nuclei of the brainstem.

Vial a glass container with a metal-enclosed rubber seal.

Virion a rudimentary virus particle with a central nucleoid surrounded by a protein sheath or capsid.

Virulence factors characteristics of certain microorganisms that cause them to be pathogenic and distinguish them from normal flora. These factors enable bacteria to destroy or damage host cells and resist destruction by the host's cellular defenses.

Virus, viral a minute parasitic microorganism much smaller than a bacterium that, having no independent metabolic activity, may replicate only within a cell of a living plant or animal host.

Viscosity, viscous the ability or inability of a fluid solution to flow easily.

Viscus, visceral an internal organ, pertaining to an organ.

Void to empty, or evacuate, such as urine from the bladder.

Volt, voltage the unit of electrical potential. In an electric circuit a volt is the force required to send 1 ampere of current through 1 ohm of resistance, or the difference in potential between two points on a conductor carrying a charge of 1 ampere when there is a dissipation of 1 watt between them.

Wavelength the distance between a given point on one wave cycle and the corresponding point on the next successive wave cycle.

Yeast any unicellular, usually oval, nucleated fungus that reproduces by budding.

Bibliography

Amersham Health X-Ray Products: *Clinical references, glucophage (metformin) and iodinated contrast media,* pp 5-7 (www.us-nai.com/html/clinref.html).

ASRT Task Force on Governance Restructuring: *Recommended governance structure,* November 2002, pp 1-6 (www.asrt.org).

Ballinger P, Frank E: *Merrill's atlas of radiographic positions and radiologic procedures,* ed 9, St Louis, 1999, Mosby.

Bonewit-West K: *Clinical procedures for medical assistants,* ed 5, Philadelphia, 2000, WB Saunders (Electrocardiography).

Bracco imaging pharmaceutical products, contrast media (www.bracco.com/Bracco/Internet/Services/Medical+Profession+Services).

Centers for Disease Control and Prevention: *Part II recommendations for isolation precautions in hospitals,* February 1997, pp 1-12 (www.cdc.gov/ncidod/hip/isolat/isopart2.htm).

Centers for Disease Control and Prevention: *Synopsis of types of precautions and patients requiring the precautions,* February 1997 (www.cdc.gov/ncidod/hip/isolat/isotab_1.htm).

Centers for Disease Control and Prevention: *Exposure to blood: what health-care workers need to know,* 2002, pp 1-8.

Centers for Disease Control and Prevention: Guidelines for hand hygiene in health-care settings, *MMWR Morb Mortal Wkly Rep* 51/RR-16:1-44, 2002 (www.cdc.gov/handhygiene).

Centers for Disease Control and Prevention: Division of Health Care Quality Promotion: *Surveillance of health care personnel with HIV/AIDS as of 2001* (www.cdc.gov/hiv/pubs/facts/hcwsurv.htm).

Centers for Disease Control and Prevention: Division of HIV/AIDS: *Basic statistics,* December 2001 (www.cdc.gov/hiv/stats.htm).

Centers for Disease Control and Prevention: Division of HIV/AIDS: *Surveillance report* 13(2), December 2001, Tables 1-33 (www.cdc.gov/hiv/stats/hasrlink.htm).

Centers for Disease Control and Prevention: Division of Tuberculosis Elimination: *Core curriculum on tuberculosis,* ed 4, 2000, Chapter 4—Testing for TB disease and infection (www.cdc.gov/nchstp/tb/pubs/corecurriculum/Chapter_4_Skin_Testing.htm).

Centers for Disease Control and Prevention: Division of Tuberculosis Elimination: *2001 Surveillance report,* December 2001, Tables 1-5 (www.cdc.gov/nchstp/tb/surv/surv2001/default.htm).

Centers for Disease Control and Prevention: Trends in tuberculosis morbidity-United States, 1992-2002, *MMWR Morb Mortal Wkly Rep* 52(11):217-222, 2003 (www.cdc.gov/mmwr/preview/mmwrhtml/mm5211a2.htm).

Durand KS: *Critical thinking: developing skills in radiography,* Philadelphia, 1999, FA Davis.

Elkin MK, Perry AG, Potter PA: *Nursing interventions and clinical skills,* ed 2, St Louis, 2000, Mosby.

Enrollment snapshot of radiography, radiation therapy and nuclear medicine programs, 2002, ASRT (www.asrt.org).

Furlow B: Ergonomics in the health care environment, *Journal of the American Society of Radiologic Technologists* 74(2):137-150, 2002.

Jensen SC, Peppers MP: *Pharmacology and drug administration for imaging technologists,* St Louis, 1998, Mosby.

Joyce EV, Villanueva ME: *Say it in Spanish,* ed 2, Philadelphia, 2000, WB Saunders.

Kremkau FW: *Diagnostic ultrasound: principles and instruments,* ed 6, St Louis, 2002, Mosby.

Low temperature gas plasma: a new sterilization technology (www.tyvek.com).

Mallinckrodt imaging pharmaceuticals (www.imaging. mallinckrodt.com/Products).

Merck Manual reference for clinical summaries of diagnosis and treatment of specific diseases (www.merck.com/ pubs/mmanual).

2001 Mosby's GenRx, ed 11, St Louis, 2001, Harcourt Health Sciences.

Occupational Safety and Health Administration: 2153. *Occupational Exposure to Tuberculosis-Final Rule Stage* (www.osha-slc.gov/Reg_Agenda_data/2153.html).

Occupational Safety and Health Administration: *Revision to OSHA's Bloodborne Pathogens Standard: Technical Background and Summary,* April 2001 (www.osha-slc.gov/needlesticks/needlefact.html).

Parelli RJ: *Medicolegal issues for radiographers,* ed 3, Delray Beach, Fla, 1997, GR/St. Lucie Press.

Perry AG, Potter PA: *Clinical nursing skills and techniques,* ed 5, St Louis, 2002, Mosby.

Purtilo R: *Ethical dimensions in the health professions,* ed 3, Philadelphia, 1999, WB Saunders.

Sanchez T: Care targets workplace and patients, *ASRT Scanner* 33(12):35, 2001.

Seeram E: *Computed tomography,* ed 2, Philadelphia, 2001, WB Saunders.

Shagam Yagoda, J: Interpreting critical laboratory values, *ASRT Homestudy Series* 3(4), 1998.

Sprawls P: *Magnetic resonance imaging principles, methods and techniques,* Madison, Wis, 2002, Medical Physics Publishing.

Spry C: Low temperature sterilization, *Infection Control Today,* May 2001, Sterilization (www.infectioncontroltoday.com/articles/151).

Tortorici M, Apfel P: *Advanced radiographic and angiographic procedures,* Philadelphia, 1995, FA Davis.

Index

Note: Page numbers followed by *f* indicate figures; those followed by *t* indicate tables; those followed by *b* indicate boxed material.